P9-DVV-120

Praise for Bradley Bale, MD, and Amy Doneen, ARNP

Beat the Heart Attack Gene

Beat the Heart Attack Gene

The Revolutionary Plan to Prevent Heart Disease, Stroke, and Diabetes

Bradley Bale, MD
Amy Doneen, ARNP
with Lisa Collier Cool

WILEY

Wiley General Trade, an imprint of Turner Publishing Company

424 Church Street • Suite 2240 Nashville, Tennessee 37219
445 Park Avenue • 9th Floor New York, NY 10022

www.turnerpublishing.com

Beat the Heart Attack Gene: The Revolutionary Plan to Prevent Heart Disease, Stroke, and Diabetes

The information contained in this book is not intended to serve as a replacement for professional medical advise. Any use of the information in this book is at the reader's discretion. The author and the publisher specifically disclaim any information contained in this book. A healthcare professional should be consulted regarding your specific situation.

Cover design: Maxwell Roth
Book design: Lissa Auciello-Brogan

Library of Congress Cataloging-in-Publication Data

Bale, Bradley.
  Beat the heart attack gene : the revolutionary plan to prevent heart disease, stroke, and diabetes / Bradley Bale, MD and Amy Doneen, ARNP, with Lisa Collier Cool.
    pages cm   5328743 8   2/14
  ISBN 978-1-118-45429-9 (hardback)
  1. Heart--Diseases--Genetic aspects. 2. Heart--Diseases--Treatment. 3. Cardiological manifestations of general diseases. 4. Genetic screening. 5. Heart cells. I. Doneen, Amy. II. Cool, Lisa Collier, 1952- III. Title.
  RC682.9.B35 2014
  616.1'2042--dc23
                        2013025408

Printed in the United States of America
14 15 16 17 18 0 9 8 7 6 5 4 3 2 1

To the love of my life, Pam; our children, Forrest, Brittany, and Jacob; and the twin miracles who light up our lives: our granddaughters, Adeline and Olivia. I also dedicate this book in loving memory of my parents, Joy and Garnett Bale, who inspired me with their passion for poetry and medicine and my sister, Barbara, who always believed in the reality of my dreams. I will carry them in my heart forever, as I strive to heal the hearts of my patients.
—Bradley Bale, MD

To Daren, your unwavering belief in me gives me the energy and passion to forge ahead. To our children, Sydney, Devin, and Sophie, your laughter and smiles remind me daily of my tremendous blessings. To my grandmother, Jordis Larson: at 90 years old, you continue to teach me about living with passion and focus. Last, to two gentle giants in my life with broad and supportive shoulders—my father and brother, Wallis and Brian Hubbard— you cheer me on at every turn.
—Amy Doneen, ARNP

To John, Alison, Georgia, and Rosalie, you lift my heart and spirit. In fond remembrance of my father, Oscar Collier, my first agent, editor, mentor, and inspiration. I shall not look upon your like again.
—Lisa Collier Cool

Contents

Foreword

I was shocked and devastated when my friend Tim Russert—NBC News's Washington Bureau Chief and moderator of *Meet the Press*—died in 2008 after suffering a heart attack at work. Tim was only 58.

After this tragedy, many questions were raised. Although Tim had been diagnosed previously with heart disease, he'd never had any symptoms. To control his risk factors, he was taking blood pressure pills and a statin to lower his cholesterol, worked out with an exercise bike, and was trying to lose weight.

Just weeks earlier he had passed a stress test with flying colors, and his heart function had appeared good, one of his doctors told the *New York Times*. At the time, the doctor had estimated Tim's risk of suffering a heart attack in the next 10 years at only 5 percent, based on a widely used risk calculator.

What went wrong? Did his doctors miss something—or was Tim's heart attack, which triggered sudden cardiac arrest that killed him, truly impossible to predict or prevent?

To find out, I asked the Larry King Cardiac Foundation to convene a panel of experts to discuss these questions. As we looked for the cutting-edge thought leaders in the field of heart attack and sudden cardiac arrest prevention to serve on the panel, one name kept popping up: Dr. Bradley Bale, co-founder of the Bale/Doneen Method.

I was so impressed by the expertise and insights that Dr. Bale brought to the panel, which also included the President of the American Medical Association and the head of the National Heart, Blood, and Lung Institute, that I told him I'd do anything in my power to help spread the word about the remarkably effective heart attack and stroke prevention plan that he and Amy Doneen, ARNP, have developed.

I wish my friend Tim Russert could have met these two renowned heart attack prevention specialists prior to his fatal event. Although it is too late for him, it's not too late for you to meet them. Their wisdom and science-backed prevention plan shared in these pages can help ensure that you avoid Tim's tragic fate.

As you will read in this book, the Bale/Doneen Method doesn't rely solely on indirect ways of evaluating heart health, such as stress tests and risk calculators, both of which can be tragically unreliable for some people, such as Tim. I've heard many other stories about people who pass these tests, only to later die from a heart attack.

Instead, the Bale/Doneen prevention program harnesses leading-edge genetics, along with the latest science, to identify which people harbor silent and potentially deadly plaque in their arteries, before a heart attack or stroke occurs. This book also reveals hidden causes of heart attacks, surprising red flags that can signal heart attack risk, even when everything else seems fine, and potentially lifesaving action steps, including simple but powerful lifestyle changes.

I used to think heart attacks happened to other people—until I had one in February 1987. Until then, I hadn't paid much attention to my heart, even though my father had a fatal heart attack at work when he was 43. I remember the concern on one doctor's face when I told him about this during a medical checkup.

Such was my denial that I actually lit up a cigarette as I left the doctor's office, telling myself that medicine wasn't as good back then as it is now. I'd been smoking since I was 17 and typically puffed three packs of Nat Sherman cigarettes a day. I also ate a diet that was heavy in fried food and lemon meringue pie, and I didn't exercise. I thought I was invincible.

When the heart attack hit, I didn't recognize the warning signs. It wasn't the classic Hollywood heart attack where you clutch your chest and keel over. I woke up with right shoulder pain that turned into a stomachache. I thought I might be having a gallbladder problem. I even smoked a cigarette on the way to the hospital.

When the doctor told me I was having a heart attack, I felt like I'd been hit by the Sledgehammer of Reality. In a way, having the heart attack was the best thing that ever happened to me, because if I'd kept on smoking, I would be dead now. I was very lucky to have survived, and I completely lost my desire to smoke. It was miraculous because I was so addicted that I even used to smoke in the shower.

On the way home from the hospital—after spending four days in the ICU—I threw my cigarettes into the Potomac River. If you think you can't stop smoking, I'm here to tell you that you can. And I hope it won't take a heart attack to convince you!

In December 1987, I woke up in the ICU after undergoing quadruple bypass heart surgery for severely clogged arteries. Soon after that, I was shocked to find out that I also had type 2 diabetes. As you will read in this book, that double whammy was probably not a coincidence. There is a very strong link between the two diseases.

After my heart attack, someone asked me how much my medical care cost. I didn't know because my health insurance paid the bills. But I promised myself I'd help other people get their hearts repaired if they lacked insurance and couldn't afford the procedures. That was the inspiration for the Larry King Cardiac Foundation, a charity launched in 1988.

Our goal is to save one heart a day. Along with paying for lifesaving procedures for some people, we promote heart-smart habits for everybody. Education and prevention are a huge part of our mission, including informing people about the major role of genetics in putting some people at increased risk for heart disease and sudden cardiac arrest. If your mother, father, grandmother, grandfather, sister, or brother has had a heart attack, then the odds are that you could also be at risk.

As you will read in this book, millions of Americans unknowingly carry genes that greatly increase their risk for heart attacks. In fact, more than 100 genes that play a role in heart disease have already been identified, and some of them increase risk as much as smoking does. A recent study suggests that genes play a role in at least 40 percent of heart attacks.

However, DNA doesn't have to doom people to suffer heart attacks and strokes. I used to think it was impossible to predict or prevent these events. That's not true. Actually, there are proven strategies, such as the Bale/Doneen Method, that can dramatically reduce your risk. I am much healthier now and have amazing stamina, even at age 80, because I've learned the right ways to take care of myself.

It would be a great idea if all people lived as if they had the heart attack gene. They would eat the right food, exercise every day, and never smoke—instead of waiting until a heart attack becomes their wake-up call, as I did. Why not assume that you do have the gene and take that as a powerful incentive to lead a healthy life, so that a heart attack never happens to you? In these pages, you'll find all the tools and inspiration you need to save your heart.

—Larry King,
Host of *Larry King Now*,
Founder of the Larry King Cardiac Foundation

Preface

Bradley Bale, MD and Amy Doneen, ARNP are on the cutting edge of prevention of heart attacks. They've developed a program that not only helps individual patients but also people around the world. I love the fact that they never stop studying, learning, and conducting the research to stop the number one killer of Americans: cardiovascular disease (CVD). Brad and Amy have a true passion for saving lives—and hearts.

I'm a strong, firm, and vociferous believer in their prevention plan. If you read this book and follow the lessons of the Bale/Doneen Method, the odds are on your side that you will live a much richer, healthier life. You'll find inspiration, the latest science, and all the tools you need to take control of your health.

Even if you have a family history of CVD, as I do, or have already developed plaque in your arteries, following this prevention plan can still help you avoid a heart attack. Brad and Amy have studied the reasons that people have heart attacks and the best ways to detect and treat CVD *before* life-threatening symptoms strike.

A few years ago, my friend Jake Orville, CEO of the Cleveland Heart Lab, told me about the Bale/Doneen Method, which uses simple blood and urine tests—some of which were developed by Jake's company—to check for inflammation and other hidden signs of heart attack risk. Jake said that we both needed to be examined. That sounded good to me. My father had type 2 diabetes and died at a young age from a heart attack. I didn't want that to happen to me.

Jake and I spent the whole day getting an in-depth assessment of our cardiovascular health. Brad and Amy are very patient-centered and have a fascinating way of explaining what's best for their patients. Even though I was at their clinic for hours, the time flew by. I loved feeling that I was getting cutting-edge information about how to take better care of myself. As you will learn in this book, CVD is a stealthy killer. Very often, the first symptom is a heart attack. Brad and Amy compare this disease to a cat lurking unseen in the gutter, as it stalks unsuspecting pigeons. If there is silent, deadly plaque in your arteries, you could be at risk for a heart attack or a stroke.

The wonderful news, however, is that there are proven ways to keep the cat from jumping out and causing a heart attack or stroke. Since inflammation is what sparks these events, the key is to keep your arteries "cool." During my initial visit, I was given a personalized prevention plan, which has helped me become a healthier person all-around.

Brad and Amy truly care about their patients. Despite their hectic schedules and giving lectures all over the world, they never forget to call me and ask how I'm doing. They want to know if I'm eating properly, getting enough sleep, and exercising regularly.

Since my initial visit to their clinic, I've lost weight, improved my diet, and worked out regularly. When I ran for the Senate in 2012, I convinced newspaper reporters that at age 70, I was fit for the job by kicking off my shoes, dropping to the floor, and doing 50 pushups in less than a minute.

I'm a huge believer in the power of prevention. About 75 percent of healthcare expenditures go to treating chronic illnesses: the ones we can avoid if we really want to be healthy. If you want to prevent a heart attack, stroke, or type 2 diabetes, look in the mirror and say, "Chunky is good, slim is better." Think about your diet and lifestyle. Lack of exercise, junk food, and smoking are some of the biggest causes of diseases we can avoid.

Use the inspiration from this book to live well and practice prevention to the fullest.

—Tommy Thompson,
Former U.S. Secretary of Health and Human Services,
Four-time Governor of Wisconsin

Beat the Heart Attack Gene

Part One

Fundamentals

Chapter 1

A Plan That's Guaranteed to Prevent Heart Attacks

"If healthcare (were) an airline, only dedicated risk takers, thrill seekers, and those tired of living would fly on it."

—Dr. Charles Vincent, *Patient Safety*, Elsevier 2006

New cars come with a warranty. Who would buy one otherwise? We think medical providers should guarantee that their care is effective. Since 2008, all patients we've treated every year at our clinics—the Heart Attack & Stroke Prevention Center in Spokane, Washington, and the Heart Attack, Stroke and Diabetes Center at the Grace Clinic in Lubbock, Texas—have been offered a written guarantee stating that if they suffer a heart attack or stroke, they will receive a refund of 100 percent of the fees paid during the year. To date, we've only had to give one refund.

While you might think we achieved these results by catering to already healthy people, in fact, many of the men and women we treat have major cardiovascular risk factors like high cholesterol or metabolic syndrome (a dangerous cluster of abnormalities—high blood sugar, high blood pressure, high cholesterol, and a wide waistline—that greatly magnify the threat of heart disease, stroke, or diabetes). Other patients were past or current smokers, were diabetic (which quadruples a person's risk for heart attacks or strokes), had a family history of cardiovascular disease, or were morbidly obese, including people weighing as much as 400 pounds. Many of our patients have already suffered a heart attack or stroke, putting them at a particularly high risk for having another of these life-threatening events.

In this book, we'll present the unique, personalized prevention and treatment plan that could save your life. By following our plan, called the Bale/Doneen Method, you can avoid a heart attack or stroke, even if cardiovascular disease (CVD) runs in your family. If you've already had a heart attack or stroke, we'll show you how to keep it from happening again. You'll also learn the action steps you need to take—today—to improve and protect the health of the most important muscle in your body, the heart, and the most important organ, your brain. The Bale/Doneen Method has helped thousands of people live active, healthy, and pleasurable lives, without the fear of a heart attack or stroke.

When we founded the Heart Attack & Stroke Prevention Center in 2003, it was one of the first facilities of its kind in the United States. Our goal was to bridge a deadly gap in the medical system: When we looked for experts in preventing cardiovascular disease, we couldn't find any—even though more than two million Americans suffer heart attacks or strokes each year, and of that number, 800,000 die.

Although we had thought that preventing these life-threatening events was the job of cardiologists, we found ourselves all too often referring the same patients to these specialists over and over again to be treated for recurrent heart attacks or strokes. One of Spokane's leading cardiovascular surgeons, Lloyd Rudy, MD, told us that after he'd performed several thousand open-heart operations, including bypass surgery, to treat CVD, he thought, "I have lots of patients I operate on every 10 years. What can I do to keep these people from coming back?"

We—a family physician and a nurse practitioner—have an answer: to treat the entire person, not just his or her cardiovascular disease, with a comprehensive prevention plan. Dr. Rudy became a dedicated patient of ours and a staunch supporter of the Bale/Doneen Method. We designed our approach to look at each patient as a unique individual, with brains and a life, as well as a heart. And we also arm patients with the knowledge they need to navigate the healthcare system, avoid the pitfalls, and be able to insist on getting the best medical options available. Very often, it takes more than the current standard of care to prevent heart attacks and strokes, as many of our patients have discovered. The Bale/Doneen Method is best told through the stories of these patients. Let us introduce you to Camille.

How Standard Care Can Fail Patients

When Camille Zaleski had her annual checkup, her regular doctor was on vacation. Another MD gave her good news. "After checking my blood pressure and cholesterol, and plugging the numbers into a software program on his PalmPilot, he said my chances of having a heart attack in the next 10 years were less than 1 percent," says the credit manager from Peoria, Arizona, then age 40. She went home reassured that her heart was healthy—and was almost certain to stay that way.

Five months later, shortly after arriving at work, Camille felt nauseated and light-headed, with an irregular heartbeat. "I thought I was having a panic attack, because I was under enormous financial stress. My husband and I had just bought a new house, and three days later he was laid off from his job. I was worrying all the time about how we'd pay the mortgage." At lunchtime, she felt so ill that she put her head on her desk, hoping that after a little rest the dizziness would clear up.

"By one o'clock that afternoon, I was having trouble breathing, and I felt like an elephant was sitting on my chest." But she still didn't consider her symptoms to be serious. "Three years earlier, I had the same kind of breathing problems climbing the steps to my doctor's office and passed out, falling down the flight of stairs. That time, my doctor said it was an anxiety attack and put me on anti-anxiety medication and an antidepressant."

She grew so dizzy that she lay down on the floor by her desk, afraid that she'd faint again. At three o'clock, she asked a coworker to call her husband, who rushed her to the emergency room. "By the time we got there, I had pulsating waves of pain in my left arm and it felt icy cold," she recalls. "The triage nurse put something on my finger and said my oxygen level was OK." She was left in the waiting room for 45 minutes, while a man with a foot injury was treated ahead of her.

By the time her name was finally called, she was in such agony that she could barely stand. Tests showed that Camille was in the throes of a massive heart attack. "The doctor said that if I'd waited any longer to go to the hospital, I would have died, because there was no blood flow to the right side of my heart. I was terrified, and my husband almost fainted."

Cardiologists threaded a balloon-tipped tube through her arteries, then inflated the balloon to open the blocked vessel, which was treated with a stent, a tiny, scaffold-like device that props the vessel open to restore blood flow. After three days in the cardiac ICU, says Camille, "I was sent home with a handful of pills and was told to call 911 if I ever had those symptoms again. I realized that the doctors were preparing me for my next heart attack, instead of telling me how to prevent it. At home, I was so scared that it would happen again that I couldn't sleep at night."

A Dangerously Unreliable Screening Technique

Almost everyone has heard stories similar to Camille's, in which a relatively young person with no apparent risk factors suffers a seemingly inexplicable heart attack weeks—or months—after getting a clean bill of health from a doctor. And the usual reaction is to wonder, "How can that happen?"

Let's take a closer look at how her doctor determined her risk. While the software program he used on his PalmPilot might have sounded like the latest medical technology, in truth, it was just an electronic version of a screening tool that's been around for decades, called the Framingham Risk Score (FRS). The scoring method is derived from an ongoing study of residents of Framingham, Massachusetts, that was launched in 1948.

Still employed widely as part of standard care today, the FRS system uses a formula to predict the risk of heart attack in the next 10 years based on the patient's age, gender, cholesterol level, blood pressure, and smoking status. As a nonsmoking 40-year-old woman with normal blood pressure, Camille fell into the lowest risk category according to the formula, even though her cholesterol was mildly elevated. When the physician asked if she wanted a statin to lower her cholesterol, Camille was lulled into such a false sense of security by her FRS that she said no. Why risk the side effects of a drug when a heart attack was so unlikely?

Camille's trust in this seemingly scientific scoring system nearly proved fatal. When life-threatening symptoms struck, she waited six hours to seek medical care, because she didn't perceive herself as a candidate for a heart attack. Compounding her danger was the questionable care she'd received three years earlier, when she literally collapsed on her doctor's doorstep. Instead of receiving a cardiac workup, she was labeled with an emotional diagnosis. Had she gotten that workup back then, using the tests we recommend in this book, her doctor almost certainly would have discovered that she had heart disease, which develops silently over many years. In many cases, the first symptom is a heart attack.

Not only were Camille's initial warning signs not investigated, but even when she arrived in the emergency room with classic symptoms of a heart attack, she still wasn't taken seriously—an all too common scenario for women, who typically receive less-aggressive diagnosis and treatment, because of the misconception that heart disease is mainly a man's disease. Many women, and a significant number of doctors, still believe that women are more likely to die from breast cancer than a heart attack. In fact, heart disease kills 10 times more women than breast cancer does. And each year, more women than men die from cardiovascular causes, with the survival gap continuing to widen, as we'll discuss in Chapter Five.

Undoubtedly, Camille wouldn't have found her FRS so reassuring had she been aware of the formula's high error rate, particularly for women. In one recent study, Framingham risk factor analysis missed 82 percent of women—and 66 percent of men—with coronary artery disease (CAD), clogged vessels that can lead to a heart attack. One reason the decades-old scoring system is so unreliable is that it was developed in the 1940s, an era when the risk factors for heart attacks weren't nearly as well understood as they are today. In Chapter Three, we'll look at heart attack and stroke red flags in depth, including some new ones that are likely to surprise you.

What's Wrong with This Picture?

It's not just the recently discovered or little-known heart attack risk factors that the Framingham system ignores. Its most glaring deficiency is its failure to factor in major threats to heart health that everybody has heard of. Camille's risk score—and her doctor—overlooked even something as obvious as her weight, which had climbed since she gave birth to her son eight years earlier: At the time of her heart attack, she was carrying 246 pounds on her 5'4" frame, greatly increasing the threat of a heart attack.

Some studies suggest that obesity is just as dangerous to heart health as smoking, especially when excess weight is coupled with a sedentary lifestyle. Yet according to the Framingham system, despite being overweight and so busy with her demanding office job that she rarely had time to exercise, Camille was deemed to be as low a risk for a heart attack as a female triathlete the same age—even if the other woman weighed only half as much as she did.

A relatively new 10-year-risk calculator developed specifically for women, called the Reynolds Risk Score (RRS), also fails to take obesity into account. Introduced in 2007, it uses a formula that includes the traditional Framingham factors, plus two additional factors: if the woman has a parent who had a heart attack before age 60 and the woman's level of a blood marker called high-sensitivity C-reactive protein (hs CRP).

At best, however, this formula offers only a modest improvement over the Framingham system—and then only for certain women. The researchers report that in their 10-year study of nearly 25,000 women, their system was similar in accuracy—or for many people, inaccuracy—to FRS in making predictions for women at low or high risk for heart attacks. Of those deemed to be at medium risk according to Framingham factors, the Reynolds system reclassified 30 to 40 percent at higher or lower risk than their FRS suggested.

So far, RRS hasn't been adopted widely, because relatively few healthcare providers use the hs CRP blood test in routine cardiovascular screening. And like the Framingham risk calculator, it can often miss women at high risk. For example, if Camille's pre–heart attack numbers had been plugged into the Reynolds formula, she would have been mistakenly classified as being at extremely low risk, creating the same false sense of security as did her Framingham score.

Incredibly, the still-popular Framingham system fails to take genes or family history into account. Over the past twenty years, an explosion of new research has revealed the key role that genetic factors play in determining cardiovascular risk. In Camille's case, her family history held two potent clues that she was in far more danger than her doctor's prediction suggested. The first clue was that Camille's grandfather had type 2 diabetes, a disease that runs in families. Having it greatly increases the threat of a heart attack. Not only are adults with this blood-sugar disorder at as high a risk for heart attacks or strokes as nondiabetics who have already suffered a prior heart attack, but diabetics typically experience these calamities at a much younger age than nondiabetics.

Since diabetes is extremely common in people who are overweight or obese— and a family history of the disease further elevates the threat—Camille's doctor should have checked her blood sugar. Had he ordered a simple, inexpensive blood test for diabetes that's covered by almost all health plans—the two-hour oral glucose tolerance test (OGTT)—the results would have revealed that she was prediabetic, tripling her risk for a heart attack. Despite the well-documented link between prediabetes or diabetes—particularly if these conditions go undiagnosed and untreated— and heart attacks, the FRS and RRS don't look at blood-sugar numbers.

That's a very dangerous omission. What most patients—and many medical providers—don't know is that the vast majority of heart attacks have the same root cause as type 2 diabetes: a condition called insulin resistance, in which the body produces insulin, but doesn't use it properly. Normally, this hormone, which is made by the pancreas, helps the body use glucose for energy. When people develop insulin resistance, their muscles, fat, and liver cells become insensitive to insulin, forcing the pancreas to crank out higher and higher amounts, trying to keep up with demand. Eventually, the pancreas becomes exhausted, and glucose (blood sugar) levels start to rise. Not only does this set the stage for type 2 diabetes, but it also starts to damage the arteries, which can lead to cardiovascular disease.

Insulin resistance can be detected with the OGTT, which is also the gold standard for accurately diagnosing diabetes and prediabetes. Unfortunately, doctors rarely order this test, and without the information it provides, patients don't realize they harbor this dangerous condition, which affects about 150 million Americans. As we'll discuss in Chapter Nine, it often takes decades of being insulin resistant before someone becomes diabetic. And meanwhile, the arteries are silently being damaged, which can lead to a heart attack. Even though rates of diabetes are soaring in tandem with America's obesity epidemic, millions of Americans with diabetes or prediabetes are walking around undiagnosed. All too often, like Camille, people only discover they have dangerously high blood-sugar levels after they've already suffered a heart attack.

In Camille's case, her family history also offered another red flag: Two close relatives had developed coronary artery disease so severe that they required open-heart surgery to repair blocked blood vessels. Many studies show that family history is one of the most important risk factors for developing heart disease, often at a younger-than-usual age—and the more affected relatives a person has, the greater the danger. While RRS does factor in family history, it includes only the patient's parents—and only if they had heart attacks at a relatively young age.

One of the greatest medical breakthroughs of the past decade is the identification of four specific genes (which we'll describe in Chapter Ten) that dramatically boost cardiovascular risk. Millions of Americans unknowingly carry these common genetic mutations, and the cost of tests to detect them has plummeted. For less than the price of a mammogram, Camille's doctor could have ordered a state-of-the-art genetic assessment, which would have shown that she's a carrier of two dangerous genes: 9P21—also known as "the heart attack gene" because it powerfully increases the threat of cardiovascular events—and of the KIF6 gene variant, which not only magnifies risk for heart attack, stroke, and sudden cardiac death, but also influences which particular statin could provide benefit. No doubt Camille wouldn't have been so quick to turn down statin therapy if she'd known her KIF6 status.

The Medical Mindset

Add up all of Camille's actual risk factors and her heart attack is no longer a medical mystery or a random quirk of fate. Instead, it was entirely predictable, had the clues been put together. And with the right care, it could have been prevented. Most doctors, however, are not disease detectives. They're trained to look for symptoms of active disorders and treat them, as Camille's doctor attempted to do by offering to prescribe a statin for her slightly elevated cholesterol. For the most part, healthcare providers don't delve deeply into family history to search for genetic risks that could lead to future illnesses.

Why not? Two of the biggest reasons are time and money. In today's harried healthcare environment, with insurance reimbursements shrinking, providers may each see sixty or more patients a day. Busy practitioners don't have time to educate patients about why it is in their best interest to have a two-hour OGTT when most people aren't worried about diabetes or insulin resistance and don't consider themselves to be at risk. Nor do health plans adequately reimburse providers for the time necessary to educate patients, even if such education might ultimately save the patients' lives. By far the faster and easier approach to heart attack prevention is to punch a few numbers into a computer and come up with a Framingham or Reynolds risk score.

Similarly, the economics of today's healthcare don't give physicians any financial incentive to investigate rigorously a patient's medical history, genetic makeup, and lifestyle habits. Thus they can't compile a personalized risk profile or determine which diagnostic tests would be most beneficial for that particular patient. Instead, they're forced to rely on medical guidelines that are designed for the general population. Consequently, patients are screened and treated according to the average results from large studies, receiving one-size-fits-all care instead of tests and therapies tailored to their individual needs.

Another problem is that an avalanche of new medical discoveries, including new research findings that sometimes turn the previous medical wisdom upside down, plus new screening options, technologies, and treatments, has made it increasingly challenging for doctors to keep current on the best ways to manage an individual patient's care. Frequently, it takes a decade or more for medical societies to update their guidelines for patient care, further elongating the lag time before the average healthcare provider learns about new, evidence-based tests and treatments and incorporates them into a typical medical practice.

The big loser in our healthcare system is early detection. As you'll learn in Part Two of this book, widely available, inexpensive tests can reliably identify the early signs of cardiovascular disease up to thirty years before it escalates into a silent killer. But many people with this potentially lethal disease smoldering inside their blood vessels miss out on early treatment that could stave off an impending heart attack or stroke because their doctors don't give them the right screening tests. The same is true of insulin resistance and prediabetes, both of which can often be reversed if caught early, sparing patients the dangerous—and costly—complications of developing full-blown diabetes. Yet millions of Americans with these increasingly common diseases continue to suffer irreversible—or even fatal—harm simply because they were diagnosed and treated too late.

A Campaign to Save One Million Lives

More than 100 million Americans—about half of the adult population—have one or more major risk factors for cardiovascular disease (CVD), the leading killer of men and women in this country. If current trends continue over the next five years, more than 10 million men and women will have heart attacks, and more than 4 million of them will die. In an ambitious effort to reduce this grim toll, the Department of Health and Human Services (DHHS); other federal, state, and local agencies; and private sector partners launched the "Million Hearts" initiative in September 2011, with the goal of preventing 1 million heart attacks and stroke fatalities over the next five years.

The initiative calls for healthcare providers to work harder on treating the three modifiable Framingham risk factors—smoking, high cholesterol, and high blood pressure—and to prescribe aspirin therapy for patients at high risk for heart attacks and strokes. These inexpensive measures alone, if consistently implemented by America's healthcare providers, could save 500,000 lives during the five-year initiative, the DHHS estimates. By expanding community programs aimed at getting people to lose weight, eat a healthier diet, and exercise more, the initiative hopes to save an additional 500,000 lives, succeeding in their stated aim, if these goals are met.

Preventing one million heart attack fatalities would be an admirable—and even spectacular—accomplishment. As specialists in preventing CVD, we applaud this campaign as a major step forward in combating the leading killer of Americans. But we also feel that it doesn't go far enough. What about the three million Americans whose lives *wouldn't* be saved over these five years, even if the initiative's best-case scenario is realized? Are they to be left in the tragic—and terrifying—position of a patient you'll meet in the next chapter, who considered himself a "dead man walking" because of his belief that modern medicine had no cure to offer?

We believe that something crucial is missing from the Million Hearts initiative: tailoring tests and treatments to each patient's individual needs. The initiative is grounded in the premise that everybody with Framingham risk factors is alike, so the program's key to saving lives is elevating standard care to a higher level of consistency. In this era of shrinking healthcare dollars, there's also a pragmatic purpose at work: to achieve the greatest good for the greatest number of patients at the lowest cost, through simple interventions like a low-salt diet for those with high blood pressure or brief smoking-cessation counseling for tobacco users.

The inevitable outcome of this assembly-line approach is that many unsuspecting patients who are at extremely high risk for heart attacks and strokes will miss out on crucial individualized medical care that could prevent these catastrophes, because they don't have the targeted risk factors. The DHHS predicts that if the initiative succeeds in its push for greater standardization of cardiac care, and the hoped-for goal is achieved, these tactics would prevent only one in four heart attack fatalities. Would you bet *your* life on those odds?

The Bale/Doneen Difference

At our heart attack and stroke prevention centers, we see many patients who have fallen through the cracks in standard care. Some have suffered heart attacks or strokes their doctors can't explain, or, like Camille, were sent home from the hospital with instructions to call 911 when their next heart attack hit. The scary statistic behind that advice: one in three heart attacks and one in four strokes occur in people who have already survived a previous cardiovascular event.

Other patients turned to us after their healthcare provider diagnosed them with cardiovascular disease—or one of its major risk factors—but didn't offer a comprehensive heart attack and stroke prevention plan. Because these men and women weren't told how to protect themselves, they felt like ticking time bombs rather than empowered patients armed with potentially lifesaving strategies to manage their disease. Later in the book, you'll meet a patient who actually considered himself to be "a dead man walking," because his cardiologists had given him such a dire prognosis that he believed that a fatal heart attack, like the one that killed his father, was both imminent and inevitable.

Our heart attack and stroke prevention method, which we've taught to hundreds of healthcare providers from all over the world in our American Academy of Family Physicians–accredited training program, is scientifically designed to detect and stop a silent killer: cardiovascular disease. All of the recommendations we make in this book are based on the latest research, such as the results of randomized clinical trials published in peer-reviewed medical journals. As a bonus, the treatments we advise, including lifestyle changes and action steps you can take on your own, are also highly effective at preventing type 2 diabetes. And if you're already diabetic or prediabetic, the plan we present in this book can halt further damage—or in many cases, can even reverse the early stages of the disease.

Throughout the book, you'll find the scientific evidence to support each test and treatment we advise, so you can show it to your healthcare provider and ask for optimal, personalized care. Our goal is to empower you to take charge of your medical destiny by identifying your true risks, what's *really* causing them, and the best treatments, including lifestyle changes, to overcome cardiovascular perils. As you'll discover in the next chapter, the comprehensive prevention we recommend uses inexpensive, noninvasive tests—along with information that may already be in your medical chart—to answer four crucial questions. Learning the answers—and acting on this information—could save your life.

Action Step:
Assess Your Heart Attack and Stroke Risk

More than 100 million Americans—about half of the adult population—have one or more risk factors for cardiovascular disease, the leading killer of Americans. To find out if you could be at risk, we suggest that you take a few minutes to answer the following questions, which are similar to those we ask our patients during their initial evaluation. The answers will help you identify potential threats to your cardiovascular health and areas you need to work on to prevent a heart attack or stroke.

1. How old are you?
   a. Male < 55 years old   1 point
   b. Female < 65 years old   1 point
   c. Male > 55 years old   4 points
   d. Female > 65 years old   4 points

2. Do you have a family history of early cardiovascular disease (a male relative affected before age 55 or a female relative affected before age 65)?
   a. No   0 points
   b. Yes   4 points

3. What is your waist circumference?
   a. If you're a women: Less that 35 inches   0 points
   b. If you're male: Less than 40 inches   0 points

   c. If you're a woman: 35 inches or more   4 points

   d. If you're a man: 40 inches or more   4 points

4. What's your weight range?
   a. Underweight   2 points
   b. Average   1 point
   c. Overweight   3 points
   d. Obese   4 points

5. What is your resting pulse?
   a. Less than 60 beats per minute   0 points
   b. Less than 75 beats per minute   1 point
   c. More than 75 beats per minute   2 points
   d. Don't Know   2 points

6. What is your blood pressure? (Check all answers that apply)
   a. Less than 120/80   0 points
   b. Taking blood pressure medication   2 points
   c. 120/80 to 139/89   3 points
   d. 140/90 or higher   4 points
   e. Don't know   4 points

7. What is your total cholesterol level? (Check all answers that apply)
   a. Less than 160 mg/dL   0 points
   b. Less than 200 mg/dL   1 point
   c. Taking cholesterol medication   2 points
   d. Greater than 200 mg/dL   3 points
   e. Don't know   3 points

8. What is your HDL (good) cholesterol level?
   a. If you're a woman: Less than 60 mg/dL   3 points
   b. If you're a man, Less than 50 mg/dL   3 points
   c. If you're a woman: 60 mg/dLor higher   0 points
   d. If you're a man: 50 mg/dLor higher   0 points
   e. Don't know   3 points

9. What is your LDL (bad) cholesterol?
   a. Less than 70 mg/dL   0 points
   b. Less than 100mg/dL   1 point
   c. Less than 130 mg/dL   3 points
   d. More than 130 mg/dL   4 points
   e. Don't know   4 points

10. Which of the following best describes your triglyceride level?
    a. Less than 100 mg/dL   0 points
    b. Less than 150 mg/dL   1 point
    c. More than 150 mg/dL   3 points
    d. Don't know   3 points

11. Do you have diabetes or high blood sugar?
    a. No   0 points
    b. Yes, I'm prediabetic   3 points
    c. Yes, I'm diabetic   4 points
    d. I haven't had my blood sugar tested   4 points

12. Do you have bleeding gums? (Check all answers that apply.)
    a. Never   0 points
    b. Yes, when I brush or floss   2 points
    c. I usually don't floss my teeth   2 points

13. Which of the following best describes your sleep patterns?
    a. I sleep soundly 6-8 hours a night   0 points
    b. I sleep restlessly for 6-8 hours a night   2 points
    c. I sleep less than 6 hours or more than 9   3 points

14. Do you snore?
    a. No   0 points
    b. Yes, occasionally   1 point
    c. Yes, frequently and loudly   3 points
    d. Yes, and I have sleep apnea   4 points

15. Do you have rheumatoid arthritis or any other inflammatory disease such as psoriasis or lupus?
    a. No   0 points
    b. Yes   4 points

16. Have you been checked for vitamin D deficiency?
    a. My vitamin D level is between 50-60   0 points
    b. My vitamin D level is less than 30   3 points
    c. I do not know my vitamin D level   3 points

17. Do you have a history of migraine headaches?
    a. No   0 points
    b. Yes, with no migraine aura   2 points
    c. Yes, with a migraine aura   3 points

18. How would you characterize your ability to cope with stress?
    a. I'm usually pretty laid back ..... 0 points
    b. I have healthy ways to cope with stress ..... (1 point)
    c. Sometimes people say that I seem stressed ..... 2 points
    d. I feel stressed and anxious most of the time ..... 4 points

19. Do you spend eleven or more hours a day sitting?
    a. No ..... (0 points)
    b. Yes ..... 4 points

20. How much exercise do you get?
    a. At least 30 minutes, 5 to 7 days per week ..... (0 points)
    b. At least 30 minutes 2 to 4 times per week ..... 1 point
    c. 30 minutes, once a week or less ..... 2 points
    d. I do not exercise ..... 4 points

21. Do you smoke?
    a. No ..... (0 points)
    b. I used to smoke, but have quit for at least 5 years ..... 1 point
    c. I used to smoke, but quit less than 5 years ago ..... 2 points
    d. I am exposed to secondhand smoke regularly ..... 3 points
    e. I smoke or I use smokeless tobacco products ..... 4 points

22. Do you drink regular or diet soft drinks?
    a. Never ..... 0 points
    b. Rarely drink soda (diet or regular) ..... (1 point)
    c. Once a week (diet or regular) ..... 2 points
    d. More than once a week ..... 3 points

23. Do you watch the amount of carbs in your diet?
    a. I limit my simple carbohydrate intake ..... (0 points)
    b. I know to balance my carb/protein balance ..... 1 point
    c. I never watch my carbohydrates ..... 2 points
    d. The majority of my diet consists of carbs ..... 4 points

24. (Women only): Did you experience high blood pressure or gestational diabetes during pregnancy?
    a. No ..... (0 points)
    b. Yes ..... 4 points

25. (Men only): Do have erectile dysfunction?
    a. No ..... 0 points
    b. Yes ..... 4 points

What Your Score Means

- Zero points: Congratulations! You're taking excellent care of yourself. Reading this book will help you maintain—or enhance—your cardiovascular health.

- One to 10 points: While you have relatively few cardiovascular risks, you'll benefit from learning how to optimize your heart health with the easy action steps in this book.

- Eleven to 20 points: You have definite risks for arterial disease. This book will alert you to what you should be doing *right now* to combat these health threats. We also recommend that you pay close attention to the six-step prevention plan in Chapter Two.

- Twenty to 39 points: You're at moderately high risk for cardiovascular disease. In Part One of this book, you'll learn how to identify—and overcome—hidden medical problems that may be putting your heart health in jeopardy, including the surprising, little-known heart attack and stroke red flags that we discuss in Chapter Three.

- Forty points or higher: You're at high risk for cardiovascular disease. To prevent a heart attack or stroke, we recommend getting a comprehensive cardiovascular evaluation that includes the tests discussed in Part Two of this book. In Part Three, you'll also learn which therapies and lifestyle changes are most likely to help you ward off a heart attack or stroke.

Turn the page to learn something that shocks our patients: the *real* reason that heart attacks happen. In the next chapter, we'll also reveal the best-kept secret in medicine: With the right personalized treatment plan, *all* heart attacks and strokes are potentially preventable. And that's a promise that we can confidently back in writing, with the guarantee we make to all of our patients, regardless of their risk factors, family history, weight, genes, or previous heart attacks and strokes.

What *Really* Causes Heart Attacks

"A baited cat may grow as fierce as a lion."

—Samuel Palmer, British painter and writer

Like most people, David Bobbett thought that the key to avoiding heart disease was dodging such "bullets" as obesity, high blood pressure, a couch-potato life-style, and a junk-food diet. "I'm unbelievably disciplined about following all of the standard recommendations for keeping your heart healthy," says the 52-year-old CEO of $500 million-dollar global corporation based in Ireland. "I'm 5'11" and 150 pounds. My blood pressure is 110/70, which is very good, and I don't smoke or eat meat. I run six days a week, work out on an elliptical machine set at a very heavy resistance level, and eat a Mediterranean diet that's high in fruits and vegetables."

David was equally diligent about getting an annual physical that included an exercise stress test. During the exam, he was hooked up to an EKG machine and a blood-pressure cuff as he walked at a gradually increasing speed on a treadmill to see how his heart reacted to the stress of exercise. Developed more than 50 years ago—and still widely used in standard care—treadmill tests check for signs of reduced blood flow through coronary (heart) arteries when the heart is working hard, such as chest pain, unusual shortness of breath, or blood pressure or heart rhythm abnormalities during exercise, all of which may signal blood vessel block-ages that could lead to a heart attack, if untreated.

Since David always passed his annual stress test with flying colors, he didn't worry about the one bullet he hadn't dodged: his persistently high levels of LDL (bad) cholesterol. "My LDL had been high for nearly twenty years, but I never took medication to lower it," says the dad of six kids. "I didn't think I needed a drug, when everything else was so right and I felt great."

A conversation with a business associate, however, fueled concern about another health threat. "He insisted that I get a checkup at a medical center in

Texas, because the very thorough exam and tests he'd received there picked up early stages of skin cancer that other doctors had missed." That alarmed the fair-skinned Irishman, who ran outside in the sun almost every day. Concerned that his doctor might have missed signs of skin cancer during the annual physical he'd had three months earlier, he scheduled an appointment to coincide with an upcoming family vacation in the United States.

At the center, David underwent a battery of screening tests, including coronary artery calcium score (CACS), which we'll discuss in more detail in Chapter Six. This test involves a CT scan to check for calcium in the coronary (heart) arteries. The score is based on the amount of calcium found in each major artery, with a separate score for the total amount. Since healthy arteries don't contain calcium, finding it is a major warning sign of atherosclerosis (plaque buildup in the arteries). In general, the more calcium the arteries contain, the greater the patient's risk is for a heart attack.

"My coronary artery calcium score (CACS) identified me as being in the worst one percent for in my age bracket," says David. "When I started reading about this test, I found out that I had a one in four chance of dying from a heart attack in the next 10 years. As a nonsmoker with this calcification score, I actually had a risk of fatal heart attack 10 times greater than a smoker without calcification.

"I got pretty scared and was in complete shock that an imaging test I'd never heard of was more powerful at predicting my future than all the risk factors that I'd been told were important. I was also angry that no one had advised calcium scoring before. Keeping patients in the dark about a lifesaving test is murder. It's like telling people to drive as fast as they want on the highway, without a seat belt, because you don't care if they're killed."

When he returned home, follow-up tests at an Irish hospital, including an angiogram, had even more alarming results. Not only were the blood vessels that fed his heart riddled with coronary artery disease, but one artery was 70 percent blocked in some areas and another was 100 percent obstructed by plaque. His doctors deemed him to be at such high risk for a heart attack that they advised immediate surgery to insert stents or bypass the clogged areas.

To David, "that sounded like a Hail Mary pass in American football. They were telling me, 'Hopefully, you won't be among the one in four people with your risk profile who dies in the next 10 years.'" Instead of scheduling surgery, adds the CEO, "I went online and looked for doctors whose patients don't have heart attacks."

When David consulted us in April 2012, he'd already seen several heart specialists, who had put him on an excellent medical program that included statin therapy, baby aspirin, and several supplements. He told us that he would consider the 5,000-mile trip from Ireland to our Lubbock, Texas, clinic worthwhile if he learned even one new thing that would help him avoid a heart attack.

Are You Headed for a Heart Attack or Stroke?

What does the Bale/Doneen Method offer to patients like David? The comprehensive prevention plan you'll find in this book uses inexpensive, noninvasive tests—along with information that may already be in your medical chart—to answer four crucial questions. Learning the answers—and acting on this information—could save your life.

1 Do you have vascular disease?

Unfortunately, many people do not know they have disease in the wall of the artery until it is too late. As one cardiologist we know grimly puts it, "All too often, the first symptom of heart disease is wearing a toe tag in the morgue after a fatal heart attack." That's why one of the primary goals of the Bale/Doneen Method is to detect disease *before* it becomes severe enough to spark a heart attack or stroke. We recommend screening for everyone older than 40 and for younger people with any of the red flags discussed in Chapter Three or with a family history of cardiovascular disease or diabetes.

Surprisingly, your doctor doesn't have to look directly at your heart to tell if you are at risk for a heart attack. One of safest ways to check for plaque in your arteries is an ultrasound exam of the major blood vessels in your neck. As we'll explain in more detail in Chapter Six, abnormalities that can be detected by this painless 15-minute exam, known as carotid intima-media thickness (cIMT), are strongly linked to high risk for heart attacks and strokes. The test also provides an estimate of your "arterial age." If your arteries are significantly "older" than your chronological age, it's a sign you are at risk for developing cardiovascular disease. Coronary artery calcium score (CACS), which we'll discuss in the next chapter, is another noninvasive imaging test that can detect hidden disease in the major vessels that feed the heart.

How does the accuracy of our method compare to standard care? We conducted a study of 576 of our patients to compare the two approaches and presented the results at the 2009 International Society of Atherosclerosis annual meeting. When we evaluated the patients with the Bale/Doneen Method, using cIMT, CACS, and other tests, we found that 408 of them were at significant risk for heart attacks or strokes, because they had plaque in their arteries or were diabetic, which magnifies risk just as much as having a prior heart attack. Using Framingham scores alone, however, would have missed 86 percent of the at-risk group.

2 How inflamed are your arteries?

Heart attacks and most strokes are triggered when a diseased artery becomes so inflamed, a condition we call *fire*, that it can no longer contain the plaque smoldering inside the vessel wall. Much like a volcano spewing molten lava, inflammation causes a breach in the vessel wall, leading to the creation of a clot that obstructs blood flow.

The Bale/Doneen Method uses simple blood and urine tests, described in Chapter Seven, which cost only a few dollars, to check for this fiery process. One of the best tests to check for inflammation costs just pennies, but doctors rarely use this extremely cost-effective, universally available urine test for this purpose, even though the information it provides could help prevent a heart attack.

For cholesterol to build up inside artery walls, there has to be some degree of inflammation. And the more inflamed a diseased vessel becomes, the higher your risk for a heart attack or stroke. If Camille's doctor had used the inexpensive tests we recommend, it would have been obvious that she was at risk for a heart attack despite her normal Framingham score.

Chronic inflammation is most common in people who are overweight or obese, particularly if they are physically inactive or smoke. Even if your weight is normal, however, having an apple-shaped body with a large waistline can also be a warning sign of cardiovascular danger. In Part Three, we'll tell you how to get rid of toxic belly fat—and explain why having a spare tire can triple your risk for a heart attack or stroke and quadruple it for type 2 diabetes.

3 What's causing your disease?

Many of the patients who consult us are desperate for answers, because their healthcare provider can't explain *why* their heart attack or stroke happened, or what is causing their CVD. When we met Camille, a few weeks after her 2004 heart attack, she was terrified to go to sleep, not knowing if she would wake up in the morning. Like many heart attack survivors, she felt anxious, depressed, and powerless because she didn't know how to protect herself from having another heart attack.

Heart attacks or strokes can have multiple causes, such as obesity, smoking, inflammatory disorders (including rheumatoid arthritis or other autoimmune diseases), high cholesterol, and even periodontal (gum) disease. Often it takes medical detective work, using the tests recommended by the Bale/Doneen Method, to uncover the root cause, which can sometimes be quite surprising. Later in the book, we'll tell you about a patient whose heart attack was triggered by a dental infection. You'll also learn how to keep your gums healthy, and why doing so can prevent a heart attack.

4 Are you getting the right treatment?

Many patients mistakenly assume that if their healthcare provider is treating them according to medical guidelines, they are getting the best possible care. Sadly, that's not necessarily true. The standard of care is adequate to prevent a lawsuit, but might not be good enough to prevent a heart attack. It is somewhat akin to aiming for a C rather than an A in school. In Chapter Ten, we'll show you how to get grade-A personalized care, without changing doctors.

If you have already been diagnosed with arterial disease because you've had a heart attack or stroke, this book will give you the latest medical findings on how to reverse the disease or halt its progression. Optimal medical care is just as effective for preventing heart attacks, strokes, and early death from CVD as are costly, invasive, and potentially risky procedures like balloon angioplasty, stents, and bypass surgery, according to the COURAGE clinical trial, which involved nearly 2,300 patients.

We'll show you how to work with your doctor to set optimal, personalized treatment goals to safely halt and reverse the disease in your arteries—without surgery. As you'll learn in Part Three, periodically monitoring and measuring the plaque in your arteries, combined with having blood or urine tests to check for inflammation, is an important way to tell if your treatment is working.

A Six-Step Prevention Plan

Unlike standard care, the Bale/Doneen Method doesn't rely solely on risk-factor analysis to predict which patients could be headed for heart attack or stroke and therefore need treatment. Risk factors such as high blood pressure, smoking, obesity, and high cholesterol do not block the flow of blood to your heart or brain. If you don't have plaque in your arteries, you won't have a heart attack or stroke, even if you have lots of other risk factors.

Conversely, if your arteries are diseased, you could have a heart attack or stroke, even if you have few or no other risk factors. Therefore, the goal of our method plan is to find out if you have atherosclerosis—and if so, to halt its progression with the best, evidenced-based therapies. Our method is based on six dynamic elements. Each element is a crucial component of taking charge of your health and could help save your life.

The first letters of these elements—*Education, Disease, Fire, Root* cause, *Optimal* care, and *Genetics*—form the acronym EDFROG, which is easy to remember if you think of our method as a frog named Ed. We picture Ed as a health champion who harnesses the power of solid science to defeat the world's most dangerous—and wily—adversary: cardiovascular disease. To illustrate key points about our method in presentations to healthcare providers and our patients, we commissioned an artist, Moss Freedman, to create simple cartoons that you'll see throughout the book.

What's the difference?

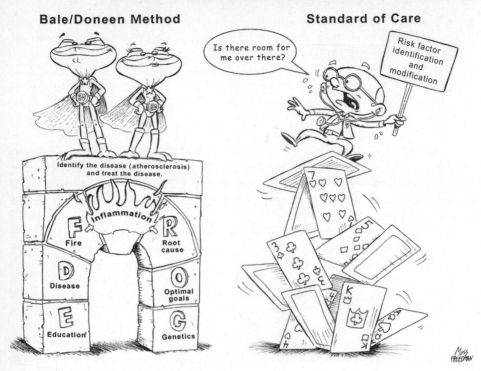

Here is a closer look at EDFROG and how the six elements of our method work together to detect and stop a wily predator: arterial disease.

1. Education: What Most Doctors Don't Tell You About Heart Attacks and Strokes

   Understanding what causes heart attacks and strokes plus the action steps needed to prevent these catastrophes empowers people to make choices that lead to recovery and wellness. Even though many of our patients have already survived a heart attack or stroke, they are shocked when we explain how these events actually occur. Most people think that heart attacks and strokes are triggered by cholesterol building up inside blood vessels, like grease clogging the drainpipe of a kitchen sink, until the vessel gets so obstructed that blood flow stops, causing a heart attack or stroke.

   That's a very common myth. More than fifteen years ago, researchers demonstrated that the blockage that triggers a heart attack or stroke is actually a blood clot, not cholesterol buildup. This potentially lethal clot occurs when a cholesterol deposit (plaque) inside an artery wall becomes inflamed, like a pimple, and causes a tear in the inner lining of the artery. The body tries to seal the crack by forming a blood clot, which can cause a major blockage of blood flow, leading to a heart attack (if the clot blocks a coronary artery) or a stroke (if the clot blocks an artery supplying the brain). We refer to this concept as "event reality."

Heart attacks and strokes aren't the only potential consequence of plaque rupture. It was recently reported that in many cases, this event can result in small clots that cause "silent" (symptomless) heart attacks or strokes, or the tear can heal, causing progressive growth of the buildup in the artery wall. In other words, the plaque deposit gets bigger and potentially more dangerous. All three of these possible consequences are serious issues.

Many doctors, however, still base diagnosis and treatment decisions on the outdated premise that heart disease is essentially a plumbing problem, a concept that's often combined with the "70 percent rule." Patients are frequently told that there's nothing to worry about unless major arteries that feed the heart or brain are 70 percent obstructed by plaque in some areas. If that's the case, you'll probably be advised, as David was, to undergo an invasive procedure, such as bypass surgery or angioplasty (inflating a tiny balloon inside the vessel to widen it temporarily, an intervention that's usually combined with inserting a stent to prop the blocked area open).

Traditionally, doctors have considered large blockages so dangerous that immediate surgery is required to head off a heart attack. The concept is that if blood vessels are too clogged, it's time to call the Roto-Rotor person (a cardiologist or cardiovascular surgeon) either to clear the blockage (angioplasty and stents) or to install new pipes (bypass surgery). That's hugely profitable for these specialists, who rake in billions of dollars from performing these procedures, but does it also pay off in better outcomes for patients?

What many people don't realize is that these costly and potentially risky procedures don't cure cardiovascular disease and also can miss potentially deadly plaque lurking silently in areas with no blockage. These hidden deposits frequently trigger the "events" we discussed earlier. Nearly 20 years ago, a study found that 86 percent of heart attacks occur in people whose coronary arteries are less than 70 percent obstructed, and 68 percent occur when the major arteries feeding the heart are less than 50 percent blocked. Yet, incredibly, areas with anything less than 50 percent blockage are usually termed "mild" by cardiologists.

That's right—most heart attacks don't strike in severely blocked areas, the ones that cardiovascular surgeons target for bypasses and stents! We recently heard about a case in which a patient keeled over from a heart attack in a hospital parking lot, on the way home after having a stent procedure that was supposed to save him from this fate. That's because the heart attack happened in a coronary artery that wasn't blocked when the stent was placed—and therefore went untreated, an all-too-common scenario when doctors practice Roto-Rotor medicine as the sole therapy for cardiovascular disease.

The problem is that invasive procedures—even ones as extensive as quadruple-bypass surgery—only treat a few inches of the more than 60,000 miles of blood vessels in the human body. It's common, however, for people with heart disease to have dozens—or even hundreds—of plaque deposits that are too small to show up in angiograms (X-rays of blood flow in heart arteries) or to cause symptoms, such as angina (chest pain sparked by resulting from reduced flow of oxygenated blood to the heart, caused by narrowing of the coronary arteries).

In fact, a startling 2004 study by Dr. Steven Nissen of the Cleveland Clinic found that only 1 percent of cholesterol plaques obstruct blood flow to the heart at all. The other 99 percent lurks silently inside arterial walls. That's why stents and bypasses failed to prevent heart attacks in many patients: 99 percent of the disease is being ignored by this approach, including the most deadly type of plaque, soft, inflamed deposits hiding inside artery walls.

Despite decades of research proving that heart attacks occur when an inflamed area of plaque bursts through an artery wall, leading to the formation of a clot that abruptly halts blood flow, the old notion that only severely narrowed arteries are dangerous persists. As one prominent cardiologist put it, once a patient is sent to the catheterization lab for heart tests, if a large blockage is found, the person often finds that he or she is trapped on a "train where you can't get off at any station along the way. Once you get on the train, you're getting the stents." Furthermore, for many patients, the express train to stent placement isn't a one-time journey: Stents are prone to clogging over time and patients often need repeat procedures.

Other heart attack truths that most healthcare providers won't tell you—or don't know—are these:

- Abnormal cholesterol levels have never been proven to cause CAD and can be a poor predictor of heart attack risk. In fact, a large study found that the vast majority of people hospitalized for heart attacks have cholesterol levels considered normal under current national guidelines, and many have "optimal" levels.

- All LDL (bad) cholesterol is *not* equally harmful. The size of the particles also matters. People whose LDL consists mainly of small, dense LDL particles—detectable with an inexpensive blood test most doctors don't order—have triple the risk of heart disease as those who have mainly large particles, studies show.

- Blood pressure reading at your healthcare provider's office may not be accurate, because some patients develop "white coat hypertension," temporarily elevated readings due to the stress of a medical visit. And the standard target of blood pressure of 140/90 mm Hg recommended by current medical guidelines may not be good enough to keep your blood vessels healthy.

- A simple measurement most healthcare providers don't check—your waist circumference—is a more accurate predictor of heart attack and stroke risk than your weight or body mass index (BMI).

- As you'll learn in this chapter, most doctors use a highly unreliable blood-sugar test that misses the root cause of 70 percent of heart attacks.

2. Disease: The Cat in the Gutter

To help our patients—and the healthcare providers who attend our continuing medical education program—understand what a sly predator cardiovascular disease is, we show them a simple cartoon. It depicts a city square in which a cat is crouched in a gutter, below ground level, preparing to pounce on an unsuspecting pigeon. The cat represents plaque deposits and the gutter is the blood vessel lining where plaque lurks. If the cat leaps out of the gutter (a plaque rupture), you could have a heart attack or stroke.

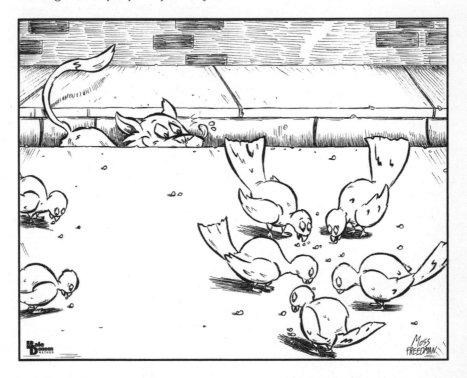

Although most people think of heart attacks as painful or fatal events, as discussed earlier, some heart attacks (and strokes) go unnoticed because they don't spark any obvious symptoms. A recent study by Duke University Medical Centers researchers found that silent, undiagnosed heart attacks are actually more common than was previously believed, affecting nearly 200,000 Americans a year. Like full-blown heart attacks, the silent ones are triggered by blood clots, not just by plaque buildup, and are more likely to occur in people with heart attack red flags, such as smoking, diabetes, or a family history of CVD.

And while these attacks typically go undiagnosed, they can have deadly consequences. When the Duke researchers tracked people who had experienced silent heart attacks for two years, those patients were up to seventeen times more likely to die from cardiovascular causes than were patients with no heart damage. Silent strokes are also dangerous because they can lead to vascular dementia, in which a series of very small strokes block the brain's blood vessels, causing memory problems, confusion, and other Alzheimer's-like symptoms. This devastating disorder is sometimes called "post-stroke dementia."

The key to finding the cat before it does irreversible or fatal harm is looking for it in the right place: the arterial wall, *not* the arterial lumen (the open corridor through which blood travels). As you've learned in this chapter, 99 percent of plaque does not obstruct blood flow—and therefore can't be detected with indirect screening techniques, such as the stress test David passed with "flying colors," three months before his coronary artery calcium score revealed his true heart attack danger.

What did the treadmill test miss? The fundamental flaw of this five-decade-old exam is that it's based on the plumbing concept: the aim is to find out if the pipes are clogged. Most patients don't know that in order to "fail" a stress test, their coronary arteries would have to be at least 70 percent blocked in some areas. And even then, as David's experience illustrates, large obstructions or even areas that are 100 percent blocked may be missed. In fact, studies show that the stress test is such an inaccurate screening tool that the U.S. Preventative Services Task Force recommends against using it to check asymptomatic patients for coronary artery disease.

Our method checks for the cat with tests that examine the arterial wall directly, such as the cIMT test we described in Chapter One. This "ultrasound of the neck" measures the thickness of the intima, the layer of the arterial wall that actually comes in contact with your blood. It's comprised of the endothelium, the smooth interior lining of your arteries, plus connective tissue. Some doctors call the endothelium "the brain" of the arteries because it plays a vital role in regulating blood pressure and other vessel activities.

Amazingly, the endothelium is only one cell thick, but qualifies as the largest organ in your body. If you removed it from your vessels and flattened it, the endothelium would cover six tennis courts! As you can see, far from being inert pipes, your blood vessels are living, multilayered tubes. If your endothelium, which we call "the tennis court," is damaged, its ability to serve as a smart barrier between your blood and your arteries is undermined. If the tennis court fails, harmful substances, such as small dense LDL cholesterol particles, can invade the vessels and form plaque. That's how these predatory cats are created.

The goal of our method isn't necessarily to get rid of the cat, which isn't always possible, even with optimal care, but rather to stabilize plaque deposits. In other words, successful treatment typically involves caging the cat so this dangerous predator can't leap out of its hiding place and attack. Periodically monitoring and measuring the plaque in your arteries is an important way to tell if your treatment is working. Medications and certain supplements are often necessary to prevent a heart attack or stroke, and without proper education about their value, patients may unknowingly refuse potentially lifesaving opportunities to halt or reverse the disease in their arteries.

The central message of our book is that even with many cats in the gutter, with the right care, you can lead a long and healthy life without fear. Heart attacks and strokes are not inevitable, even if you already have blood vessel disease or are at high risk for developing it because of your family history or other red flags.

3. Fire in the Arteries: The Hidden Cause of Heart Attacks and Strokes

Some people, like Camille, have early warning signs of an impending heart attack weeks, months, or even as long as three years before the event—clues that are often misdiagnosed by physicians or dismissed as stress related, a study has shown. Other people have no symptoms at all prior to going into cardiac arrest. In either scenario, what fuels these catastrophes is chronic inflammation, a manifestation of other abnormalities in the body such as obesity, stress, high cholesterol, poor diet, arthritis, insulin resistance, and infection.

Most of the time, inflammation, which we call *fire*, is a lifesaver and combats diseases such as bacterial and viral infections. We've all experienced the typical signs of redness, warmth, and swelling around a wound. But in some people, particularly those who are overweight, inactive, eat poorly, or are migrating toward diabetes, this fiery process becomes chronic. The body responds as if normal cells are alien invaders and attacks them.

Think of plaque as kindling. Inflammation is what lights the match, causing the plaque to rupture explosively. That tears the blood vessel lining, leading to the formation of a clot. The clot chokes off blood flow to the heart, igniting a heart attack. Inflammation is the key player in destabilizing plaque, explaining why some people with relatively little buildup have heart attacks and strokes, while others with substantial plaque deposits never suffer these events.

Our method uses a "fire panel" of inexpensive blood and urine tests to check for this fiery process and treatments designed to cool inflamed vessels. Statins, for example, aren't just cholesterol-busters. They also appear to combat inflammation and reduce the risk of cardiovascular events. One large study led by Dr. Paul Ridker at Brigham and Women's Hospital in Boston, involving about 12,800 patients in 26 countries, found that treating patients who had high levels of C-reactive protein (CRP), an inflammatory marker, but normal cholesterol with statins trimmed heart attack risk by 54 percent. Stroke risk fell by 48 percent, compared to the control group.

Inflammation is one of the most cutting-edge areas of medical research. It's now believed to be one of the causes of coronary artery disease and has recently been linked to a wide range of other disorders. One surprising 2010 research finding is that people who take low-dose aspirin for heart attack prevention also have a lower risk of several types of cancer, including of the breast, colon, and esophagus. It's likely that aspirin therapy reduces cancer risk by combating inflammation, offering a potential new insight into how some types of cancer develop that could lead to improved treatments.

4. Root Cause: Finding the Hidden Trigger of Cardiovascular Disease

To put out the fire inside blood vessels, it's essential to know what's causing it. If you have already had a heart attack or stroke, identifying and treating the root cause of the inflammation, along with determining genetic predispositions, is crucial to preventing a recurrence.

In Camille's case, the tests we performed a few weeks after her heart attack showed that the double whammy of genes and insulin resistance, which is extremely common in people who are overweight or obese, was the culprit. Because she had been insulin resistant for such a long time, she was on the brink of diabetes. Receiving a diagnosis that explained the heart attack was a profound relief for Camille, since she finally understood *why* it had happened. Armed with that knowledge, she no longer felt powerless over her disease.

We were also able to solve the mystery of why David had developed widespread heart disease, despite his impressively healthy lifestyle. Even though he was lean and physically fit, his blood sugar tested in the prediabetic range, as measured by the highly accurate two-hour oral glucose tolerance test (OGTT). The Irish CEO was astonished, and dismayed, by the diagnosis, since an earlier test by another healthcare provider had near-normal results.

It turned out that the other provider had used an unreliable screening tool called the AIC blood test. Since this test doesn't require fasting before the blood is drawn, it's convenient for busy patients. However, it frequently yields misleading results, our research shows. In a study we presented in 2011 at the 4th International Congress on Prediabetes and Metabolic Syndrome in Spain, we found that of 527 patients who were checked with various blood-sugar tests, using the A1C test alone would have missed 259 of those with prediabetes. That alarmingly high error rate, along with published data from other researchers demonstrating the same thing, is why we recommend against this test.

About 150 million Americans have insulin resistance—essentially a prediabetic condition—and most of them don't know it, because their doctors haven't done the OGTT advised by the Bale/Doneen Method and endorsed by the American Diabetes Association as the "gold standard" in diagnosing diabetes and prediabetes. Our method also uses the results of this test to uncover insulin resistance years—or even decades—before it progresses to diabetes.

Although David was dismayed by this diagnosis, he also found it empowering. "It was an unbelievably important part of the evaluation to learn that I was on the route to diabetes. Getting that insight was very valuable, because this is an incredibly preventable disease. The lesson was that I'm sugar-sensitive and have to be very controlled about what I eat," said the CEO, who is working with a dietician to further improve his usually highly disciplined eating habits.

One key change is forgoing sweet drinks, such as the ice-cream smoothies he sometimes indulged in prior to his prediabetes diagnosis. Like many people, he was unaware of how dangerous these beverages can be: A recent study found that sugar-sweetened drinks were the culprits in 14,000 new cases of heart disease, 75,000 new cases of diabetes, and 7,000 premature deaths over the past decade. And a recent Harvard study also reported that drinking just one or two sugar-laden drinks a day magnifies diabetes risk by 26 percent.

Uncovering the root cause of David's cardiovascular disease helped us fine-tune the treatments his other doctors had prescribed, by adding an ACE (angiotensin converting enzyme) inhibitor. These medications widen blood vessels to improve the amount of blood the heart pumps. Not only do they lower blood pressure, but research shows that for prediabetic patients like David, they also reduce the risk of progressing to full-blown diabetes by 34 percent.

Our method also uses the OGTT test results to catch insulin resistance long before it progresses to prediabetes or diabetes. Finding out if you have this dangerous condition, which is the root cause of 70 percent of heart attacks and strokes, and getting the right treatment, could help you lead a longer and healthier life, by protecting you from three of the leading killers of Americans: heart attacks, strokes, and diabetes.

5. Optimal Goals: The Key to Cardiovascular Wellness

All patients deserve optimal care, but sadly, the standard medical guidelines—a do-the-bare-minimum approach—for assessing heart attack risk failed to discover Camille's true danger before her heart attack, and standard management of her care after the attack would have left her at risk for having another heart attack, because her doctors hadn't identified and treated the root cause. Our comprehensive assessment of both her risk factors and the disease present in her arteries revealed that her doctor was on the right track by advising a statin, but she also needed a beta blocker and a diabetes drug to improve her body's sensitivity to insulin. Similarly, David needed an additional medication to lower heart attack risk—and halt the progression toward diabetes.

Instead of simply asking if Camille wanted these medications—or telling her she must take them to save her life—we helped her make an informed decision by explaining our rationale for advising these therapies and presenting the pros and cons (in Chapter Eleven, we'll discuss these and other common heart and diabetes drugs, as well as natural supplements, in depth). Without this knowledge, patients like David and Camille may refuse potentially lifesaving treatments, believing that they aren't necessary or out of fear of potential side effects that are far less concerning than the threat of a fatal heart attack.

And while practitioners of standard care probably would have told Camille that she should lose weight and exercise more, overweight, out-of-shape people who are recovering from a heart attack or stroke already know that. What's lacking in usual cardiac care are achievable goals and the specific action steps outlined in Part Three of this book, showing you what to do every day to promote a healthier lifestyle and bring your disease under control.

Like many other people with CVD, Camille had struggled with her weight for her entire life, particularly after she became a busy mom juggling child-care and a full-time office job. While it would have been great if she could have achieved the ideal weight for her frame, research shows that if overweight people in the early stages of diabetes shed as little as 5 to 10 percent of their body weight (12 to 24 pounds, in Camille's case), the risk of progressing to full-blown diabetes falls dramatically. Empowered with the knowledge that losing even a few pounds could make a major difference to her health, she cut down on calories and starting walking, then jogging.

6. Genetics: The Ultimate in Personalized Care

Care that's personalized to the individual, rather than treating everybody according to the average results from a large study, is the best way to prevent heart attacks and strokes. As you'll learn in Chapter Eight, millions of Americans unknowingly carry common genetic mutations that boost their cardiovascular threat, including one mutation that can raise heart attack risk by up to 102 percent. Basing your medical care and lifestyle choices on your unique genetic makeup is truly the ultimate in personalized medicine. That's why the Bale/Doneen Method has used genetic testing for more than a decade.

Genetic testing used to cost thousands of dollars. Now the cost is about $100 per gene tested. At present, there are four genes known to play a major role in heart attack and stroke threat for which the Bale/Doneen Method recommends tests. This risk assessment costs less than a mammogram or colonoscopy. And unlike other medical tests, genetic tests only need to be done once, since your genes don't change. Testing is sometimes covered by insurance, particularly if you have a family history of CVD.

David's genetic tests revealed another root cause of his heart disease. Like Camille, he was also a carrier of the 9P21 "heart attack" gene, an independent predictor of risk even when such confounding factors as diabetes, high blood pressure, and obesity are taken into account. As is the case for about 25 percent of Americans (including Camille), he was homozygous for this gene, meaning that he had inherited copies of the gene from both parents. Studies link this genetic profile to a 102-percent rise in risk for suffering a heart attack or developing heart disease at an early age, compared to noncarriers of the gene, and a 74-percent jump in risk for aortic abdominal aneurysm, a weak, ballooning area in the heart's largest blood vessel. About 50 percent of Caucasians and Asians have one copy of the 9P21 gene, which the same studies calculate as conferring half as much risk of each of the outcomes above.

The genetic tests we ordered also showed that David had a variant in his ApoE gene that both increased his heart attack risk and influenced how his body broke down nutrients, making some foods that are heart-protective for most people the wrong choices for him. In Chapter Twelve we'll describe how your diet can be tailored to your DNA for increased protection against heart attacks and strokes. We'll also alert you to a variety of easy actions, some of them surprising and fun, that enhance heart health.

Had his primary care doctor ordered genetic tests, and discovered the hidden threats lurking in David's DNA, the MD should have ordered a thorough cardiac workup, instead of relying on the dangerously unreliable treadmill test that even missed the 100 percent obstruction in one of his coronary arteries. Similarly, had Camille's doctor discovered through genetic testing that she was a carrier of both the 9P21 and KIF6 genes, he should have insisted on comprehensive tests and aggressive management of her cardiovascular threats to prevent a heart attack.

By following the personalized treatment plan that we recommend in this book, one year after her heart attack, Camille had lost 45 pounds through diet and exercise, and was so fit that she competed in a 12K race and later a half-marathon. "I got a medal and felt very proud of how hard I'd worked turn my health around," says Camille, who changed jobs to a different position in her field. In her old job, she worked a 10-hour day under the supervision of a very demanding boss. The new job isn't as stressful and the hours are shorter.

Although Camille has continued to struggle with her weight (she now weighs 188 pounds), the healthy changes she's made have actually reversed her prediabetes so effectively that she no longer needs a diabetes drug. "Learning the right way to take care of myself has been life-altering," Camille told us during a recent checkup. More than seven years after her heart attack, she remains in excellent health. "And now I sleep like a baby, because I'm not worrying about when the next thunderbolt will strike."

And while David was already at an ideal weight for his height, he's now working out seven days a week and has gotten his secret sweet tooth under control. Our comprehensive exam also uncovered that he had another cardiovascular risk: periodontal disease, a bacterial infection of the gums. Nearly 75 million Americans have unhealthy gums, which can nearly double the risk of a heart attack—and like David, many of them don't realize it, because an oral infection is painless in the early stages. Gum disease can also be a red flag for stroke danger—and not just for the elderly. Another little-known fact: Good oral health and getting regular dental care can help lower diabetes risk. There seems to be a two-way link: Periodontal disease worsens insulin resistance, and having insulin resistance raises the threat of developing gum disease too.

Since oral infections and insulin resistance each spark inflammation, having both disorders packs a one-two punch that further magnifies risk for diabetes. Using the state-of-the-art therapies we advise later in the book, David is working with a periodontist to extinguish the inflammation in his gums, which in turn, is helping put out the fire in his blood vessels.

Although David has only been following our program for a few months, he no long fears that cardiovascular disease will cut his life short, forcing his six children to grow up without a father. And he's avoided a trip to the OR for bypass surgery, despite severe blockages. "My blood sugar and LDL levels are already way down and I no longer have the arteries of an 87-year-old man, as my initial cIMT results showed. I feel extremely fortunate that I now have the tools to manage my health, based on empirical evidence," he says.

David realizes that he gained much more than one additional insight through his 5,000-mile trip to our clinic. Despite his prior consultation with two other excellent experts in heart attack prevention, he was still able to add to the comprehensiveness of his evaluation and personalized treatment using the Bale/Doneen Method to ensure he lives a long, productive life without suffering a cardiovascular event. "It's a crime that everyone isn't getting this type of lifesaving care," adds David, who has lost four close relatives to fatal heart attacks, including an uncle who died at age 55.

He reports that his doctor had never asked about his extended family history. "In Ireland, you're typically only asked at what age your parents died. Since my father was in excellent health up until his heart attack at age 85, and my mother also lived into her eighties, I had no reason to suspect that I'd developed widespread heart disease at age 52. Had I not discovered through testing that I was in the worst 1 percent for heart attack risk—and found doctors who have come forward with a solution—there's no doubt that I would have dropped dead."

In the next chapter, we'll alert you to red flags that signal increased heart attack and stroke risk, including several that are little-known and very surprising. You'll also meet a 37-year-old dentist who suffered a seemingly inexplicable stroke, which turned out to be triggered by a truly shocking, recently recognized risk factor—and find out how to protect yourself from this common cardiovascular menace.

Action Step: Compile Your Family Medical History

As genetics is explaining more and more diseases, including many cases of cardiovascular disease, gathering a complete, accurate family medical history is key to managing your health. While the Reynolds Risk Score for women only deems the death of a parent because of cardiovascular disease before age 60 significant, we advise patients of both sexes to compile data on your immediate and extended family—specifically your parents, grandparents, aunts, uncles, and siblings for a fuller picture of potential danger that may be lurking in your DNA. Alert your doctor if these relatives have any history of the following conditions:

- Cardiovascular Disease at Any Age

  Since CVD often progresses slowly, over decades, if anyone in your extended family was affected by it, try to determine the *earliest* age at which it was first detected. For example, if your grandfather or another close relative died of a heart attack at age 85, it's also important for your doctor to know if the disease was initially diagnosed at 60, since that might increase your risk for developing CVD at a younger-than-usual age.

  Gather as much medical data as possible on close relatives who experienced any of these events: a diagnosis of heart disease, undergoing bypass surgery or other heart procedures, or suffering a stroke or ministroke (also known as a transient ischemic attack, or TIA). Also ask about factors that may have increased the affected relative's risk, such as smoking, obesity, or high blood pressure (which can also have an inherited component).

- Diabetes or Prediabetes

  As you learned in Chapter One, insulin resistance is the root cause of 70 percent of heart attacks and is also the culprit in many strokes. Any family history of diabetes or prediabetes in close relatives raises your risk of developing high blood sugar, particularly if you are also overweight, and indicates that you should be checked with a two-hour oral glucose tolerance test, as should anyone over age 40, regardless of family history.

- Alzheimer's Disease or Dementia

  Sometimes referred to as "senility," cognitive impairment is not a normal part of aging. Frequently, blood vessel disease, which can include a series of small strokes or TIAs that may not cause any noticeable symptoms, causes or contributes to dementia. Damage from these silent stokes, which typically result in blood clots that temporarily dam flow though the brain arteries, leading to confusion and memory loss.

  As you'll read in the next chapter, even full-blown strokes usually aren't painful. Because public awareness of the warning signs is alarmingly low, people who suffer them frequently delay seeking medical care or make the tragic, even fatal mistake of thinking that they'll feel better after a good night's rest. And you may be startled by some of the red flags that can signal that even a young person may be at higher risk for a heart attack or stroke than he or she thinks.

Chapter 3

Red Flags— Are You at Risk?

"Each patient carries his own doctor inside him. They come to us not knowing that truth. We are at our best when we give the doctor who resides within each patient a chance to go to work."

—Albert Schweitzer, MD

When strange symptoms struck, Lauralee Nygaard, DDS, MS, says, "I had just enough medical knowledge to be dangerous." It was late afternoon, near the end of a hectic day at her dental clinic. Then 37, the periodontist from Spokane, Washington, had been feeling unusually tired and listless for months, but thought, "This is what midlife looks like."

Or maybe she was juggling too much. Between working long hours at her periodontal clinic and trying to keep up with her two kids—a toddler and an energetic six-year-old—at home, there were many days when she didn't have time even to floss her teeth. Usually a quick brushing in the morning was all she could manage before rushing off to the dental clinic.

Between patients that afternoon, Lauralee took a quick break to eat a candy bar. With one more gum surgery to perform before heading for home to cook dinner for guests, she really needed a quick energy boost. Besides, the extra calories were nothing to worry about. Even after two kids, she could still fit into her size-two skinny jeans. And although she wasn't exercising as much as she used to, friends always told she was the healthiest-looking person they knew.

The gum surgery went smoothly, but just as she was about to put in the final stitch, something strange happened. "I looked through my magnifying loupe. All of a sudden, I couldn't see. Everything was a blur." Suspecting that something might be wrong with the magnifying lens, she put it down and peered at the patient's chart. It was equally blurry.

"I was starting to have trouble with my motor skills, but somehow I managed to tie the final suture so I could leave the patient," she recalls. "From the medical training I'd received in dental school, I intuitively knew I was having a stroke. I walked into my office and chewed two aspirin. The neurologist told me later that I'd probably saved my life by doing that.

"There was no pain or even tingling. That's what makes strokes incredibly dangerous. You don't feel like anything serious is happening. The whole experience just seemed surreal—everything looked like it was covered with white fuzz, like the snow on an old TV screen."

So deep was her denial that she could be facing a potentially life-threatening medical emergency at age 37 that it didn't occur to her to call 911 or even tell her staff about her symptoms. Instead, she calmly walked across the clinic to see the final patient of the day. "When I said, 'Hello,' my speech was so slurred that my dental hygienist asked, 'What's wrong? You sound like you're drunk.'"

But Lauralee still didn't consider her symptoms alarming. "My eyes felt weird, but I wasn't stumbling, my blood pressure was fine, and just to look at me, you wouldn't have known that anything was wrong. But I was acting oddly, so my staff drove me home."

By the time she got there, her vision and speech had returned to normal. Other than her unusual exhaustion, everything seemed fine. She ate dinner with guests who were staying with her, then went to bed early, unaware that delays in getting medical care for a suspected stroke can be a very dangerous—or even fatal mistake.

The next morning, at her husband's insistence, she consulted her family physician. "He patted me on the shoulder and said he was pretty sure that I'd had a migraine headache," a problem she'd never experienced in the past. Lauralee demanded that the doctor order a brain MRI, which showed that she had indeed suffered a stroke.

She was referred to a neurologist, who ordered a battery of high-tech tests, including two additional MRI scans. "The neurologist said that in someone under 40, a stroke was usually caused by a genetic defect or a clotting disorder, but he'd check for everything."

Three months and thousands of dollars in medical bills later, she was diagnosed with "cryptogenic stroke," meaning that the cause was a medical mystery. "The neurologist said, 'I don't know why it happened, but I hope we never have to see each other again. It's a miracle that you have no neurological impairments from the stroke.'"

Like Camille Zaleski, she was advised to remember her symptoms and call 911 if they ever happened again. "I wasn't able to accept that the medical community couldn't explain why I'd had a stroke when I wasn't even 40 years old. I had young children and thought, 'I have to live to see them grow up. There's no way this just randomly happens.'"

Brain Attack

Every year, nearly 800,000 Americans have strokes—and for 25 percent of those who do, it's a repeat event, leaving them at extreme risk for serious or fatal complications. Stroke is the third leading cause of death worldwide, killing more than five million men and women a year. Scarier still, researchers recently predicted that this grim toll will double by 2020, largely due to an aging population combined with our increasingly unhealthy lifestyle.

Also known as "brain attack," *ischemic stroke* (the most common type of stroke) is basically a heart attack that occurs in the brain. Like a heart attack, this type of stroke is usually triggered by a rupture of an inflamed cholesterol plaque inside the artery walls, leading to the formation of a blood clot that cuts off blood flow to part of the brain. With an *embolic stroke,* a clot (embolism) forms in a blood vessel in another part of the body (often the heart), then travels to the brain. Clots spark about 90 percent of strokes.

A *hemorrhagic stroke* occurs when a blood vessel inside the brain bursts. The leading risk factor is high blood pressure, which can stress arteries until they develop a weak, ballooning area known as an aneurysm. If untreated, the aneurysm can eventually rupture, allowing blood to spill into brain tissue, often causing serious or even fatal damage.

Because stroke symptoms can be subtle and are rarely painful, they often don't seem alarming. Lauralee is unusual in that she correctly diagnosed herself. Surveys show that most people can't even name two symptoms of this killer condition. Later in the chapter, we'll tell you an easy way to remember the warning signs and a quick test you can do if you suspect someone is having a stroke.

During a stroke, two million brain cells die each minute. The longer someone waits to get care after the onset of stroke symptoms, the greater the risk of permanent brain damage, lifelong disability, or death. Only 10 percent of stroke survivors make a full or nearly full recovery. The rest are left with varying degrees of impairment, which can include brain damage, paralysis, memory loss, confusion, difficulty talking or swallowing, and, in some cases, chronic pain.

Stroke is the number-one cause of chronic disability in adults—a frightening statistic that highlights the urgent need for optimal medical care to prevent brain attacks. Most people, however, don't receive that level of care, even after they've already suffered one or more strokes.

Deadly Misconceptions

One of the most dangerous medical myths still widely prevalent among doctors, including some neurologists, is the belief that certain strokes are impossible to prevent or even explain. Patients like Lauralee are left in a terrifying position: Because they're told that their stroke was just random bad luck—like being struck by lightning on a cloudless day—they feel powerless to protect themselves from the next, possibly fatal thunderbolt that might loom in the future.

In reality, all strokes and heart attacks are potentially preventable with optimal medical care, which includes correctly identifying and treating the root causes of the patient's cardiovascular disease. In this chapter, we'll also alert you to some surprising—and little-known—red flags that signal increased risk for a heart attack or stroke, including migraine headaches, psoriasis, and even snoring.

Thirty-seven percent of Americans have two or more major risk factors for cardiovascular disease, such as a couch-potato lifestyle, obesity, smoking, high blood pressure, diabetes, and high cholesterol. And while most women consider themselves to be at considerably lower risk for stroke than men are, in reality, the opposite is true. Nearly two-thirds of all fatal strokes occur in women. As we'll discuss in Chapter Five, women often receive less-aggressive care for CVD, because women themselves—and many doctors—underestimate their risk.

Another common misconception is that strokes are primarily a threat to the elderly. In reality, 33 percent of strokes—and 45 percent of heart attacks—occur in people under age 65. A recent study found that the warning signs of stroke are frequently misdiagnosed in people under age 50, as occurred in Lauralee's case, when her symptoms were initially attributed to a migraine headache.

Stroke Triggers

When Lauralee consulted us, she was convinced that even after an extensive battery of tests—including MRIs and other imaging exams—her physicians had missed something. A slender nonsmoker, she was one of the healthiest-looking patients we'd ever seen in our practice. She didn't have high blood pressure, which magnifies stroke risk by four to six times, or insulin resistance, the root cause of 70 percent of heart attacks and strokes.

Her medical records showed that she'd received a standard workup for an unexplained stroke. According to her test results, she didn't have any of these stroke triggers:

- A Hole in Her Heart

    About 40 percent of people who suffer unexplained strokes—particularly patients under age 55—have a small hole in the heart called a patent foramen ovale (PFO). Everyone has a PFO before birth: This opening between the two upper chambers of the heart allows a fetus's blood to bypass the developing lungs. After birth, the PFO normally closes.

    In about 25 percent of people, the PFO fails to seal shut. The flap-like opening typically acts like a swinging door, only opening when there's increased pressure in the chest, which can occur when the person coughs, sneezes, or strains during a bowel movement. A PFO makes it possible for a blood clot that forms elsewhere in the body to travel to the brain, where it can block a blood vessel and cause a stroke.

    A PFO can be diagnosed through imaging tests such as an echocardiogram. Stroke patients who have a hole in their heart are often put on blood-thinning medications to reduce the risk of recurrence, while people with a PFO who haven't had a stroke don't need treatment unless the condition is causing other problems, such as a transient ischemic attack (ministroke).

- Abnormal Heartbeats

    Nearly three million Americans have atrial fibrillation (AF), the most common heart arrhythmia. AF occurs when rapid, disorganized electrical signals make the heart's two upper chambers (atria) contract very rapidly and irregularly (fibrillation). AF is a major risk factor for stroke, making people who have it five times more likely to suffer a stroke than those without it. That's because the irregular beat allows blood to pool in the atria, boosting the danger that a clot will form and then be carried to the brain.

Although AF can strike at any age, it's most common in the elderly, affecting about 5 percent of those ages 65 and older. Often, it doesn't cause any noticeable symptoms, but some people who have it experience racing, pounding, or fluttering in their chest, known as "the butterflies." About 20 percent of strokes are linked to AF.

One way to tell if you might have AF is to check your pulse for 60 seconds and see if you notice any irregular beats. If so, consult your doctor for further evaluation, which may include an electrocardiogram. Also be aware that some people experience asymptomatic AF that requires longer-term evaluation with an "event monitor" to track heartbeats for up to 30 days.

- Blood-Clotting Disorders

    A number of inherited conditions, such as Factor V Leiden, raise the risk of developing blood clots. Warning signs that you might have a clotting disorder include developing clots in your legs (deep vein thrombosis) and livedo reticularis (areas of skin with a mottled, purplish discoloration. Women who have suffered more than one miscarriage are also at increased risk for blood clots.

    Other risk factors for developing clots include recent surgery, a broken bone or other injuries, taking birth control or hormone replacement therapy, obesity, and making long airplane or car trips. If you're prone to blood clots or have a clotting disorder, your doctor may prescribe blood-thinning medication. During travel, it's advisable to get up and move around every two or three hours to keep your blood flowing and reduce the risk of forming a clot.

- Blood Vessel Blockages

    Using an ultrasound test called carotid duplex, Lauralee's doctors checked for narrowing and blockages in the carotid arteries, two large blood vessels on each side of the neck that supply the brain. This test can be valuable for stroke patients, but it also has a major limitation: The exam only looks at one aspect of blood vessel health, the rate of blood flow through the carotids much like police using a radar gun to see how fast cars are traveling on the highway.

    Since no blockages were found, her healthcare providers concluded that she didn't have cardiovascular disease, the number-one cause of ischemic strokes. What most patients—and many doctors—don't know is that it's possible, and even common, to have CVD that's severe enough to cause a heart attack or stroke *without* blockages in the vessels. In fact, the vast majority of plaque deposits—including highly inflamed areas (the kind that ignite heart attacks and strokes)—do *not* obstruct blood flow at all. Therefore, lack of blockages is *not* proof that a patient is free of CVD.

The Bale/Doneen Method doesn't rely on the results of a single test, but rather a comprehensive, personalized assessment of blood-vessel health, including the patient's red flags, family and medical history, a physical exam, and laboratory and imaging findings. In Lauralee's case, cardiovascular disease remained the top suspect as we continued our evaluation.

Family History: The #1 Heart Attack and Stroke Red Flag

Lauralee had major risk factors for CVD, including a huge red flag: her family history. Two of her uncles had had strokes. Her grandfather had died from heart disease, a few years after undergoing quadruple-bypass surgery for severely obstructed arteries, and her father had survived a heart attack when he was in his fifties. Several large studies show that having a parent who suffered a heart attack or other cardiovascular event at a younger-than-usual age can double or even triple a person's risk.

Like her mom, Lauralee developed very high cholesterol while in her twenties. Initially, she told us, the problem went untreated. "My family doctor said, 'Oh, it's a false positive.' He didn't seem concerned at all. When I had it checked again, a few years later, it was much higher, and so were my triglycerides. I was told to try diet and exercise, but after three months of following a vegan diet and working out, the numbers were even worse, so I was put on a statin. When I had the stroke, I'd been taking Lipitor for about a year. At my last checkup, I'd been told that my cholesterol numbers looked fine."

Understandably, Lauralee assumed the problem had been solved. Like most patients—and some healthcare providers—she wasn't aware that cholesterol numbers aren't the whole story. Studies show that many heart attack and stroke patients have normal or even "optimal" cholesterol levels, yet still have potentially deadly plaque in their arteries. That's why it's also important to look at the *quality* of cholesterol—not just the quantity—using the advanced cholesterol test we recommend in Chapter Seven.

Had her physician ordered this comprehensive cholesterol test, which is covered by all major insurance plans, he would have discovered that one of her numbers was actually dangerously high. Lauralee had elevated levels of lipoprotein (a), a subtype of LDL (bad) cholesterol that's also known as Lp(a). Not only do elevated levels triple a person's risk for heart attacks, three large studies recently found, but Lp(a) also boosts risk for blood clots that can trigger a stroke. Lifestyle doesn't influence Lp(a) levels, which are mainly determined by genes. Nor are statin drugs an effective treatment for elevated Lp(a). Instead, the best therapy is niacin (vitamin B3).

Like Camille, Lauralee was lulled into a false sense of security based on an incomplete risk assessment, since the standard cholesterol test doesn't check Lp(a) levels. Given her family history, her healthcare provider should have investigated her high cholesterol more thoroughly with the advanced cholesterol panel, a simple blood test that costs about forty dollars. Had he done so, and then added an inexpensive vitamin to her treatment, her cardiovascular danger would have been dramatically reduced.

The Health Threat in Your Mouth

When we examined Lauralee's mouth, we discovered a very surprising—and rather ironic—red flag for heart attack and stroke risk: the young dentist had periodontal disease, the very condition that she specialized in treating at her clinic. People with periodontal disease—a bacterial infection of the gums, connective tissue, and bone supporting the teeth—have double or even triple the risk of a heart attack or stroke, recent research suggests.

"Like most dental practitioners, I was so busy taking care of other people that I wasn't very good about taking care of myself," admits Lauralee. "I probably flossed twice a week, if I remembered, and got my teeth cleaned every year or two. In hindsight, I recall my hygienist asking me if I was pregnant, because my gums looked completely inflamed. I thought that was a silly question, but it turned out to be a red flag that I wasn't savvy enough to recognize at the time."

Almost 75 percent of Americans have some degree of gum disease, the most common chronic infection in the United States, many of whom don't know they have it, because in the early stages, the disease is painless. When the infection is relatively mild, it's called gingivitis and when it's more severe, it's known as periodontal disease (PD). At age 30, there's a 50 percent probability that you have periodontal disease and by the time you're 65, risk rises to 70 percent.

The leading warning sign of PD is bleeding gums. Contrary to what many patients assume, it is *not* normal to experience any bleeding, even slight amounts, when you brush or floss. Other symptoms of periodontal disease include bad breath, puffy or receding gums, teeth that look longer (due to receding gums), loose teeth, pockets of pus between your gums and teeth, or a change in your bite. Risk factors for developing periodontal disease include poor oral hygiene, smoking, diabetes, and the hormonal upheavals of pregnancy. Periodontal disease is more likely to strike men than women and disproportionately affects people of certain ethnicities, such as Mexican-Americans.

If you have any of these warning signs, alert your dentist or dental hygienist and ask to be screened for PD. Screening is painless and typically involves:

- A visual inspection and exam of your gums, using a mirror and periodontal probe, to check for redness, puffiness, or other signs of oral infection.

- Positioning the probe at six specific points of each tooth where it's attached to the gum, to measure pocket depth. Pockets measuring three millimeters or more indicate disease.

- Checking for tooth movement. Loose teeth are another sign of gum disease and loss of bone support for the teeth.

When the first studies linking oral infections to higher risk for CVD appeared nearly a decade ago, the Bale/Doneen Method immediately began advising healthcare providers to check patients for periodontal disease. Today, scientific evidence that healthy gums help prevent heart attacks and strokes is so powerful that the editors of *The American Journal of Cardiology* and the *Journal of Periodontology* issued a consensus statement recommending that:

- Doctors and dentists warn patients with moderate to severe gum disease of their potential cardiovascular danger.

- Patients with gum disease should get a complete physical exam and blood pressure measurement annually.

- These patients should also be checked for diabetes, high cholesterol, and a family history of early deaths from CVD.

- People with gum disease and one or more other CVD risk factors, such as blood pressure or high cholesterol, should be treated with lifestyle changes and if necessary, medication, a topic we'll explore in more detail in Chapter Fourteen. In Part Two of this book, we'll discuss additional ways to evaluate your oral health, including a saliva test to check for dangerous oral pathogens that may also harm heart health. This high-tech test uses genetic information and can alert to you to an oral health problem *before* you develop the signs and symptoms of gum disease described in this chapter.

The Inflammation Connection

What's the link between periodontal disease and CVD? Very sophisticated studies have demonstrated a strong similarity between the amount of inflammation in our gums and the amount of inflammation in the major arteries of the neck and the heart's largest artery, the aorta. That's dangerous because inflammation is the key player is destabilizing plaque in the artery walls, explaining why some people with relatively little buildup experience plaque rupture and subsequent strokes or heart attacks, while others with substantial deposits never suffer these events. Studies are now revealing that most plaques in the carotid artery actually contain many of the germs known to cause PD.

Ultimately, our tests showed that Lauralee did have CVD—solving the apparent mystery of her so-called "cryptogenic" stroke, a diagnosis that the Bale/Doneen Method doesn't accept. With the right tests and evaluation, there's no such thing as a medically unexplainable stroke or heart attack. However, the cholesterol plaque in her arteries didn't show up in the carotid duplex test she'd received because it's designed to look for blockages, not vulnerable plaque hidden in artery walls. What her story illustrates is how dangerous even small deposits can be if they become inflamed, in much the same way as being careless with matches can accidentally set a house on fire.

Gum disease isn't the only inflammatory disorder that can raise your heart attack or stroke risk. Inflammation is cholesterol's partner in crime, multiplying CVD risk. When elevated levels of LDL start to burrow inside the blood vessel walls, it sparks an inflammatory response, which is believed to accelerate cholesterol buildup. This in turn triggers more inflammation, creating a vicious cycle as the two villains work in cahoots to create more and more plaque, if the disease goes untreated.

Hidden Risk Factors for CVD

Several surprising disorders have also been linked to a greater threat of CVD. *Even if you don't have any noticeable symptoms of heart disease and don't consider yourself to be a candidate for a stroke, if you have any of these conditions, you're at risk and need to take action now to protect yourself. And the more of them you have, the greater the threat of a heart attack or stroke.*

Early recognition of these red flags coupled with appropriate treatment could save your life. You'll find detailed guidance about medical and natural therapies, including healthy lifestyle changes, to reduce risk—or even reverse—CVD and diabetes in Part Three of this book.

- Migraine Headaches

  Women who have migraines with an aura (visual disturbances, such as flashing lights) at least once a week are more than four times more likely to have a stroke. Migraines also raise CVD risk for men, though not by as much. One intriguing theory: There's evidence that these headaches may be linked to PFO, which affects one in four Americans. Women with migraines shouldn't use birth control pills, which increase stroke risk. And while there are a variety of effective treatments for migraine headaches, it's not yet known if using them will also lower stroke risk.

- Rheumatoid Arthritis

  Having rheumatoid arthritis (RA), an autoimmune disease that causes painful inflammation of joints and surrounding tissues, raises heart attack risk by about 45 percent. However, if you have RA and hyperlipidemia (high levels of lipids, such as cholesterol or triglycerides), heart attack danger soars by a whopping 700 percent—a compelling reason to track your cholesterol with the advanced test advised by the Bale/Doneen Method. If you have RA and plaque in your arteries, we also recommend having your inflammatory markers checked every three months with the tests discussed in Chapter Seven.

- Gout

  A form of arthritis that occurs when uric acid builds up in the blood, gout magnifies your risk for insulin resistance—the leading cause of heart attacks.

If you have even intermittent attacks of gout, we advise getting your blood-sugar level checked with the two-hour oral glucose tolerance test to check for IR, since discovering and treating this very common condition is key to heart attack prevention.

- Lack of Sleep

  Skimping on shut-eye increases the danger of dying from CVD. But until recently, experts weren't sure why. The latest research shows that people who average six hours of sleep an night have significantly higher levels of inflammatory markers than those who snooze for eight. Chronic sleep deprivation is also tied to worse health, as well as to higher rates of smoking, obesity, and high blood pressure, offering additional explanations for its toll on the heart. And getting less than six hours of slumber more than quadruples risk for prediabetes.

  The best defense: Rest one extra hour a night. In a five-year study of healthy volunteers in their forties, that reduced risk of calcium buildup in heart arteries—a predictor of future heart disease risk—by 33 percent. This may be because blood pressure drops during sleep, reducing wear and tear on vessels. It's possible, however, to get too much of a good thing, since nine hours of slumber a night is also tied to higher risk of CVD. Seven to eight hours is optimal.

- Erectile Dysfunction

  Difficulty maintaining an erection sufficient for sex is one of the leading warning signs of heart disease in men. Understanding this link is important for the thirty million American men affected by erectile dysfunction (ED). Research shows that men with ED are 1.4 times more likely to suffer a serious cardiovascular event, such as a heart attack or stroke. Age also plays a role, since ED is much more frequently associated with cardiac issues in men in their forties than it is in men in their seventies.

  If you have ED, discuss a cardiovascular workup with your doctor. Vascular disease doesn't just affect the heart and brain—it can also affect blood vessels in the penis. While drugs like Viagra may strengthen erections, these therapies don't protect against heart attacks and strokes, so it's important to investigate and treat the underlying cause of the dysfunction. Although some men find it embarrassing to discuss sexual matters with their doctors, a frank conversation could help you avoid life-threatening illness.

- Depression and Anxiety

  Depression can literally break hearts, Columbia University researchers recently reported. While doctors already knew it can hit after a heart attack or stroke, worsening outcomes, the study, which tracked 63,000 women with no history of heart trouble over a twelve-year span, revealed that gloom could also trigger heart disease in the first place. Compared to women who weren't depressed, sufferers had more than twice the rate of sudden cardiac death (SCD), abrupt loss of heart function.

What's more, a study of male twins found that depression is just as dangerous as obesity, high blood pressure, and high cholesterol. And another study, involving 50,000 men, reported that those suffering from anxiety (diagnosed by a psychiatrist during the initial medical exam) had more than double the risk of developing heart disease or a heart attack over the next 37 years, compared to men without anxiety.

Yet both depression and anxiety often go untreated because people don't recognize the symptoms or they try to tough it out on their own. Sufferers may overindulge in comfort foods, leading to weight gain and even greater heart disease risk—another reason to get treatment if misery becomes chronic. Medication and/or therapy helps 80 percent of people with depression feel better, often within weeks.

- Sleep Apnea

Frequent loud snoring may trumpet obstructive sleep apnea (OSA), a dangerous disorder that can trigger a stroke or heart attack. Bouts of interrupted or irregular breathing during sleep cause blood pressure to spike, damaging arteries over time. Since some people with OSA don't snore, other warning signs to watch for include often waking in the night for no apparent reason and unexplained daytime drowsiness. Women with a neck diameter of 16 inches or more, or men with a diameter of 17 inches or greater are at increased risk for having it.

If you fit this profile, your doctor may order a sleep study, which involves spending the night in a lab, hooked up to monitors. There are also home sleep-study systems that can effectively diagnose OSA. Because OSA mainly strikes the obese, treatment typically includes weight loss. You may also need continuous positive airway pressure (CPAP), a device that gently blows moist, heated air into your nose and mouth while you sleep.

- Vitamin D Deficiency

Having low levels of the sunshine vitamin doubles the risk of heart attack and stroke, several studies show. Skimping on vitamin D may also boost the risk of developing high blood pressure and blood vessel inflammation, which may explain the link to CVD. A 2011 study of more than 10,000 patients found that those with low blood levels of D were twice as likely to have diabetes, 40 percent more likely to have high blood pressure, and about 30 percent more likely to suffer from cardiomyopathy (a diseased heart muscle) than those with normal levels.

Deficiency is extremely common, affecting up to half of seemingly healthy Americans. Compounding the problem, vitamin D is found in relatively few foods, such as sardines, salmon, egg yolks, and fortified milk and cereal. If a blood test shows that you are deficient in the sunshine vitamin, it can easily be treated with supplements, reducing your risk for both CVD and type 2 diabetes.

- Psoriasis

Here's the real heartbreak of psoriasis: It hikes risk for heart attacks, stroke, and peripheral artery disease (clogged vessels in the legs) as much as smoking does. Marked by red, sore, flaky, and often itchy patches, and in some cases, painfully swollen joints, psoriasis has also been linked to increased risk for high cholesterol, high blood pressure, obesity, and diabetes.

A recent study also reported that 40 percent of psoriasis sufferers meet criteria for metabolic syndrome—a dangerous cluster of heart attack risk factors. Although most people have never heard of it, metabolic syndrome affects 50 million Americans, many of whom are unaware of their risk. As you'll learn in the next chapter, metabolic syndrome is so easy to detect that you can diagnose yourself by checking five numbers that should be in everyone's medical record.

Think F.A.S.T. to Stop a Stroke

To raise awareness of the warning signs, the American Stroke Association and other groups have mounted a public health campaign to teach people to do the "F.A.S.T. test" if they suspect someone might be having a stroke:

F = Face

Ask the person to smile. A stroke may cause one side of the face to droop. Abrupt dimming of vision or a sudden, severe headache with no known cause can also be symptoms.

A = Arms

Ask the person to raise both arms. If one arms drifts downward, that could signal a stroke, which can also trigger weakness, numbness, or paralysis of an arm or leg.

S = Speech

Ask the person to repeat a simple sentence. During a stroke, people may slur their words, have trouble speaking or understanding speech, or not be able to talk at all.

T = Time

Observing any of these warning signs means it's time to call 911 or take the affected person to the nearest hospital. Stroke is a life-or-death emergency and every minute counts. To have any hope of reversing a stroke, treatment must be started quickly.

Action Steps

Step 1: Take Care of Your Teeth

A habit that takes five minutes a day can add years to your life and also reduces risk for heart attacks, strokes, diabetes, colds, flu, and even arthritis. A 2012 study found that one of the simplest—and cheapest—ways to a long life is brushing and flossing your teeth daily. Conversely, neglecting your chompers can actually be fatal, the researchers reported.

Just how much impact does good oral health have? California researchers tracked 5,611 seniors for 17 years, and found that:

- Never brushing at night boosted the risk for death during the study period by 20 to 25 percent, compared to brushing every night.

- Never flossing hiked mortality risk by 30 percent, versus daily flossing.

- Not seeing a dentist in the previous 12 months raised the risk of death by up to 50 percent, compared to getting dental care two or more times a year.

Another startling finding: One major predictor of early death was missing teeth, even after other risk factors were taken into account, the study reported. That's powerful motivation to see your dentist regularly and fight heart disease with a toothbrush and floss. Later in this book, you'll find detailed tips about how to take your dental health to an even higher level, including a state-of-the-art DNA test to check for the most dangerous oral bacteria.

Step 2: Recognize Your Red Flags

If you have any of the arterial health threats described in this chapter, alert your doctor and discuss an appropriate cardiovascular workup. In Part Two, you'll learn which tests to ask for and what your lab results mean. Once you've identified your cardiovascular risks, you can start to reduce—or even reverse—them by gradually making healthy changes in your life, using the Bale/Doneen Method.

In Part Three, we'll present an easy-to-follow action plan that includes ways to become more active, improve your diet, and get rid of toxic belly fat. We'll also show you how to manage the stress in your life and what the best supplements to improve heart health are, as well as offer guidance on medications that can make a dramatic difference for those who need them.

In the next chapter, you'll find out which simple measurement you can take at home to get a better predictor of your heart attack and stroke risk than your weight or your body mass index. We'll also reveal another of the best-kept secrets in medicine: Even if you've already had a heart attack or stroke or have been told that you've run out of treatment options, it's never too late to turn your health around, as our patient Dead Man Walking discovered.

Chapter 4

The Best-Kept Secret in Medicine

"Superior doctors prevent the disease. Mediocre doctors treat the disease before it is evident. Inferior doctors treat the full-blown disease."

—Huang Dee Nai-Chang, from the first known Chinese medical text, ca. 2600 B.C.

Because many doctors cling to a dangerously outdated, flawed concept of how heart attacks happen, millions of Americans with coronary artery disease are either overtreated or undertreated. They're overtreated with stents and bypasses many of them don't needed, and undertreated because potentially lethal disease is not detected. As discussed in Chapter Two, 99 percent of plaque lurks inside arterial walls. Therefore, these hidden deposits can't be found with imaging tests that check blood flow to the heart, such as angiograms, or that look for indirect signs of clogged arteries, such the exercise stress test.

Under the current standard of care, cardiovascular disease remains the leading killer and disabler of Americans. And many, until they survive their first heart attack or stroke, are completely unaware of their risk, because of the failure to identify and manage all of the precarious, unseen plaque inside the arteries. As you learned in an earlier chapter, about one-third of the heart attacks that occur each year are in people who have already survived one or more heart attacks, and about one-quarter of annual strokes occur in people who have had a previous stroke.

What's the solution? In the first known Chinese medical text, written more than 4,700 years ago, Huang Dee Nai-Chang nailed the answer: The best doctors prevent the disease. Today, the best-kept secret in medicine is that with the right care, all heart attacks and strokes are preventable. For many patients, the current standard of care isn't enough, so instead of just treating 1 percent of arterial disease, the Bale/Doneen Method is designed to treat the entire patient, to stop—or even reverse—its progression.

We've been called "disease detectives" because we investigate each patient thoroughly for the presence of plaque, even the silent, deadly kind. If it's found, then our mission is to solve the mystery of *why* our patients have cardiovascular disease by tracking down the root causes, including genetic influences. Think of a heart attack, stroke, or severely diseased arteries as a crime scene. How satisfied would you be if the police just rounded up the usual suspects (large blockages) and declared the case closed, when the real villain (deadly plaque hiding in the arterial walls) remained on the loose, leaving the victim at risk for repeat crimes?

That's what happened to Joe Inderman and Henry Nugent when their coronary artery disease was treated with standard care. As you'll learn from their stories, Joe actually had an extremely common, but little-known syndrome that puts more than 50 million Americans at elevated risk for heart attacks. And it doesn't take a disease detective to find out if you have it: In fact, you can actually diagnose yourself, using the information in this chapter. You'll also find out which three action steps you need to take right now to protect your health.

A Tale of Two Patients

Joe Inderman and Henry Nugent have never met, but they have a lot in common, including nearly identical symptoms and scars from a surgery they never thought they'd need. And although they both thought they'd been cured, each faced a new, even-more-terrifying medical crisis after the operation.

In Henry's case, the initial symptoms—angina, shoulder discomfort, and unusual shortness of breath—struck when the then-66-year-old retired Air Force pilot from Billings, Montana, was trying to improve his fitness: it was during a training run for the seven-and-a-half-mile Bloomsday road race in Spokane, Washington. Assuming that the symptoms meant he wasn't in as good shape as he thought, Henry cut his jog short and tried again the next day, only to have the same thing happen.

Like Camille Zaleski, Henry didn't consider his symptoms significant. But when they hit yet again during a long walk, his wife insisted that he go to an urgent care center to find out what was wrong. After signing what he thought was a consent form for an angiogram to check blood flow through his arteries, he woke up three hours later to discover that he'd undergone open-heart surgery and a quadruple bypass.

"I felt like somebody had dropped a ton of bricks on me, and I gave the doctor hell for operating on me," says Henry, who then discovered that fine print in the consent form authorized the doctor to perform any procedures deemed necessary, based on the angiogram results. Without realizing it, he'd gotten on the express train to a bypass.

Joe's angina also started during exercise. Three weeks later, he was wheeled into the OR for quadruple-bypass surgery. Then 57, the retired real estate broker was almost exactly the same age that his father had been when the older man had needed a quadruple bypass for coronary artery disease. After Joe's bypass operation, he spent six weeks in cardiac rehabilitation. These programs are customized with exercise, nutritional counseling, and education addressing healthy lifestyle changes to aid in the recovery from a heart attack or cardiac surgery.

Joe was determined to avoid the same fate as his father, who had died at age 62, five years after a quadruple bypass. He quit smoking, dramatically improved his diet, and started working out regularly. "During cardiac rehab, I asked the nurse if it was possible to reverse heart disease, or if the best I could hope for was that I didn't get even worse. She told me that physicians used to think that all they could do was keep patients from getting worse, but there was a doctor and nurse practitioner in Spokane who had success in reversing this disease. She said she was planning to send her own mother to these specialists because the standard treatments weren't helping her.'"

Initially, however, a healthier lifestyle seemed to do the trick. Before long, Joe, an avid nature photographer, felt well enough to resume his favorite activities: hiking, kayaking, and training his three German short-haired pointers for bird-dog field competitions—challenging events that required following the fast-moving dogs on horseback through rough terrain to find hidden birds.

But the seemingly miraculous improvement only lasted 18 months. Not only did his angina return, but it soon became so severe, despite treatment with nitroglycerin tablets and other medications, that even the slightest exertion—such as walking to his car—triggered excruciating pain.

A physically fit nonsmoker with acceptable LDL (bad) cholesterol levels, Henry Nugent wasn't given any medication, cardiac rehabilitation, or specific treatment recommendations. Therefore, he assumed he was already cured. Six months later, however, his symptoms returned. He was rushed back to the OR to have stents placed in the same arteries that had previously been treated.

"I got very upset and told the cardiologist, 'Listen, I'm in the same situation I was in before having heart surgery six months ago. I need a plan to make sure my plumbing doesn't clog up again,'" says Henry. The cardiologist responded that several specialists had discussed Henry's case at a hospital meeting and no one knew why his disease was so aggressive.

"The doctor said that my cardiac condition was probably hereditary, and that there was nothing more that could be done to prevent another event in three to six months." Henry was despondent, remembering that his father had died from coronary artery disease. He'd always thought that his dad's fatal heart attack was caused by a long battle with type 2 diabetes.

Joe also feared that he was on the same tragic trajectory as his father. "The cardiologist kept trying stress tests and told me I had new blockages, which I kind of knew. Then he sent me to the hospital for an angiogram," says Joe, who still gets choked up remembering what happened next.

"When the cardiologist came into my room with the results, my two sons and their wives were with me," he recalls. "I was told that two of the vein grafts from my bypasses had basically collapsed or failed. Then the cardiologist—with a heart surgeon standing beside him—said that if they tried going in with stents, it could actually cause a heart attack and I might not even survive the surgery. They felt that I needed to consider a heart transplant.

"That really shook me, and my family started crying," says Joe. "After the cardiologist and the heart surgeon left the room, I told my sons, 'Maybe that's what it boils down to, but I'm not stopping here. I want a lot more answers before this goes any further.'

"I felt that the cardiologist wasn't looking at why I'd gone downhill so fast after the quadruple bypass. My blood pressure was staying at 150/90 and I'd done enough research to know that wasn't normal. But he'd just say, 'For your age, that's a decent number. You can live with that.' I felt I was just being herded along, like sheep in a pen, from one intervention to the next. Basically, he was telling me, 'You've drawn a bad hand of cards in life and all we can do is put in a new heart.'"

Henry was also desperate for answers—and a treatment plan to prevent a heart attack. He consulted a second specialist who gave him the same bleak prognosis. "I felt like I was being handed a death sentence. I got very depressed and started drinking more, trying to drown my sorrows," he said in an interview.

Considering himself "a dead man walking," Henry set off on a trip across the United States to sell real estate he owned and say his last good-byes to dear friends, his three children, and six grandkids. "I thought I had to accept that my time was limited and put my affairs in order before my wife was left a widow."

A Surprising Risk Factor Most Doctors Don't Check

During Dead Man Walking's farewell journey, his best friend, who happens to be one of our patients, told him we might be able to help. We stayed late at our clinic to see him that evening. As he told his story, Henry kept lifting his wire-rimmed glasses to wipe away tears. His beautiful wife, Mickey, sat next to him, hunched over in a posture of abject despair and helplessness.

In medical school, students are often taught that if they listen long enough, the patient will tell them what's wrong. Henry's case proved the wisdom of this approach. After we'd listened for 30 minutes and asked a few pointed questions, we learned that there was something significant that the other specialists he'd consulted hadn't investigated. "Since I was 20, I've told every doctor I've ever seen that my father was a type 2 diabetic," Henry said. "I've always felt that was very important, but no one ever paid any attention."

Like many of our patients, Henry was surprised when we measured his waist as part of our physical exam. None of his other healthcare providers had ever done that. Most patients, and many doctors, don't know that waist circumference is actually a better predictor of heart attack and stroke risk than weight or BMI (body mass index, a number calculated from height in inches and weight in pounds, using a mathematical formula: weight is divided by height squared, then multiplied by 703).

Traditionally, BMI has been used to check for obesity, usually considered to be a BMI of thirty or higher. At 5'11" and 195 pounds, Henry, a physically fit non-smoker, had a BMI of 27, putting him in the mildly overweight category. Although he didn't look heavy, he had a large waist. Studies show that for a man, a measurement of more than 40 inches, as was the case with Henry, is strongly linked to greatly increased risk for heart attack and strokes—even if the person's weight and BMI are normal.

Having a large waist and apple-shaped body boosts the threat of developing type 2 diabetes, metabolic syndrome, sleep apnea, and some forms of cancer. Research even shows that a spare tire around the middle can shorten life expectancy. And a big belly is also the number-one warning sign of insulin resistance. Based on Henry's family history of type 2 diabetes—and his waist measurement—we told Henry that we thought we knew *why* he had heart disease, and if we were right, there was a lot more that could be done to save his life.

Henry and Mickey looked up with the first glimmer of hope, as we explained that we needed to do one more test—a two-hour oral glucose tolerance test (OGTT)—to confirm our suspicion. Although Henry's blood sugar had been checked with other, less reliable tests, with seemingly normal results, he'd never had an OGTT, the gold standard in accuracy for identifying diabetes. Performed after an overnight fast, this simple, universally available blood test involves drinking a sugary liquid to challenge the pancreas, as blood samples are taken over the next two hours to see how fasting glucose (sugar) levels change. It's also a critical test to identify prediabetes or insulin resistance.

By the end of the visit, Dead Man Walking was as excited as a death row inmate who'd just gotten word that he was about to get a reprieve. In our practice, we've seen that look many times in the eyes of men and women who fear they've turned to us too late, because they've already had a heart attack or stroke, or have undergone repeated bypasses or angioplasties, only to have their coronary artery disease continue to progress and their symptoms worsen.

Some, like Dead Man Walking have even been told that their days are numbered and they've run out of treatment options. What fuels our passion for prevention is the opportunity to deliver a powerful message of hope: It's never too late to optimize your care, solve the mystery of why you're not responding to your current treatment, and even save your life. Often, a few simple lab tests are all it takes to discover the root cause of your illness and open the way to additional treatments.

Henry's intuition that his family history was the key to understanding his health turned out to be on target. As was the case with Camille Zaleski and David Bobbett, the results of his OGTT revealed that he was prediabetic and insulin resistant (IR). That's not just a coincidence, as we'll explain in Chapter Nine. Essentially a prediabetic condition, IR is the hidden cause of most heart attacks and most cases of cardiovascular disease. It's also the condition that leads to type 2 diabetes if it goes undiagnosed and untreated.

Although most healthcare providers don't check patients for this extremely common condition, the good news is that once insulin resistance is properly diagnosed, it's highly treatable with medications and a healthier lifestyle. In fact, it can almost always be reversed, thus preventing both heart attacks and the gradual progression of IR to type 2 diabetes.

A Dangerous Disorder You Can Diagnose Yourself

When Joe arrived at our clinic for his appointment, his chest pain was so excruciating that he was unable to walk across the exam room without stopping to take a nitroglycerin tablet to temporarily quell the angina. Despite being so sick, however, he had a surprisingly upbeat attitude. After the nurse at the cardiac rehab program had told him about the Bale/Doneen Method, he attended one of our lectures and felt optimistic that we could help him.

When we reviewed his medical records, we quickly found a glaring red flag: the results of a blood-sugar test performed a few years earlier. "How long have you been prediabetic?" we asked. Joe looked puzzled and then angry that none of his doctors had ever told him that his blood sugar was too high. Like one-third of the 79 million Americans with prediabetes, he was walking around undiagnosed and untreated, while the disease was silently damaging his blood vessels. Without treatment, most people with prediabetes progress to full-blown diabetes within three to ten years.

Joe was also unaware that he had a dangerous disorder that's so easy to detect that he could have even diagnosed himself: metabolic syndrome. Later in this chapter we'll tell you how to check yourself for this extremely common cluster of five specific risk factors for heart attacks, strokes, and diabetes that often strike in tandem. All you need is a few basic numbers—including waist circumference, blood pressure, and cholesterol levels—that every patient should know. Here's why it's important to know if you had metabolic syndrome: it triples risk for a heart attack and quintuples it for type 2 diabetes.

Simply by measuring Joe's waist and looking at his medical records, we were able to diagnose him with metabolic syndrome during his initial visit—without doing even one lab test. To meet the medical criteria for this condition, patients must have at least three of the risk factors. But incredibly, Joe had all five, yet none of the specialists he'd consulted—including two cardiologists—had ever put the glaring red flags in his medical record together.

That's not as unusual as you might think. Most Americans (85 percent) have never heard of metabolic syndrome or can't name even one of the five abnormalities that comprise this condition, a national health survey found. For example, while smoking is bad for your heart, it's not a sign of metabolic syndrome. And of the more than 211,000 people polled, less than 1 percent thought they had the condition themselves. While that may make it sound extremely rare, actually, metabolic syndrome affects nearly 26 percent of adults—more than 50 million Americans.

Why is awareness of such a common—and dangerous—disorder so stunningly low? Part of the problem is that it has more aliases than a career criminal. Over the years, it's also been known as Syndrome X, insulin resistance syndrome, obesity syndrome, and hypertriglyceridemic waist. Another issue: Some people confuse metabolic syndrome with better-known conditions linked to metabolism, like diabetes or obesity. And since patients don't ask doctors if they have it, glaring red flags in their medical records may be overlooked, resulting in the condition going undiagnosed.

Five Cardiovascular Villains

What are the telltale signs of metabolic syndrome? Like Henry, Joe had a wide waist, the ringleader of the gang of five metabolic villains that define the syndrome. Because the condition typically strikes people who are overweight, like Joe, who was carrying 215 pounds on his 5'10" frame, rates of metabolic syndrome have soared in tandem with America's obesity epidemic.

It's also possible, however, to have metabolic syndrome if you're not overweight, since the key player is abdominal obesity, not overall body fat. A recent Mayo Clinic study of 16,000 patients with heart disease found that those with high levels of waist fat (an apple-shaped body) were at 75 percent higher risk for premature death—even if their weight was normal—than patients with smaller waists.

The next red flag was Joe's persistently high blood pressure reading of 150/90, which his cardiologist had declared "decent" for his age and something he "could live with." Actually, high blood pressure is the leading risk factor for stroke and also a major contributor to heart attacks. Far from being a condition that people can "live with," it's a silent killer that needs to be managed with the right medications and lifestyle changes to head off life-threatening cardiovascular events. Joe urgently needed treatment to lower his blood pressure.

Joe's lipid levels revealed two more metabolic red flags: Specifically, his level of HDL (good) cholesterol was abnormally low, while his level of blood fats called triglycerides was too high. The fifth red flag was his fasting blood sugar, which was in the prediabetic range. What this cluster of abnormalities revealed was that Joe not only had metabolic syndrome, but that he also had insulin resistance, the root cause of most cardiovascular disease. That's true for everyone with metabolic syndrome, so checking for this easily diagnosed condition is one of the easiest ways for patients to tell if they have IR.

However, while everyone with metabolic syndrome, by definition, is insulin-resistant, the opposite is not always true. About half of people with IR don't have metabolic syndrome. For example, Henry didn't meet the criteria for metabolic syndrome since he only had two of the abnormalities: a wide waist and low levels of HDL cholesterol. That's why we needed to do the oral glucose tolerance test, which confirmed our suspicion that he was insulin resistant.

In both cases, our discovery that Joe and Henry—like many of our other patients—were resistant to their own insulin was a major turning point in their treatment. This diagnosis helped explain *why* both men's coronary artery disease was continuing to progress, despite quadruple-bypass surgery and other treatments. The diagnosis proved extremely important, because it opened the way to additional therapies that hadn't previously been considered, including medications, certain over-the-counter supplements, and specific lifestyle changes. There were lots of therapies left to halt their previously unrelenting arterial disease.

We also uncovered genetic factors that predisposed to them to heart attacks, offering additional insight into the best therapies to prevent these potentially fatal events. But just as heart disease develops over many years, halting and reversing it also takes time. The Bale/Doneen Method isn't an instant miracle cure, but stabilization of the disease can occur quickly. Sixty-five-year-old Henry (aka Dead Man Walking) would die—someday—but we could confidently promise him that it wouldn't be soon and the cause wouldn't be a heart attack or stroke.

Joe's excruciating angina wasn't going to disappear in a day, a week, or a month, but over time, he could expect improvement. We were able to reassure him that he did not require someone else's heart in his chest to continue living.

Rating Your Risk

Do you have metabolic syndrome? Because the syndrome's cluster of disorders frequently doesn't spark any obvious symptoms, it's easy for people to go undiagnosed, especially if they don't get regular physicals. And most healthcare providers don't routinely measure patients' waists, an obvious indication that doctors aren't on the lookout for this disorder.

The good news is that you don't need an alert healthcare provider to find out if you have this dangerous syndrome. In fact, you can diagnose yourself by checking this list of the five warning signs. Making the call is a bit like baseball: three strikes and you're out. If you have three or more of the diagnostic criteria then you have metabolic syndrome—and therefore, also have insulin resistance:

1. A large waist

   A simple way to tell if you might be at risk: Check your waist circumference. You can check your waist circumference by wrapping a tape measure around the top of your pelvic bones, found where love handles grow. Take the measurement at the end of a normal expiration. Do not assume your belly button marks your waist, as its position can vary significantly from one person to another.

   There are ethnic differences in "failing" scores. A waist measurement above 35 inches for a woman, or above 40 inches for a man, is one "strike" for Caucasians, African Americans, and Hispanics. For Asians, however, the abnormal numbers are 31 inches and 35 inches for women and men respectively, and for Japanese the numbers to watch for are 31 inches for women and 34 inches for men.

   Fifty-three percent of people with the syndrome are carrying excessive belly fat, a study by the Centers for Disease Control and Prevention found. The researchers also found that the higher the study participants' BMI, the greater their threat of metabolic syndrome. Among men, only 7 percent of those who were underweight or normal weight had three or more of the risk factors, compared to 30 percent of overweight men and 65 percent of obese men. Obese women were 17 times more likely to have three or more risk factors than their slimmer sisters.

2. High blood pressure

Also called *hypertension*, high blood pressure affects one in three Americans. Not only does it damage blood vessels, increasing risk for coronary artery disease and heart failure, but it can also lead to kidney failure. High blood pressure is the leading risk factor for stroke.

Your blood pressure reading, which should be checked at every medical visit as an important vital sign, consists of two numbers: "Systolic" describes the pressure of your blood when it is pumped out of the heart to start its journey through your body. "Diastolic" is the lower number and describes the pressure of your blood right before the heart pumps it out again. You can reliably check your blood pressure at many stores or with home equipment.

What is considered a failing score may shock you. If your pressure is 130/85 mmHg or higher, you have a strike. Many healthcare providers still consider this pressure acceptable despite decades of data showing this level of pressure damages arteries placing individuals at higher risk for heart attacks, strokes, and kidney failure.

You need to know your numbers. You cannot rely on the healthcare provider's often simple response to the question, "How is my blood pressure?" A blood pressure of 130/85 will usually garner a response of: "It is fine." If you are on a treatment for high blood pressure, it is also considered a strike even if the treated pressure is below 130/85, according to the definition of the disorder used by the American Heart Association, the National Heart, Lung, and Blood Institute, and the Bale/Doneen Method.

3. Low HDL cholesterol

Although most of us think of cholesterol as a villain, it also plays two helpful roles in our body. Your cells use this waxy substance, produced by the liver, to waterproof their protective outer membranes. Without cholesterol, the cells would die. Cholesterol is also a building block for certain hormones, including sex hormones.

HDL (high-density lipoprotein) is the "good" cholesterol. A HDL level below 50 mg/dL for women, or under 40 mg/dL for men, is another strike for metabolic syndrome. Many people who are headed for arterial disease and diabetes will run low HDL levels. Some healthcare providers are so hung up on LDL (low density lipoprotein), or "bad" cholesterol, as the only value to worry about that "failing" HDL levels are not even discussed with the patient. If you are being treated for HDL, you have a strike even if the levels are above the numbers given here. In Chapter Eight, we discuss cholesterol in detail, including the optimal levels for cardiovascular health, and alert you to a surprising cholesterol number that predicts heart attack risk.

4. High triglycerides

   Like cholesterol, triglycerides are a type of fat (lipid) found in your blood. When you eat, your body converts calories that aren't needed for immediate energy into triglycerides, which are then stored in fat cells for later use. If you regularly consume more calories than you burn, your triglycerides may be high. Many people who are headed for arterial disease and diabetes will run high levels.

   High triglycerides are often a warning sign of other disorders that can boost the threat of heart attacks and stroke, including obesity and poorly controlled diabetes. High levels also increase risk for cardiovascular disease. If your triglyceride level is 150 mg/dL or above, you have acquired another strike. If you are being treated for high triglycerides, it is a strike even if the level is below 150 mg/dL.

5. High fasting blood sugar

   The glucose (sugar) in your blood comes from the carbs in your diet, the body's main source of energy. Fasting means you have not consumed anything with calories for at least 10 hours. A level of 100 mg/dL or higher during a fast counts as a strike. Fasting blood sugar levels of 100 mg/dL to 125 mg/dL indicate that you're prediabetic. If the level is above 125 mg/dL, you actually have diabetes.

It's Never Too Late to Turn Your Health Around

Finding out that you have metabolic syndrome (or insulin resistance without metabolic syndrome) may seem frightening, but all of the risk factors are highly treatable, often with simple steps. If you have a large waist (central obesity), you may be surprised to learn that dropping as few as seven to ten pounds can not only improve heart health, but also dramatically cut your risk of developing type 2 diabetes, even if you're already prediabetic.

To prevent or reverse IR, however, the treatment that trumps all others is regular exercise. It's even more important than how much you weigh or what you eat, crucial as both of these are for optimal cardiovascular health. Working out for 30 minutes a day at least five days a week has been proved to prevent prediabetes from progressing to diabetes 60 percent of the time and has similarly powerful benefits for preventing metabolic syndrome. Later in the book, we'll also look at the best diet to ward off this cluster of heart attack, stroke, and diabetes risks.

For Joe and Henry, treatment also included dietary supplements and medications. Medication is usually a last resort for insulin resistance that doesn't respond to lifestyle changes, but for some patients, the right medication can dramatically reduce the risk that prediabetes will progress to full-blown diabetes. Joe and Henry also needed additional therapies for their heart disease and risk factors, including Joe's poorly controlled high blood pressure.

How did our method work out for these two men?

Eight years after Dead Man Walking set off on farewell journey, he celebrated a day he never thought he'd see: his 73rd birthday. To his amazement, he'd out-lived his father, who had died at age 72 from undiagnosed heart disease. Soon after that milestone birthday, Henry told us, "I'm 170 pounds. I go to the gym four to five times a week. Two days ago, I got back from Hawaii, and I'm about to take a trip across the beautiful United States to visit family and friends—for pleasure.

"It's just criminal that I was handed a death sentence and told nothing could be done when that wasn't true," he added. "And why didn't any of the general practitioners, internists, and cardiologists I saw over the years ever do a glucose tolerance test, particularly after finding out that I had plugged-up pipes? The Bale/Doneen Method isn't magic: Simple, inexpensive treatments saved my life and I don't understand why every doctor in America doesn't practice this way."

Joe, now 63, has also outlived his dad. "While I never gave up hope that I would get back to leading a normal life, I certainly had my doubts when the cardiologist said I needed a heart transplant. But I decided to ignore his advice and stick to the Bale/Doneen Method. It isn't a quick fix, and it took a solid year before I saw sig-nificant improvement. Gradually, I began to need the nitroglycerin less and less. Over the past four years, I've gone from taking more than 100 tablets a month to needing them only occasionally, because the angina is almost gone. I feel like I really understand what my problems are, and know how to take care of myself over the long-term."

And he's literally back in the saddle again. "Yesterday, I spent all day on horse-back, working my three bird dogs, which is definitely something I couldn't have done a few years ago. My son and I have won two back-to-back national bird-dog championships, and this year, I was a judge at the National All-Ages Champion-ship. I was in the saddle eight to ten hours a day throughout the entire five-day event, riding over very rough terrain—and didn't have any angina symptoms at all."

Joe no longer has to live with high blood pressure. He's now on two medica-tions that have brought the numbers down to the normal range, plus a diabetes drug to lower his blood sugar. "In my case, I could have made all the lifestyle changes in the world, but without the proper medications, I don't think the pro-gression of the disease would have been stopped. I also feel that a positive atti-tude has made a huge difference: When you're faced with the same disease that killed your father, you can either give up—or you can decide to fight it with every-thing you've got."

Action Steps

Step 1: Know Your Numbers

Healthy numbers—from your waist measurement, to your blood pressure, cholesterol levels, and blood sugar—are an important part of preventing heart attacks and strokes. Unhealthy numbers can reveal if you have metabolic syndrome or insulin resistance. The four key numbers you should know are:

- Your blood pressure.
- Your lipid levels, including total cholesterol, HDL, LDL, and triglycerides.
- Your waist size.
- Your blood sugar, if you are age 40 or older with no diabetes risk factors or under 40 with risk factors.

Step 2: Compile Your Medical History

Part of being an empowered patient is collecting and studying your medical records. You'll need them if you change healthcare providers, consult a specialist, or face a medical crisis. It's also important to check for errors that might cost your medical coverage—or in the case of medication allergies, even your life.

Under the federal Health Information Portability and Accountability Act (HIPAA), you're legally entitled to your records, including the results of heart and other tests you've had, doctors' summaries, hospital and emergency room discharge summaries, and radiology reports. Generally, your doctor has to provide the records within 30 days after a written request. Medical offices may charge a fee for making photocopies, which varies by state.

The easiest way to start compiling your medical history is to ask your doctor for your results and summaries during your next medical visit and begin by building a file of current records, then work on gathering the older ones. Also tuck a personal health information card in your wallet, listing such crucial information as the names and dosages of your medications, any adverse reactions to drugs, medical conditions you've been diagnosed with, and your emergency contact information. There are also phone apps to store medical and emergency data.

Step 3: Get Your Test Results

While people often assume that no news is good news, it could also mean that your doctor hasn't checked the results, has lost them, or has misinterpreted the findings. A shocking study recently published in *Archives of Internal Medicine* found that in more than 7 percent of cases, primary care doctors failed to notify patients of abnormal test results, including those that revealed potentially life-threatening conditions. Scarier still, some of the doctors studied made this dangerous mistake up to 26 percent of the time.

Make sure the doctor tells you the results of every test and gives you a copy of the findings for your personal medical records. Later in the book, we'll discuss how to understand your lab results and the numbers you want to see on each of the tests we recommend. For some tests, as we'll explain, results that are considered "normal" under standard medical-practice guidelines may not be good enough to prevent heart attacks and strokes, which is why the Bale/ Doneen Method sets optimal goals based on the latest science.

Until recently, most of the knowledge, treatments, and research on heart disease focused on men. And even today, women's cardiovascular disease remains underdiagnosed and undertreated, leading to worse outcomes and a deadly gender gap in survival after a heart attack. In the next chapter, you'll learn which unique risk factors women need to watch for, why women's heart disease and heart attack symptoms are more likely to be misdiagnosed, and why prevention is important at every age—not just for older women.

Chapter 5

Women and Heart Disease

"A woman's heart is a deep ocean of secrets."

—Rose Dawson Calvert in the film *Titanic*, 1997

It was nearly 7:00 A.M. and Juli Townsend was rushing to get ready for work. As the customer service representative from Spokane, Washington, was putting the finishing touches on her makeup, the first pain hit. It started in her chest, then shot down her right arm, making her fingers feel numb and tingly. Suddenly, she was struggling to catch her breath.

Thinking a little fresh air might help, she took a few steps, only to collapse on her bedroom floor, overcome by waves of intense pain and nausea. "Honey, I need help," she shouted to her husband, Matt, who was in the next room with the couple's three-year-old daughter, Selah.

As Matt drove her to the ER, with Selah in the backseat, Juli tried to figure out what might be triggering her terrifying symptoms. "I thought, 'There's no way I could be having a heart attack at 37,' but that's what I thought it would feel like," recalls the young mom. "I told myself it was probably a panic attack, because I was hurrying so much that morning, worried that I'd be late for work."

After a long time in the emergency department's waiting room, she was given an EKG. "The doctor said it was normal and told me that if it were a heart attack, the pain would be on the left side of the body, not the right arm. Then he asked if I got anxious. I said, 'Every day, but not like this.' I was still in a lot of pain, and I vomited while they were checking me," adds Juli, who was diagnosed at the time with bacterial pneumonia. "The nurse gave me a five-day supply of antibiotics and told me, 'This will take care of your cough.' I said that I didn't have a cough, but I was told to take the medication and get a checkup after I finished taking the pills."

The treatment seemed to help. "When I went to the urgent care center five days later, I felt fine. The doctor listened to my lungs and said everything was good." But that night, as Juli was clipping grocery coupons, with Selah sitting in her lap, similar symptoms struck again. This time, however, the pain was in her back and jaw, and accompanied by nausea and pressure in her chest. Assuming that her bacterial pneumonia had flared up again, she went to bed early.

During the night, she woke several times as the pain intensified. Matt wanted to take her to the ER, but Juli worried about the expense under their high-deductible health plan. She took an aspirin and told him that she'd try to sleep it off until the urgent care center opened, at 8:00 A.M.

When Matt drove her to the center in the morning, she adds, " I felt like I'd been hit by a truck. On the way, we prayed for a medical mastermind like the TV character Dr. House to figure out what was wrong. When the physician started asking me questions, I could see him shaking his head in disbelief, because he wasn't buying the bacterial pneumonia diagnosis."

The doctor ordered blood tests, which revealed an abnormally high level of cardiac enzymes. "The doctor told me that my heart had been damaged and he wanted to call an ambulance." Again concerned about cost, and uncertain what her test results meant, Juli asked her husband to drive her to the ER, where the physician told her a cardiologist would be standing by to provide immediate care.

Instead, the young mom ended up sitting in the ER waiting room for two hours, still in excruciating pain, while other patients were treated ahead of her. When she was finally seen, she received another EKG and an hour later was told that it was normal. "After that, suddenly everybody came running in with these frightened looks on their faces, because they'd just gotten my blood test results. That's when I found out what elevated cardiac enzymes meant: You've had a heart attack."

In fact, as she soon learned, it was actually her second heart attack, since she'd been misdiagnosed during her previous ER visit five days earlier. What's more, the antibiotic that was mistakenly prescribed, azrithromycin, was an extremely dangerous treatment for someone in the throes of a heart attack. This medication was shown in a recent study of 347,795 patients to nearly triple cardiovascular mortality during the five days of treatment, compared to the rate for a group of patients who didn't take the antibiotics. While deaths associated with use of azrithromycin are rare, by far the highest rate was seen in people with cardiovascular disease, while no increase in CV mortality was seen in users of other common antibiotics, such as Cipro.

The elevated enzymes signaled that some of Juli's heart muscle cells had died due to lack of oxygenated blood in the blocked area, ER physicians explained. Then she was asked to make a terrifying decision. "The doctors wanted me to say yes to angioplasty, but it could be dangerous: I could die if the blockage was knocked loose during the procedure." In a haze of fear and pain, she signed the consent form.

The procedure went smoothly, and three days later she was released from the hospital with prescriptions for a beta-blocker and a high-dose statin pill. "The only advice I received was to get a checkup in two weeks. I asked why I was on such a high dose of statins when I'd been told that my cholesterol levels were perfect. The answer I got was, 'That's what we do after a heart attack.' "

At a follow-up appointment, she adds, "I was sitting next to a 60-year-old man who had smoked his whole life. I looked around the waiting room and thought, 'What am I doing here? I'm only 37. I don't smoke, I go to the gym, and my blood pressure is normal.' " And the young mom was at an ideal weight for her 5'6" frame.

During her recovery, she recalls, "I was an emotional wreck because nobody was concerned about why I'd had a heart attack. I felt very lost and was constantly checking my body for problems. Every time I felt a pain or tightness somewhere, I'd think, 'Is this another heart attack?'"

Medical Neglect and Misdiagnosis Put Women's Lives at Risk

What happened to Juli isn't as unusual as you might think. Of the 435,000 American women who have heart attacks each year, 83,000 are under age 65 and 35,000 are under age 55. Another frightening fact: Women with heart disease, especially younger women, are far more likely than men to be misdiagnosed. One study that looked at more than 10,000 patients (48 percent women) who went to the emergency room with heart attack symptoms found that women younger than 55 who went to the emergency room with heart attack symptoms were *seven times* more likely to be misdiagnosed and sent home untreated than men of the same age.

One key factor that contributes to women being misdiagnosed is the lingering myth that heart disease strikes mainly men. Many women—and even their physicians—still think that breast cancer is the leading threat to women's health. An American Heart Association (AHA) survey found that 43 percent of women didn't know that CVD is the number-one killer of women, claiming 10 times more female lives each year (432,700) than breast cancer (40,800). Only 8 percent of primary care doctors—and 17 percent of cardiologists—knew that more women than men die from heart disease, the AHA survey found.

This appalling lack of awareness often results in women receiving less-aggressive diagnoses and treatment from their healthcare providers, resulting in worse outcomes:

- After a heart attack, women are almost twice as likely to die than men—and since 1984, the gender gap in survival has continued to widen.

- Compared to men, a smaller percentage of women receive beta-blockers, ACE inhibitors, and even aspirin after a heart attack—therapies known to improve survival. Undertreatment is a key reason for the higher rate of post–heart attack complications in women than men, even after adjusting for age.

- Women who are eligible candidates for life-saving clot-buster drugs are far less likely than men to receive them.

- Women's hearts respond better than men's to healthy lifestyle changes, yet women are less likely to be referred to cardiac rehabilitation programs that provide this type of education.

- Women with heart disease receive fewer heart procedures such as balloon angioplasty and bypass surgery. Getting more of these procedures wouldn't necessarily be better for women, however, since they also have a higher risk for complications or death after bypass surgery. Women between ages 40 and 59 are up to four times more likely to die from bypass surgery than men.

- Women are much less likely than men to be referred for angiography, an invasive test that's widely used to diagnose people at high risk for heart attacks. And when women do receive angiography for chest pain, about half of them don't have major blockages, prompting doctors to write off their symptoms, even though, as you learned in earlier chapters, small blockages that this test can miss are just as dangerous as large ones.

- Women only comprise 24 percent of participants in all heart-related studies, so far less is known about which procedures and therapies can best help prevent or treat their heart attacks. And since most tests for diagnosing heart disease were studied mainly in clinical trials of male patients, the results can be misleading for women's care. For example, the exercise stress test is far less accurate for women than for men, as we'll discuss in more detail in the next chapter.

Six Heart Attack Warning Signs Women Ignore

Heart attack symptoms aren't always unisex. Women are less likely to experience the classic Hollywood heart attack characterized by crushing chest pain (often described as feeling like an elephant is sitting on your chest) that may radiate down the left arm. Instead, women have a higher rate of so-called atypical symptoms that may not include any chest pain, but are also serious warnings that a blocked artery is cutting off blood flow to the heart.

Remember how ER doctors dismissed Juli's symptoms as unrelated to her heart because her pain was in the "wrong" arm? One shocking 2005 study reported that a stunning 30 to 50 percent of women's heart attack symptoms go unrecognized by emergency and medical professionals. And while you'd expect women's cardiovascular care to have improved since then, a 2012 study published in the *Journal of the American Medical Association* involving more than 1.1 million heart attack patients reveals that women are *still* being misdiagnosed at far higher rates than men.

The researchers in the 2012 study also reported that of heart attack patients under age 55 who had atypical symptoms, those who are female are less likely to seek care. And when women do go to the hospital, their symptoms often go unrecognized, causing them to miss out on potentially lifesaving treatment until it's too late. Almost 15 percent of the women studied died in the hospital after a heart attack, compared to 10 percent of men. Younger women with no chest pain had a 20 percent higher risk of death after a heart attack than their male counterparts.

After a heart attack, every minute counts, so it's vital to call 911 if you or someone you know is having any of the warning signs listed below. As Dr. John Canto, a cardiologist at the Watson Clinic in Lakeland, Florida, and lead author of the 2012 study published in the *Journal of the American Medical Association,* puts it, "Time is muscle and muscle is life. When an artery is blocked, the heart muscle begins to die after 30 to 60 minutes. We call it the golden hour of heart attacks. Every minute you wait after that golden hour, more heart muscle will die. And once you lose it, it's not coming back."

Act fast if you or someone you know is having the warning signs listed below—with or without chest pain:

- Shortness of breath: During a heart attack, or in some cases, in the days or even weeks before the attack, 58 percent of women report panting or the inability to carry on a conversation.

- Non-chest pain: Instead of an explosive pain in the chest, women may develop less-severe pain that resides in the upper back, shoulders, neck, jaw, or arm. And contrary to what Juli was told, the pain may be on either side of the body.

- Unusual fatigue: In one study of women who had survived a heart attack, 71 percent of the women had flu-like symptoms and unusual fatigue in the weeks before the attack. The fatigue can be so extreme that women are too tired to make their bed, lift a laptop, or walk to the mailbox.

- Heavy sweating: Women may be suddenly drenched with sweat for no apparent reason and their faces may become pale and ashen. Unfortunately, many women dismiss this symptom as related to menopause or hormonal fluctuations.

- Nausea or dizziness: During an attack, women often vomit or feel like they're going to pass out. A sudden, unexplained fall can also be a warning sign.

- Anxiety: Many women experience a feeling of impending doom or fear before a heart attack. That's their bodies telling them to pay attention—and listening to that urgent inner instinct can be potentially lifesaving. In some cases, as occurred with Camille, warning signs of an impeding heart attack can occur up to three years before the actual event, a study of 515 female heart attack survivors reported.

Regardless of your age, if you notice any of these symptoms, it's imperative to demand a thorough cardiac workup. While cardiovascular disease is more common after menopause, it can and does strikes younger women—even in the absence of typical risk factors, as Juli's case vividly highlights.

New Thinking About Hormone Replacement Therapy

Over the past decade, many women have been scared away from using hormone replacement therapy (HRT), because of a widespread perception among women and their healthcare providers that the dangers far outweighed the benefits. This avalanche of alarm was fueled by 2002 data from the Women's Health Initiative (WHI), a large clinical trial conducted by the U.S. government that suggested that women who used estrogen-and-progesterone replacement therapy faced a significantly higher threat of several dangerous conditions, compared to the placebo group, including:

- A 41 percent increase in strokes

- A 29 percent rise in heart attacks

- Double the rate of blood clots

- A 22 percent increase in total cardiovascular disease

- A 26 percent increase in breast cancer.

At the time, the findings were deemed so frightening that the estrogen-and-progesterone arm of the trial was halted in July 2002, three years earlier than planned. (Another arm of the study, in which women received estrogen-only HRT, was also halted for safety reasons in 2004.) Prescriptions for estrogen replacement therapy, once believed to be an elixir to keep women healthy, youthful, and sexy long after menopause, plummeted by 71 percent in the U.S. between 2001 and 2009, according to the North American Menopause Society. In England, the number of women on HRT dwindled from a peak of 1.5 million to fewer than half that. Recently, however, new analyses of the same data have prompted several of the original study investigators to either reverse their views or declare the 2002 warnings unwarranted for many women.

In fact, the authors of a 2012 reappraisal of WHI data concluded that mass fear fueled by the 2002 findings has resulted in millions of women suffering needlessly from menopause symptoms that in many cases could have been relieved safely by HRT. A 2011 examination of the data reported that HRT may be a good option for most healthy postmenopausal women in their fifties, depending on their family and medical history, symptoms, and health concerns.

Understandably, the conflicting findings have left many women confused and concerned as they face a vexing decision after menopause: Should they use HRT or not? Up to 80 percent of postmenopausal women experience hot flashes, sometimes for years—a problem that can severely disrupt sleep and adversely affect energy, mood, and mental function. Other common symptoms affecting quality of life include night sweats, mood swings, depression, memory problems, vaginal dryness, reduced libido, bladder-control symptoms (such as frequent or urgent urination), and pain or discomfort during sex. Loss of estrogen also raises heart attack and stroke risk and causes bones to thin, boosting the likelihood of osteoporosis and fractures later in life.

While there's still no simple answer that's right for every postmenopausal woman, the latest research offers important new insights that can help women partner with their healthcare providers to make an informed choice about HRT. To help you sift through the confusion and controversy, here are four key takeaway messages offered by the Bale/Doneen Method, and supported by our friend and colleague, Marina Johnson, MD, F.A.C.E. A board-certified endocrinologist and pharmacist, Dr. Johnson is a leading national expert on HRT and the author of the book *Outliving Your Ovaries: An Endocrinologist Reviews the Risks and Rewards of Treating Menopause with Hormone Replacement.*

1. There is a critical "window of opportunity" after menopause.

    The recent reappraisals of the original WHI data show that the benefits of HRT outweigh the hazards if the therapy is started soon after menopause. In the WHI, the risks mainly affected women who started taking estrogen-and-progesterone therapy long after their periods stopped. In fact, the average woman in the study was 12 years past menopause when the treatment began.

    "Information that has emerged over the last decade shows that, for most women starting treatment near the menopause, the benefits outweigh the downsides, not just for relief of hot flashes, night sweats, and vaginal dryness, but also for reducing the risks of heart disease and fractures," said Robert Langer, MD, who was the principal investigator at the WHI center at University of California, San Diego, in a May 2012 statement.

    A series of articles published in a special June 2012 issue of *Climacteric*, the peer-reviewed journal of the International Menopause Society, highlights the new thinking about HRT. The latest medical evidence supports the "window of opportunity" concept: Overall, women who begin HRT before age 60 (or within 10 years of menopause) may have a *reduced* risk of heart disease. What's more, if treatment begins during this critical window of opportunity, HRT may actually be more beneficial to the heart that taking statins or aspirin, a 2012 study reports, while starting treatment later significantly increases risk.

    Taken together, these findings suggest that what's hazardous to the heart is a prolonged dip in hormonal levels after natural or surgical menopause, followed by a sharp rise when a woman begins taking HRT years after her ovaries stop producing estrogen. A sudden jolt of estrogen long after menopause begins appears to worsen or accelerate the progression of vascular disease in women who already have it, thus explaining the increased heart attack and stroke risk observed in older women who started the therapy long after entering menopause.

2. The HRT risk/benefit analysis needs to be personalized for each woman, based on her age, medical and family history, and health concerns.

Reflecting the new, more nuanced view of the potential risks and benefits of HRT, one ob/gyn remarked, at a recent meeting of the North American Menopause Society, "Every patient is like a Rubik's cube, and you have to find the right solution for her. Hormones are neither a panacea nor a weapon of mass destruction." Personalized care—rather than treating all patients according to the average results of large clinical trials like the WHI—is a cornerstone of the Bale/Doneen Method. Here's a look at important considerations to discuss with your healthcare provider to help you decide if HRT is right for you.

- Heart health

   For younger, healthier women, the latest research suggests that HRT may actually help ward off atherosclerosis. Estrogen replacement has also been linked to higher levels of HDL (good) cholesterol. *However, while there's emerging evidence suggesting some potential benefits to the heart, HRT should never be taken solely for prevention of heart disease, since it also has potential risks. A 2012 analysis by the U.S. Preventative Services Task Force recommends against using it for this purpose, or for the prevention of fractures or dementia.*

   We recommend that if you do decide to use HRT for symptom relief, after weighing the risks and benefits discussed in this section, treatment should start early in menopause to maintain steady hormonal levels. We also advise taking the lowest dose that keeps your symptoms at bay, for the shortest time possible, and discussing non-pill options with your healthcare provider.

   Bear in mind also that menopause isn't itself a medical condition. Not all women experience symptoms, and for those who do, HRT is simply one option. Regular weight-bearing exercise can be an excellent alternative that also helps keep their hearts and bones healthy after menopause: A 2012 study found that when women who had recently entered menopause followed an aerobic exercise program for six months, they had significantly lower rates of night sweats, mood swings, and irritability than those who didn't exercise.

   Several other studies show lower rates of hot flashes and other symptoms in women who exercise regularly, at least four times a week, choosing such activities as walking, jogging, biking, or lifting weights. One theory is that working out may help postmenopausal women regulate their body temperature better, leading to fewer hot flashes. Exercise helps improve mood by raising the level of feel-good brain chemicals called endorphins. Exciting new evidence has also shown that exercise enhances a cellular process called "autophagy." This is a mechanism by which our cells maintain their health: It helps keep us 'young' and assists in combating infections and cancerous changes.

If you smoke, here are even more reasons to quit: Women who smoke have up to *twice* as many hot flashes as nonsmokers do. Smokers also hit menopause about a year earlier than women who don't light up, possibly because smoking may reduce estrogen levels. Early menopause is linked to higher risk for a wide range of dangerous disorders, including cardiovascular disease, diabetes, Alzheimer's disease, osteoporosis, and obesity.

Need additional motivation to snuff out the habit? Here are five more reasons to stop playing with fire:

- Women who smoke risk having a heart attack 19 years younger than nonsmoking women. Puffing even one cigarette a day hikes the threat of a heart attack by 63 percent, and smoking 20 or more cigarettes daily more than quadruples it.

- Cigarette smoking doubles or even triples women's risk of dying from heart disease. Secondhand smoke also puts the health of your children and spouse at risk.

- Lung cancer is now the leading cause of cancer death in American women, with 80 percent of cases in women linked to smoking.

- Postmenopausal women who smoke have lower bone density and higher rates of hip fracture than nonsmoking women the same age. Smoking is also a major risk factor for osteoporosis.

- Women who smoke also have an increased risk for developing cancers of the oral cavity, pharynx, larynx (voice box), esophagus, pancreas, kidney, cervix, and bladder.

- Strokes and blood clots

  Taking HRT soon after menopause has been linked to a "modest" increase in risk for ischemic stroke, while starting hormonal therapy long after menopause elevates the threat of a stroke significantly. Oral HRT has been shown to raise the threat of blood clots—the cause of both ischemic stroke and most heart attacks—and this increased risk may be further magnified by obesity and increasing age, according to another new report. "When choosing HRT, giving estrogen topically—as patches, gels, creams, or mists—avoids blood clots and strokes seen with oral estrogen," Dr. Johnson advises, citing evidence from recent studies.

  If you're considering HRT, it's crucial to first find out if there's a cat in the gutter waiting to pounce (atherosclerosis), using the tests to check for plaque and inflammation discussed in Chapters Six and Seven. Inflammation has recently been shown to *cause* heart attacks and strokes, so if there's inflamed plaque in your arteries, a therapy that "modestly" raises stroke risk in the average patient could be dangerous for you until the fire in your arteries has been extinguished with the treatments discussed in Part Three, including simple lifestyle changes.

- Cancer

   What about breast cancer? "Women should not deny themselves HRT because of fear of breast cancer," says Dr. Johnson, pointing out that reappraisals of the WHI data show that concern about higher rates of the disease in HRT users has been greatly overblown. "The risk is rare, less than one in a thousand."

   In addition, evidence from the WHI and other trials shows that current HRT users have a 40 percent *lower* rate of colon cancer. That's a valuable benefit, because the disease, also known as colorectal cancer, ranks as the second-most-common cancer in women. Every year, it strikes about 103,000 Americans and kills about 50,000. And 90 percent of cases occur in people over age 50.

- Fractures

   After menopause, loss of natural estrogen also causes bones to thin, putting middle-age and older women at increased risk for osteoporosis (bone loss) or osteopenia (bone thinning), the brittle-bone disease that can lead to fractures, disability, and deformity. About 10 million Americans, including 8 million women, have osteoporosis and another 34 million have low bone density.

   After age 50, about one in two women (and one in four men) will suffer an osteoporosis-related bone fracture during their remaining lifetime. In the WHI study, taking estrogen plus progesterone reduced the rate of hip fracture by 33 percent, compared to the placebo group, and lowered the total fracture rate by 24 percent. A recent scientific paper reports that HRT has greater bone benefits than many drugs commonly used for prevention and treatment of osteoporosis, such as biphosphonates.

3. If you choose HRT, discuss non-pill options with your healthcare provider.

   HRT is now available in a wide variety of forms, including sprays, gels, skin patches, vaginal rings, tablets, and suppositories. Applying HRT topically reduces the systemic (whole-body) effects of the medication, by lowering the amount in your bloodstream, and may therefore decrease risk for side effects.

   Dr. Johnson also recommends opting for pharmaceutical bioidentical (natural) hormones. Bioidentical hormones are defined as being chemically equivalent in molecular structure as to those that a woman's body naturally produces. Some bioidentical hormones are made by drug companies, approved by the FDA, and are sold in standard doses. Other bioidentical preparations are made in special pharmacies called compounding pharmacies, which formulate the preparations for each patient.

   Which type is best? "Bioidentical pharmaceutical hormones meet stricter standards for quality control and efficacy than compounded hormones," she reports. The main hormone that's lost after menopause is estradiol, which is available in many FDA-approved bioidentical pills, patches, creams, and gels from traditional pharmaceutical manufacturers. These are made from the same plant sources that compounding pharmacies use but cost much less.

Compounded preparations are not regulated by the FDA and may vary widely in potency, with one shocking study reporting that only one in ten compounding pharmacies provided progesterone vaginal suppositories that were within the range required for FDA-approved products of this type. What's more, the FDA-approved estradiol products are typically covered by insurance plans, while the more expensive compounded versions are not.

Increasingly, doctors are prescribing estradiol instead of Premarin, a type of HRT derived from urine of pregnant mares. Premarin was the drug used in the WHI study. Discuss the potential risks and benefits with your health-care provider. Also be aware that there are two main types of HRT:

- Estrogen and progesterone

  Also called combination therapy, this form of HRT combines doses of two hormones that regulate women's menstrual cycles before meno-pause. Combination therapy is the only form of HRT that's appropriate for women who haven't had a hysterectomy. That's because taking estrogen alone raises risk for endometrial cancer (cancer of the uterine lining) by causing an overgrowth of endometrial cells that can lead to cancer, while the addition of progesterone prevents this problem.

- Estrogen therapy

  Women who had had a hysterectomy usually don't need to take pro-gesterone, so are typically treated with an estrogen-only therapy.

  The delivery method should be tailored to the symptoms being treated. Pills and skin patches, for example, are helpful for a wide range of meno-pause symptoms, including hot flashes. If your main concern is meno-pause-associated vaginal and sexual changes, however, then low-dose vaginal HRT—inserted in the form of a cream, tablet, or ring—could be an excellent option to consider.

  Here's why vaginal HRT helps relieve sexual and vaginal symptoms of menopause: when you're in your forties, your vagina is bathed in estro-gen, keeping the tissue moist, plump, and elastic. Folds and furrows allow the walls to stretch like a rubber band during lovemaking or childbirth. In fact, this is the one area of your body where it's good to have wrinkles!

  After menopause, waning hormone levels cause about 40 percent of women to develop vaginal dryness, the leading cause of painful sex. Com-pounding the problem, the vagina's folds and creases gradually disappear over time, reducing elasticity, and the walls thin with age, changes known as vaginal atrophy. The vagina may also shrink slightly.

  If sex hurts, you may do it less often, which leads to a double whammy: The vagina becomes even less flexible, making sex even more painful. Vaginal estrogen therapy, provided at dose much lower than that used for oral HRT, can actually have a rejuvenating effect. Over a few months, women typically notice a gradual increase in the thickness and elasticity of vaginal tissue, along with improved lubrication, both of which help increase sexual pleasure.

Since the medication is absorbed through the walls of the vagina, very little of it enters the bloodstream. And less-systemic absorption appears to equate to lower risk for blood clots—or associated heart attacks or strokes—new studies suggest.

4. Whether you take HRT or choose not to, heart disease is *not* inevitable after menopause.

While women's heart attack and stroke risk rises sharply during the years after menopause, loss of estrogen by itself doesn't *cause* vascular disease. It can, however, lead to cardiovascular changes that contribute to the increased risk women experience after their periods stop. Until menopause, estrogen helps keep your heart and blood vessels healthy and cholesterol in balance, key reasons why women, on average, develop heart disease 10 years later than men do. Afterward, arteries tend to become stiffer and less flexible, which may lead to a rise in blood pressure.

As women approach menopause, many of them have strikingly adverse changes in their lipids levels. One study that tracked 1,054 women over 10 years, before and after menopause, found that on average, their total cholesterol rose by 6.5 percent during the two-year window surrounding their last period, while LDL (bad) cholesterol jumped by 9 percent. Other research reports that levels of protective HDL fall after menopause, while other blood fats (triglycerides) typically increase.

It's also common for women to gain weight after menopause, particularly around the waist. Often, hormonal changes alone aren't the sole culprit, since menopausal women tend to exercise less, on average, than younger women do. In addition, muscle mass naturally decreases with age, so if you don't step up your workouts, your body composition will shift to a higher ratio of fat to muscle. Middle-age spread has serious implications for your cardiovascular health, since a wide waist is the leading warning sign of insulin resistance, which in turn can magnify heart attack and stroke risk.

While this tag team of postmenopausal risk factors probably sounds pretty scary, the heart-healthy lifestyle and therapies we recommend help counteract cardiovascular vulnerabilities that may become more noticeable after menopause. Remember, however, that risk factors alone don't cause a heart attack or stroke: the cat in the gutter does. That's why prevention with the Bale/Doneen Method is vital at every age to keep this wily predator at bay.

Action Step: Find Out If Your Arteries Are Diseased

Cardiovascular disease doesn't spring out of nowhere the day after a woman's periods stop: It develops slowly over many years, and even young, seemingly healthy, premenopausal women like Juli can harbor hidden disease that may go dangerously undetected, unless they're screened with the Bale/Doneen Method. And while Juli lacked the traditional risk factors, such as high blood pressure, she had two red flags discussed in earlier chapters.

An alert healthcare provider could have identified these warning signs without doing any lab tests: An examination of Juli's mouth would have revealed that she had periodontal disease and measuring her waist would have shown that despite her normal weight, she was in cardiovascular danger zone, since her waist circumference was greater than 35 inches. These two warning signals meant that despite her young age, she was a candidate for evaluation with our method, which we recommend for everyone older than age 40 and younger people with one or more red flags discussed in earlier chapters, or a family history of cardiovascular disease. In Part Two of this book, we'll reveal why Juli's heart attack happened—and which tests can tell if *you* might be at risk for a heart attack or stroke.

And here's news that may make your heart skip a beat: As you'll learn in the next chapter, one of the most commonly used tests that doctors rely on to check patients for heart disease is so unreliable that it misdiagnoses up to 40 percent of patients, with the highest error rate in women. We'll also tell you about a painless fifteen-minute ultrasound exam that can accurately determine if there's danger lurking in your arteries, even if you have no outward symptoms or risk factors. And you'll may be surprised to learn why your chronological age isn't nearly as important as how "old" your arteries are.

Part Two

Medical Detective Work

Chapter 6

Tests That Could Save Your Life

"A man is as old as his arteries."

—Thomas Sydenham, English physician,1624–1689

Wesley Robinson may not be able to leap tall buildings at a single bound, but to us, he will always be Superman. We gave him that nickname during his first visit to our clinic because the brawny 6'1" Texan with six-pack abs looked more like a movie superhero than a patient seeking evaluation of his heart health.

Like the comic book "Man of Steel," Wesley considered himself "invincible." In fact, the 44-year-old CEO of a satellite telecommunications company had only consulted us at the urging of his wife, who feared that he might have the cardiovascular equivalent of kryptonite in his arteries because of his mildly elevated cholesterol levels and alarming family history: His father had been disabled by a stroke at age 55, and then suffered a heart attack at 58. His maternal grandfather had died from a heart attack at age 60.

Still, Wesley found it hard to believe that he was in any danger of a similar fate: "I was living the life—skiing, snowboarding, and hunting—ate a healthy diet, and felt great." But with two young sons to raise, then ages 18 months and five, Wesley reluctantly concluded that his wife was right: With his frightening family history, it would be wise to get a thorough cardiovascular assessment to make sure that he'd be around to see his children grow up. He was confident, however, that we'd find nothing wrong.

Suzanne Dills was another reluctant patient. When her annual physical showed that her cholesterol levels were significantly higher than the year before, she thought her family doctor was overreacting when he referred her to Heart Attack & Stroke Prevention Center. After all, she didn't smoke and had no family history of CVD. "My blood pressure was 90/60, my resting heart rate was 38, and my EKG was normal, all of which indicate good heart health," says the then-60-year-old nurse, who was so physically fit that she was a national swimming champion in her age group.

When she arrived at our center for her appointment, this wonder woman of the water immediately felt out of place. "I looked around the waiting room and all the other patients were really overweight or were smokers." In fact, she was so convinced that a cardiovascular assessment was unnecessary that she actually apologized for "wasting" our time, telling us, quite emphatically, "I don't belong here."

An Epidemic of Denial

Up to 90 percent of adults rate their hearts as healthy, according to surveys by the American Heart Association (AHA) and other groups. For many, however, this belief is based on a false sense of security: a recent study by the Centers of Disease Control found that less than of 8 percent of Americans age 25 or older can now be considered at genuinely low risk for heart disease, based on such factors as their weight, blood pressure, smoking history, cholesterol levels, and diabetes, a finding that the researchers called an "ominous trend." Compounding the danger, millions of Americans have the cardiovascular red flags discussed in Chapter Three.

Other research suggests that the overwhelming majority of men and women overestimate their own healthy behaviors, while being in denial about their risks. Amid a growing obesity epidemic, surveys show that up to 66 percent of people polled tell their doctors a big fat lie, by fibbing about their weight. Another recent survey found only 12 percent of Americans exercise regularly, eat the recommended amounts of fruits and vegetables (nine servings daily), and practice good oral hygiene (defined in the survey as brushing twice a day and flossing at least once).

The leading excuse is that we're too busy to take care of our health. Superman was a case in point: the hard-charging CEO thought he could get away with averaging four to five hours of sleep a night as he juggled a stressful career and caring for his young children.

Since CVD is a silent disease, Superman couldn't see plaque creeping into his blood vessels and becoming progressively more inflamed. Nor did he recognize his risk: After all, he was "invincible," at least in his own estimation. A recent study shows the dangers of denial: supposedly "healthy" middle-aged Americans are up to three times more likely to suffer a fatal or nonfatal cardiovascular event than to die from noncardiovascular causes, largely because arterial disease often goes undiagnosed until an event occurs.

As a nurse, Suzanne was familiar with dangers of CVD, since she'd worked in the coronary care unit with heart attack survivors. But because she didn't look like her typically overweight, out-of-shape patients, the svelte swimming champion had convinced herself that she was immune to the disease that ranks as leading killer of women. Like many other women, she viewed cancer as her number-one health threat.

Are You at Risk for a Heart Attack or Stroke?

Superman's Framingham Risk Score predicted that over the next 10 years, his chances of having a heart attack were only 1 percent. The Reynolds Risk Score for men—which includes the Framingham factors, plus two additional factors: the man's blood level of the inflammatory marker high-sensitivity C-reactive protein, and if the man has a parent who suffered had a heart attack before age 60—rated Superman's 10-year heart-attack risk at 3 percent. In Suzanne's case, both scoring systems calculated her 10-year risk as less than 1 percent.

Based on these risk prediction systems, most practitioners of standard care would have patted both patients on the back and encouraged them to continue their excellent lifestyle. And Superman's worried wife would have been assured that there was no cause for concern: Despite her husband's frightening family history, he was every bit as healthy as he looked and almost certainly would stay that way over the next decade.

But those assumptions would have been dead wrong: Using a 15-minute ultrasound test—carotid intima-media thickness (cIMT), which we'll describe later in the chapter—we discovered that Suzanne had small areas of silent but potentially lethal plaque inside the walls of her arteries, while Superman had huge plaque deposits in his neck arteries. Superman's deposits weren't cats in the gutter— they were lions! And without appropriate treatment, they could have killed him, because having plaque in the wall of *any* artery—not just those that supply the heart—greatly increases the risk of a heart attack, stroke, or death from cardiovascular causes in the next 10 years.

The landmark 2001 CAFES-CAVE study revealed the danger of *not* treating plaque. Ten thousand low-risk, healthy men and women, ages 35 to 64, were screened for plaque, using both cIMT and a similar test (femoral IMT) that checks the intima-media thickness of leg arteries. Even if plaque (disease) were found, the participants weren't given any medical therapy known to be helpful, such as low-dose aspirin or statins. After 10 years of follow-up, the researchers correlated the rate of cardiovascular events (heart attacks and strokes) and deaths with the participants' IMT findings at the start of the study, which were classified in four categories, with these results:

- Class I (normal arteries). The 10-year rate of CV events in this group of study participants was 0.1 percent, with no deaths.

- Class II (wall thickening). Nearly 9 percent of this group had CV events during the study, also with no fatalities.

- Class III (plaque deposits that didn't obstruct blood flow). Nearly 40 percent of this group suffered heart attacks or strokes, including fatal events.

- Class IV (obstructive disease). Eighty-one percent of these people had heart attacks or strokes and of all CV-related deaths among the study participants, the overwhelming majority occurred in this group.

Based on the CAFES-CAVE study, the largest investigation of this kind ever conducted, Suzanne's true risk for a heart attack or stroke in the next 10 years was *nearly 40 times higher* than her FRS and Reynolds risk scores predicted, if she'd gone untreated. And without treatment, Superman's actual risk was also nearly 40 times than his FRS predicted, even though he had no symptoms of disease.

Just as his wife feared, this muscular man of steel really did have kryptonite in his arteries.

Only through vascular screening did Superman and Suzanne learn they were in potentially life-threatening danger, despite their apparent outward good health and reassuringly low Framingham and Reynolds risk scores. Nearly 70 percent of heart attacks occur in men and women who have never been diagnosed with CVD, so the value of *screening tests* (which check people who don't have symptoms) is that they can detect silent, but deadly plaque, so it can be treated in time to prevent life-threatening heart attacks and strokes. If you do have symptoms, *diagnostic tests* are used to find out what's triggering them.

Do *You* Have Kryptonite in Your Arteries?

If you're older than 50, you've probably received unsolicited letters in the mail touting "a simple, potentially lifesaving screening to assess your risk for stroke, abdominal aortic aneurysms, and other vascular diseases." Or you may have received brochures in which a celebrity urges you to "take the first step to safeguard your health" by buying a package of four ultrasound screening tests, offered at a senior or community center near your home.

Some of these ultrasound scans are extremely valuable screening tools—and can indeed be lifesaving, by detecting vascular disease before a heart attack or stroke occurs. These ads, however, can also be misleading. Typically, the package of scans marketed by these direct-to-consumer companies, such as Life Line Screening, do not include cIMT, despite studies showing that this ultrasound exam of the neck arteries is one of the best—and safest—ways to check for the cat in the gutter.

Instead, these companies usually offer a test that sounds similar, but has a completely different purpose: carotid duplex ultrasound. Its purpose is to find out if the lumen of the artery (the channel through which blood flows) is blocked. It's frightening to realize that based on this "purpose," Superman and Suzanne would have been told they were fine, since the plaque in their neck wasn't obstructing blood flow. Although this scan can be valuable to diagnose people with certain symptoms and conditions, as discussed later in this chapter, the United States Preventative Task Services Force, a group of public health doctors who issue evidence-based guidelines for healthcare providers, recommends against using carotid duplex as a screening test.

The rest of this chapter provides a guide to vascular disease screening tests that can save your life by finding hidden disease before it triggers a heart attack or stroke, as well as other imaging tests your healthcare provider may order if you have certain symptoms or medical conditions. The goal of all of these tests is to find out if you have vascular disease.

Some of the tests, however, like cIMT, directly examine the arterial wall—and therefore can diagnose plaque—and others, like carotid duplex, look for indirect evidence of disease (reduced blood flow through your arteries). In other words, some of the tests can find the cat in the gutter (indicating that you are at increased risk for a heart attack or stroke, if your disease goes untreated), while others can only tell you if there *might* be a cat. We will go over why each test is used, how it feels, and the pros and cons. This will help you think like a disease detective as you learn how to interpret the test results, and then get the right diagnosis and the most effective treatment, if you need it.

Because each patient is unique, we don't support the concept of a one-size-fits-all package of tests to evaluate blood-vessel health. The tests one patient undergoes may be significantly different from those we advise for another patient, depending on his or her age, medical history, and genes. And again, we want to emphasize that there is no one specific test that provides a complete evaluation of your cardiovascular health. That's why this chapter and the rest of Part Two of this book focus on the best tests to provide a *comprehensive, personalized* assessment of your overall heart attack and stroke risk.

The Ultrasound Advantage

On August 24, 2011, the Joint Commission issued a Sentinel Alert reporting that over the past 20 years, Americans' exposure to ionizing radiation (X-rays) through medical tests has nearly doubled, creating potential health threats, including increased risk for cancer. The commission recommended that healthcare providers use other types of imaging, including ultrasound, whenever those tests "will produce the required diagnostic information at a similar quality level."

Ultrasound is a very safe, inexpensive, and painless way to check for vascular disorders, including peripheral artery disease (PAD), aortic abdominal aneurysm, and plaque that could trigger a heart attack or stroke. Unlike X-rays, which can only detect hard, calcified plaque (stable plaque that contains flecks of calcium), the carotid intima-media thickness ultrasound scan discussed in this section can also detect soft, vulnerable plaque—the kind that can cause heart attacks and strokes.

Disease

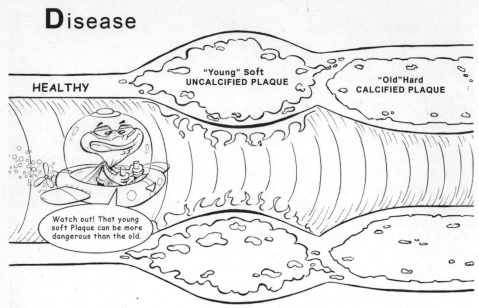

Plaque formation is an active process and its consistency changes over time.
Some technologies (X- rays) can only see hard calcified disease, while others like
ultrasounds can spot soft disease.

Here's a look at five common ultrasound tests.

Carotid Intima-Media Thickness (cIMT)

What It Checks for:

Carotid intima-media thickness (cIMT) is a FDA-approved test that measures the thickness of the two inner layers—called the intima and the media—of the carotid arteries, the major arteries of the neck, which carry oxygenated blood from the heart to the brain. Most important, the cIMT can identify actual atherosclerosis (cholesterol plaque growing in the wall of the artery, between the intima and the media), which is often undetectable with tests that only examine the arterial "pipes" through which blood flows.

A cIMT scan can also be used to find out how "old" your arteries are. As you age, it's normal for your artery wall to gradually get thicker, but in some people, arterial aging is accelerated, particularly if they smoke or have high blood pressure, high cholesterol, or diabetes. Therefore, your "arterial age" can be compared to your chronological age, based on norms for your age and gender developed through large studies of healthy people.

The Procedure:

The test is typically performed in a healthcare provider's office or at a medical center as you lie on an examining table. After applying gel to your neck, the sonographer glides an ultrasound transducer over the right and left side of your neck, as images are taken of the carotids so the thickness of the walls can be measured. The measurements are then analyzed for the mean common carotid wall thickness (which reveals your arterial age) and most important, for the presence of atherosclerosis. The exam takes about 15 minutes.

Who Should Get the Test:

We recommend cIMT for anyone with traditional cardiovascular risk factors or the red flags discussed in Chapter Three. If you've already been diagnosed with vascular disease, the test is also valuable for monitoring your response to treatment over time, to see if the therapy is working. Coauthor Amy Doneen, ARNP, recently served on a Society of Atherosclerosis Imaging and Prevention (SAIP) expert committee, which developed appropriate-use guidelines for cIMT including:

- Screening patients whose 10-year risk for coronary heart disease (CHD) is moderate (6 to 20 percent).

- Screening patients ages 30 or older who have metabolic syndrome.

- Screening patients with diabetes or a family history of early CHD.

- Screening people with two or more of the following risk factors: low HDL (good) cholesterol, high LDL (bad) cholesterol, diabetes, age (being over age 45 for a man and over 55 for a women), and a family history of early CHD.

Pros and Cons:

While checking the neck may seem like a surprising way to tell if you might be headed for a heart attack (or stroke), the carotids, which are just below the surface of the skin on each side of your neck, offer an easily accessible "window" to blood-vessel health, without exposure to X-rays. A recent study of more than 13,000 men and women found that adding intima-media thickness and the presence of plaque to traditional risk factors significantly improved the accuracy of 10-year predictions of heart attack and stroke risk. In fact, 22 percent of patients were reclassified as higher or lower risk than their FRS predicted when cIMT and plaque were taken into account. The study compared initial predictions with the patients' CV events over a 10-year period.

Since cIMT requires special ultrasound software, it's less-widely available than older technologies, such as carotid duplex. And your health plan may not cover the cost. A few states, however, have recently passed or proposed laws mandating insurance coverage of cIMT and coronary artery calcium score (discussed later in this chapter).

What the Results Mean:

Superman was horrified to learn that inside his brawny 44-year-old body, he had the arteries of a 62-year-old man, while Suzanne was equally aghast to discover that at 60, she had an arterial age of 78. Having arteries that are eight or more years "older" than you are is a sign of trouble, since it's evidence that you're headed for vascular disease in the future, while finding plaque means that you already have atherosclerosis.

Although any amount of plaque is dangerous, size does matter. One recent study found that plaque buildup measuring 1.5 mm or larger significantly raises risk for both heart attack and stroke, compared to people with less plaque or none. Another study linked areas of plaque measuring 2.33 mm or greater in the common or internal carotid with a 75 percent lifetime risk for stroke. Superman had two large plaques in his left carotid artery: 3.0 mm and 2.6 mm. Either one alone would cause significant risk for a cardiovascular event.

If cIMT detects plaque in your neck arteries, data from large studies indicates that you are not only at risk for a stroke, but also for a heart attack. In Part Three, we'll discuss the four cornerstones of treatment to halt or reverse the progression of vascular disease. The one that trumps all others is the personalized heart-healthy lifestyle recommendations you'll find later in this book, along with a guide to the best medications and supplements, if you need them.

Should you breath a sigh of relief if no plaque or evidence of accelerated arterial aging is found? Unfortunately, as is true of all other medical tests, a normal cIMT result isn't conclusive proof that you *don't* have disease, since the test, while highly accurate, only checks one of many arterial beds. It's also possible to have *no* plaque in your carotids, but to still have it other parts of the body, such as the coronary arteries.

Therefore, we recommend that patients with normal cIMT results be considered for further evaluation with the coronary artery calcium score test discussed later in this chapter, which uses a different imaging modality to check directly for plaque. These patients may also be candidates for peripheral artery disease testing along with ultrasound examination of the aortic artery. Both tests are described later in this chapter.

Carotid Duplex Ultrasound

What It Checks for:

Unlike cIMT, which directly examines the arterial wall for plaque, the carotid duplex test looks for indirect evidence of disease by measuring blood flow through the carotids. In other words, it's based on the plumbing concept of cardiovascular disease and checks for blockages in the "pipes."

The Procedure:

The test is performed in a similar manner to cIMT, but uses sound waves to assess the velocity of blood as it moves past the ultrasound probe, much like the police using a radar gun to find out how fast cars are moving on the highway.

Who Should Get the Test:

Carotid duplex is typically performed on patients with symptoms of reduced blood flow to the brain, such as temporary blindness in one eye or brief loss of the ability to talk, understand speech, or move. It's also an appropriate test for stroke survivors like Lauralee Nygaard and for monitoring the effects of surgical procedures to improve blood flow through the carotids, such as stent placement. As noted earlier, it is *not* recommended for screening patients for atherosclerosis.

Pros and Cons:

Like all ultrasound tests, it's safe, painless, and noninvasive. Carotid duplex can determine if life-threatening blockages are present in the carotid arteries. If performed inappropriately as a screening tool, however, patients like Suzanne and Superman, whose plaque was not obstructing their arteries, could gain a false sense of security. A 2007 study reported no evidence that this type of screening is beneficial to asymptomatic patients and it could even be harmful, since an abnormal result could lead to invasive tests, such as angiogram, that may not be necessary.

What the Results Mean:

Carotid duplex results are expressed as percentages, indicating the extent to which the diameter of the artery is narrowed (stenosis). Each lab sets its own range of "normal" results. For example, University of Massachusetts's clinical vascular service defines 1 to 29 percent stenosis as the "normal" range, while higher numbers are considered increasingly abnormal.

One hundred percent stenosis (also called "occlusion") means that the vessel is completely blocked, with no blood flow. Severely obstructed carotid arteries are usually treated with surgical procedures, such as balloon angioplasty and stent placement or endarterectomy, an operation to remove plaque buildup.

Ankle-Brachial Index (ABI)

What It Checks for:

This test is used to diagnose peripheral artery disease (PAD), a circulatory problem in which plaque buildup narrows arteries, reducing flow of oxygenated blood to your extremities (usually the legs). About eight million Americans have PAD, including up to 20 percent of people older than age 60. If you have coronary heart disease, there is a one in three chance that you also have PAD. And if you smoke, here's yet another reason to snuff out the habit: Smokers have up to six times higher risk for PAD. Nearly half of the people who develop this debilitating disorder are current or former smokers.

The classic symptom is leg pain or cramps when you're walking that improve with rest. Other warning signs include smooth, skinny skin, atrophy of leg muscles, cold, numb toes, and sores or ulcers on the feet or legs that don't heal. However, up to 40 percent of people with PAD—a serious, but treatable condition—have no symptoms, so the disorder often goes undiagnosed and untreated. That's dangerous, since having PAD quadruples or even quintuples the risk for heart attack or stroke.

The Procedure:

Ankle-brachial index is a painless exam that compared the blood pressure in your lower legs to the blood pressure in your arms. A technician or healthcare provider measures the pressure in your arms, using a standard blood pressure cuff, and then measures the pressure in arteries near your ankles using a blood pressure cuff and an ultrasound probe (or stethoscope). Blood pressure readings may be taken while you're at rest and again after you've walked on a treadmill. The test takes about 10 to 15 minutes.

Who Should Get the Test:

We recommend ABI if you are 50 or older, even if you don't have symptoms, or at any age if you do. We also advise being screened for PAD at age 40 if you have any of these risk factors: diabetes, high blood pressure, high cholesterol, atherosclerosis (plaque in your arteries), abdominal aortic aneurysm (AAA, discussed in the next section of this chapter), a family history of cardiovascular disease, or the 9P21 gene.

Sometimes called "the heart attack gene," because it's an independent predictor of risk for developing extensive coronary artery disease at an unusually young age, as happened to David Bobbett, the 9P21 gene also boosts the threat of PAD and AAA. In Chapter Eight, you'll learn which potentially lifesaving test can determine if you're a carrier of this extremely common gene or other variants that magnify heart attack and stroke danger, along with the right steps to tailor your personalized prevention plan to your DNA.

Pros and Cons:

The ABI can reliably diagnose PAD. Since the disorder often causes no symptoms until it reaches an advanced stage, in many cases, screening is the only way to catch the disease early, before it triggers dangerous or fatal complications. If severe enough, PAD can lead to leg infections and in the most serious cases, gangrene, and lower limb amputation. PAD is frequently a sign of widespread atherosclerosis, signaling that you could be a high risk for a heart attack or stroke without proper treatment.

Some older patients, or those with a history of kidney disease or diabetes, may develop rigid blood vessels that don't compress easily with a blood pressure cuff.

As a result, the ABI can be inaccurate. For those people, a toe-brachial index (TBI) is sometimes used instead of the ABI, since blood vessels in the toe rarely become rigid.

What the Results Mean:

To calculate your ankle-brachial index, the doctor divides the highest blood pressure recorded in your ankle by the highest pressure in your arm's brachial artery. The normal range is between 0.9 and 1.4. Any number lower than 0.9 indicates some degree of decreased blood flow to the feet, meaning that you have PAD, while a measurement higher than 1.4 indicates stiff arteries (often due to buildup of plaque that's hardened by calcium, known as calcified atherosclerosis).

PAD can often be treated with lifestyle changes, including quitting smoking, exercising more, and eating a healthy diet. You may also need medication, such as drugs to help prevent blood clots, such as daily aspirin therapy or Plavix.

Abdominal Aortic Aneurysm Scan

What It Checks for:

About 1.1 million Americans ages 50 to 84 have abdominal aortic aneurysm (AAA, pronounced "triple-A"), a weak, bulging area in the lower portion of the body's largest artery, which supplies blood to the abdomen, pelvis, and legs. Like a balloon, the larger the aneurysm becomes, the more likely it is to burst, causing massive bleeding that's fatal in up to 90 percent of cases. Ruptured aortic aneurysm kills about 30,000 Americans a year.

Although abdominal aortic aneurysm is often stereotyped as a disease of male smokers, about 22 percent of the people who develop it are nonsmokers and 40 percent of AAA fatalities occur in women. While the exact cause isn't yet known, many of the same conditions that accompany heart disease are contributing factors, including smoking, obesity, diabetes, high cholesterol, high blood pressure, and genetics.

Not only can the AAA scan reliably detect an aneurysm, if you have one, but it can also identify calcification (atherosclerosis) in the artery wall that signals increased risk for heart attack or stroke.

The Procedure:

Like the other tests in this section, the AAA scan is an ultrasound test, performed as you lie on an examination table. Not only can the test reliably detect an aneurysm, but it can also identify calcification (atherosclerosis) in the artery wall that signals increased risk for heart attack or stroke. To obtain the best images, you must avoid eating or drinking anything for four hours before the test.

Who Should Get the Test:

We recommend this scan for everyone older than 50, or at age 40 if you are a smoker, have a family history of AAA, or are a carrier of the 9P21 gene, particularly if you have two copies of the gene (inherited from both your mother and father).

Pros and Cons:

The test is painless, noninvasive, and relatively inexpensive. It is also extremely reliable for detecting AAA with close to 100 percent accuracy, or for determining that you don't have this disorder. Most of the time, an aneurysm doesn't cause any symptoms prior to rupture and is often difficult for doctors to detect during a physical exam, unless you are relatively thin, with a large aneurysm.

The downside is that Medicare only covers the scan (on a one-time basis, with a 20 percent copayment) for men ages 65 or older who have smoked more than 100 cigarettes in their life and for men and women with a family history of AAA. Some private plans only pay for men age 65 or older to be screened, while women may not be covered at all, regardless of their age or family history.

What the Results Mean:

If an aneurysm is detected, your healthcare provider may advise a watch-and-wait approach (monitoring the aneurysm with periodic ultrasound scans to see if it's getting bigger) or refer you to a vascular surgeon, depending on the size of the bulge. An aneurysm measuring 1.6 inches in diameter is classified as small, medium aneurysms measure 1.6 to 2.2 inches, and large ones exceed 2.2 inches. Surgery generally isn't recommended for small aneurysms, since the risks of the procedure outweigh the risk of rupture.

Finding calcified plaque means that you have the cat in the gutter and therefore could be in danger of having a heart attack or stroke. In the next section of this chapter, you'll learn which imaging test can pinpoint how much calcified plaque is in your coronary arteries—and what the results reveal about your true heart attack risk, even if you have no outward warning signs or symptoms.

Calcium in the Crosshairs

Atherosclerosis (also called "hardening of the arteries") begins with fatty streaks that develop very early in life. Incredible as it sounds, studies of premature babies show that fatty streaks can even develop before birth, particularly if the mom had high cholesterol. As cholesterol and other fatty materials continue to build up in the arteries, they initially form soft plaque. In a study in which the arteries of teenagers were examined under ultrasound, 17 percent of kids studied already had small plaques.

One of the ways the body tries to heal the damage from plaque is by depositing calcium in the injured area, resulting in calcified plaque. In fact, calcium can account for up to 20 percent of the volume of some plaque deposits. Calcium deposits are what put the hardness in "hardening of the arteries."

Since X-rays can detect calcifications in the arteries, one of the ways we can diagnose plaque in our patients—without doing any tests—is by reviewing their medical records. X-rays of any part of the body can potentially diagnose arterial disease by identifying calcium in arteries in the area that was imaged, if the deposits are large enough, thus revealing which patients are at increased risk for heart attack or stroke. These include dental X-rays, chest X-rays, mammograms (breast X-rays), and X-rays of the arms or legs, among others.

If X-rays taken for other medical purposes don't show any arterial calcifications (which aren't always noted on X-ray reports), or you haven't been X-rayed, the high-tech imaging test discussed below can detect even very tiny calcium deposits in your coronary arteries, thus diagnosing calcified plaque.

Coronary Artery Calcium Score

What It Checks for:

Also known as cardiac calcium score or coronary calcium scan, coronary artery calcium score (CACS) uses an electron beam tomography (EBT) or computed tomography (CT) scanner to look for flecks of calcium in coronary artery walls. The reason EBT or CT—rather than conventional X-rays—is required to find them is that the heart is in constant motion, so the images have to be taken very quickly. This challenge has been compared to trying to photograph a strand of spaghetti as it shimmies in rapidly boiling water, since the coronary arteries are relatively small and take many twists and turns as they travel through the beating heart muscle.

The amount of calcium is called a "calcium score" and is a strong predictor of heart attack risk, regardless of your risk factors. A 2012 study of patients with no symptoms of heart disease found that those with calcium in their arteries (as diagnosed by CACS) had more than double the risk for heart attack or stroke—even if their cholesterol levels were low, compared to people without calcium in their arteries.

The Procedure:

You are hooked up to electrodes as you lie on an examining table. The electrodes are monitoring the heart and allow high-speed X-ray images to be taken at a certain point in the heartbeat. As the table slides into the tunnel-like scanner, the CT machine rotates around your body taking extremely fast pictures of the heart. Calcium shows up as white spots in the arteries of the heart. Since your head remains outside of the machine during the scan, it's unlikely that you'd feel claustrophobic during the scan. The procedure takes about 10 minutes.

Who Should Get the Test:

Evidence-based guidelines developed by the Society for Heart Attack Prevention and Eradication (SHAPE) task force advise vascular screening with either CACS or cIMT for almost all men ages 45 or older and almost all women ages 55 or older. The only exception is men or women in these age groups who are at extremely low risk for heart attack or stroke because they meet *all* of the following criteria: They don't smoke, have total cholesterol below 200 and blood pressure below 120/80, don't have diabetes, and have no family history of CVD.

Among the studies the SHAPE task force reviewed are a major study called the Multi-Ethnic Study of Atherosclerosis, which reported the predictive power of traditional risk-factor prediction models, such as the Framingham Risk Score, is greatly improved with the addition of CACS, particularly in people who are considered at intermediate risk for future cardiovascular events. The SHAPE strategy, which the Bale/Doneen Method recommends, is designed to detect people who currently suffer heart attacks without ever having previously been diagnosed as high risk.

Pros and Cons:

The value of detecting calcium is that it can diagnoses plaque and therefore can help your healthcare provider determine if you are at higher risk for a heart attack or stroke, if the disease goes untreated. A 2012 study also linked buildup of calcified plaque in arteries outside of the brain with an elevated risk for dementia CACS is painless, noninvasive, and relatively inexpensive. Because CACS involves exposure to a low level of radiation, pregnant women should avoid taking the test.

Health plans usually don't cover the test, but laws recently have been passed or proposed in some states to mandate insurance coverage for both CACS and cIMT. Although CACS is reliable for detecting small amounts of calcium, it doesn't pick up softer, noncalcified plaque—the most dangerous kind. Because of the cost, the health risks of repeated exposure to radiation, and the inability to find soft plaque, CACS is not recommended to monitor your response to treatment over time.

What the Results Mean:

If your calcium score is 4 or higher, you have arterial disease and greater danger of a cardiovascular event. The higher the score, the more calcified plaque has been detected in your coronary arteries. A score above 400 indicating extensive disease. Although low scores are sometimes termed "mild" coronary artery disease, in reality, "mild CAD" is an oxymoron. It's as ridiculous as saying that someone is "a little bit pregnant." *Again, having* any *plaque in your arteries means that without aggressive prevention, you could have a heart attack or stroke.*

A calcium score of zero, however, doesn't rule out CAD, since you could have uncalcified (soft) plaque that this test is unable to detect. CACS is less reliable in younger patients.

Tests That Check for Blockages

While some tests directly check artery walls for evidence of vascular disease (i.e., the cIMT, CACS, and AAA scan), other tests look at blood flow and signs of blockages in the arteries. The problem is, 99 percent of plaque does *not* obstruct blood flow, yet can still cause a heart attack if it becomes inflamed and ruptures (think of a volcano in your artery). That eruption can result in a blood clot that causes a heart attack or stroke.

So, it's important to remember that the final three tests presented—angiograms, stress tests and the Heart SPECT scan—check only for blockages and therefore offer a less-comprehensive assessment of vascular health.

Coronary Angiogram

What the Test Checks for:

An angiogram has a simple mission: to determine if your arteries are blocked. Healthcare providers use data from an angiogram to decide if a patient needs invasive procedures, such as an angioplasty (a "balloon" inserted into the blood vessel to reopen the clogged area) or bypass surgery. This is the test that identified David Bobbett as having 100 percent blockage in one area of a coronary artery, and 70 percent blockage in another. He was advised to have surgery, but opted for aggressive medical management.

The Procedure:

Before the test, you'll be asked to fast for eight hours. You'll receive a mild sedative to help you relax. An angiogram is a special X-ray test in which radioactive dye is injected into the coronary blood vessels in a procedure called cardiac catheterization (threading a thin tube called a catheter through an IV in your arm, neck, or groin through your blood vessels up into the heart, under real-time X-ray guidance). A series of images (angiograms) are taken, providing a detailed look inside the vessels. An angiogram is an invasive test and therefore carries risk of complications. Although the test itself should take less than 30 minutes, patients are usually asked to lie quietly for a few hours after the test is completed.

Who Should Get the Test:

Angiograms are typically ordered for people with symptoms that could signal reduced blood flow through the coronary arteries, such as crushing or squeezing chest pain, pressure or tightness (angina), shortness of breath, dizziness, fainting or unusual fatigue during exertion, and excessive sweating. The test may also be performed to evaluate patients with heart failure, heart attack symptoms, chest injury, heart valve disorders, or congenital heart defects. *Because an angiogram is an invasive test with small, but serious risks, it is generally not advised to evaluate asymptomatic patients like David Bobbett.*

Despite this knowledge, angiograms are a common scenario when an asymptomatic patient consults a cardiologist after a noninvasive scan, such as cIMT (or the coronary artery calcium score test discussed in the next section of this chapter), shows plaque buildup. Very often, instead of investigating *why* an otherwise healthy patient like David—who could run on a treadmill at high speed without any chest pain or other cardiac warning signs—has diseased arteries, the doctor will instead order an unnecessary angiogram to find out how big the blockages are. This frequently leads to patients being told they urgently need a stent or bypass, when their disease could safely be managed without surgery.

Pros and Cons:

For people with symptoms of heart attack or blood vessel blockages, the angiogram gives an excellent look at the coronary arteries. The potential benefits, however, should always be weighed against the risks, which include a small chance that the catheter might injure a blood vessel or dislodge clotted blood or fat from an artery, which could block blood flow—or even trigger a heart attack or stroke. Other rare, but scary complications include excessive bleeding, infections, blood clots, and allergic reactions to the dye.

During an angiogram, patients are also exposed to a relatively high amount of radiation, equivalent to about 200 chest X-rays, which could increase their overall risk of cancer. A recent study estimated that up to 45,000 future cancers could be related to radiation exposure from medical scans performed in the United States in 2007 alone, with chest angiography being a significant contributor to cancer risk. Additionally, angiograms are relatively expensive, but may be covered by insurance.

What the Results Mean:

Normal results suggest that blood is flowing freely, with little or no narrowing of the vessels. Many patients with "normal" results, however, have dangerous atheromas (cats in the gutter) in their coronary arteries, and abnormal results indicate some obstruction in arterial lumen.

If the obstruction is less than 50 percent, patients are usually told they have "mild" disease. This is despite the knowledge that 68 percent of heart attacks arise from plaques less than 50 percent obstructive. If the blockage is greater than 70 percent, it is usually assumed to be related to the symptoms and invasive intervention is considered.

Heart SPECT Scan

What the Test Checks for:

Heart SPECT (Single Photon Emission Computed Tomography) is the most common "nuclear" heart scan used to look for indirect signs of heart disease, by evaluating blood flow though the coronary arteries. It can also detect damaged heart muscle—say, from a prior heart attack or infection—and measures how well your heart is pumping blood to the rest of the body. It's similar to turning on a string of Christmas lights to see which ones aren't working; if one area of the heart isn't getting enough blood (perfusion), this test will show it.

The Procedure:

Before the test, you'll be hooked up to an IV and receive an infusion of a harmless radioactive dye. You'll then receive two SPECT scans, one taken after you've been sitting quietly and the other after a treadmill stress test, to compare blood flow when the heart is at rest and when it's working hard. The scanner acts like a Geiger counter, tracking the movement of the radioactive dye through your coronary arteries. Each scan takes about 15 minutes.

Who Should Get the Test:

You're a candidate for this test if you have symptoms of coronary artery disease or failed an exercise stress test. It might also be reasonable for patients who have indirect evidence of significant coronary artery disease such as a very high calcium score. We also recommend this test for anyone with type 2 diabetes, even if he or she is asymptomatic. By the time someone develops diabetes, that person may have so much nerve damage that even if the heart is not being adequately supplied with blood, he or she may not have symptoms.

A recent study of 1,430 diabetic patients who received a SPECT scan reported that in 39 percent of cases, evidence of silent coronary artery disease was detected. The researchers also reported that the patients with abnormal results had a 5.4 percent rate of cardiovascular events over the next year, compared to a rate of 1.9 percent in patients with normal results. Moreover, SPECT scan results were a much stronger predictor of short-term risk than the patient's blood pressure or symptoms, such as angina (heart pain during exercise) or shortness of breath.

Another recent study of symptom-free patients with type 2 diabetes had even more dramatic results, reporting that those with moderate or large areas of inadequate perfusion were *six times* more likely to suffer a cardiovascular event, such as a heart attack or stroke, and were at *25 times* higher risk for cardiac death. A SPECT scan can also be a good diagnostic test for anyone with suspected circulation problems; its images are so clear that it shows how efficiently each heartbeat sends blood out from the heart's lower chambers.

Pros and Cons:

An abnormal SPECT scan result reveals hidden risk for heart attack or stroke, by detecting indications of inadequate flow of blood to part of the heart muscle. This possibility would need investigating further with an angiogram. The test can also identify patients who may be in so much danger that they should be treated with surgical procedures, such as a bypass operation, to improve blood flow, help prevent heart damage, and potentially head off a potentially life-threatening cardiovascular event. Therefore, basing the treatment approach on abnormalities found in SPECT scan could greatly improve the patient's short- and long-term prognosis, or even save his or her life.

This noninvasive test can also help people avoid unnecessary surgery. One of our patients was advised to have bypass surgery or a stent procedure after an angiogram showed that one of his coronary arteries was 100 percent obstructed and three others were 70 to 90 percent blocked, including the left anterior descending (LAD) artery. Traditionally, blockages in the LAD artery are deemed so deadly that it's known as "the widow-maker." A SPECT scan, however, revealed that this patient had excellent perfusion to this area of his heart through other arteries. That meant he didn't need surgery.

Our bodies are amazing. When an artery slowly (over years) becomes blocked, signals go out to make new smaller arteries to take over supplying that part of the body blood (angiogenesis). In some cases by the time the large artery gets totally blocked, there are plenty of smaller ones delivering plenty of blood to the affected area, as was the case with this patient.

Similarly, David Bobbett, despite 100 percent blockage in one of his coronary arteries, had adequate flow to the heart through other arteries and therefore didn't need the emergency bypass or stent procedure that specialists he consulted had recommended. For patients like these, a SPECT scan can be a valuable way to find out if they really do need to go under the knife.

The drawbacks of the SPECT scan are that it's relatively expensive and involves significant exposure to ionizing radiation. In rare cases, patients have reported allergic reactions to the radioactive tracer used in the SPECT scan.

What the Results Mean:

Images captured by the SPECT scan show colors, brighter areas, and dark spots, which a radiologist interprets. Abnormal results identify areas of the heart that aren't getting adequate blood, which is usually a sign of blockages caused by coronary artery disease—indicating potential heart attack risk that urgently needs treatment, either through surgical interventions and/or medical management, using the personalized prevention plan presented in Part Three of this book.

As is also the case with all of the other indirect techniques of evaluating heart and blood-vessel health discussed in this chapter, it's possible to get normal SPECT scan results and still have significant disease in your arteries, since this test can't detect nonobstructive plaque.

Stress Test

What the Test Checks for:

Stress tests, also called exercise stress tests or treadmill stress tests, look at how well the heart works during exertion and helps healthcare providers evaluate patients with symptoms that only emerge when the heart is forced to pump harder and faster than usual. A stress test can also detect irregular heartbeats or blood pressure abnormalities during exercise.

The Procedure:

Stress tests take four basic forms. They all aim to "stress" the heart and examine it while it's not at rest:

- The *exercise stress test* usually involves exercising on a treadmill or a stationary bike, with electrodes attached to your chest, legs and arms. The electrodes are connected to an electrocardiogram (EKG) machine that monitors your heart beat, while a blood pressure cuff measures blood pressure during the test. You begin by walking or bicycling slowly, then the exercise gradually becomes more strenuous. The aim is to work the heart hard for 10 to 12 minutes.

- In a *nuclear* or *thallium* stress test, as in the exercise stress test, you exercise on a treadmill or bike. In this version, however, thallium is injected into a vein before the test and, after a 15- to 45-minute wait, a special camera scans the chest. Then you use the treadmill or bike while your heart is monitored. While it's working hard, thallium is again injected and another scan is taken. Comparing the two sets of images helps the healthcare provider find out if blockages in the arteries are reducing the flow of oxygenated blood to the heart muscle.

- *Pharmacological stress testing* involves mild exercise, but a small amount of radioactive chemical is first injected into the vein. A special camera called a gamma camera takes computer images of the heart before and during a slow treadmill walk. Pharmacological stress testing is typically used for patients who are not able to exercise; they rest during the entire test.

- *Stress echocardiography* improves on the basic exercise stress test by adding ultrasound imaging to the process. Images are taken before the patient begins exercising and at various points during the test.

Who Should Get the Test:

While stress tests are often included in annual physicals to screen healthy people for heart disease, most people don't realize that in order to "fail" the test, their coronary arteries must be at least 70 percent obstructed in one or more areas. *A number of studies indicate that the stress test is a highly inaccurate vascular screening tool, prompting the U.S. Preventative Services Task to recommend against using it to check the heart health of low-risk people who lack symptoms.*

The test can be helpful to evaluate people with chest pain, cardiovascular disease (to assess severity or response to treatment), irregular heartbeats (arrhythmias), heart failure, and congenital heart disorders, and to check the cardiovascular health and fitness of sedentary people prior to participating in exercise or sports programs.

Pros and Cons:

One of the greatest benefits of this test involves measuring physical fitness, as determined by analyzing the intensity and amount of exercise performed, along with heart rates during the workout and the heart rate recovery during rest. If there is a narrowing of 70 percent or more in one of the coronary arteries, stress test results may indicate that a portion of the heart is inadequately perfused during the exercise portion of the exam.

The downside is that stress tests have a high rate of "false positives" (healthy people being told they have disease), leading to anxiety, fear, and unnecessary additional tests, as well as false negatives (missing disease, as occurred with David Bobbett, who passed his annual stress test with "flying colors" despite having 100 percent blockage in one area of his coronary arteries and 70 percent blockage in another area). Overall, the stress test misdiagnoses up to 40 percent of patients, with the highest error rate in women.

The stress test is relatively expensive, but very well covered by insurance, a combination that contributes to inappropriate use of the test for screening low-risk people, while depleting healthcare resources that would be more wisely allocated to screening tests better supported by scientific evidence, such as cIMT.

What the Results Mean:

Abnormal results may indicate arrhythmia or a possible blockage in your arteries. A normal result, however, may not be as reassuring as it sounds, since a study published in *Journal of the American Academy of Cardiology* reports that "patients who have normal imaging stress tests frequently have extensive atherosclerosis."

Tim Russert, NBC News's former Washington bureau chief and moderator of *Meet the Press,* is a famous case in point. Just weeks after passing a stress test in 2008, he suffered a fatal heart attack at work, at age 58. Like 50 percent of men and 64 percent of women who die suddenly from a heart attack, he had no previous warning signs. His tragic story is a grim reminder of the importance of getting a comprehensive, personalized evaluation of cardiovascular health, rather than just relying on a single test, particularly one that's as dangerously unreliable for screening symptom-free patients as the treadmill test.

Action Step: Find Out If You're on the Fast Track to Arterial Disease

Even if the tests in this chapter don't find any plaque or reduced blood flow in your arteries, you're not necessarily in the clear. Chronic arterial inflammation can put you on the fast track to developing vascular disease by speeding up the aging of your arteries. New research shows that inflammation actually causes vascular disease and is at the root of many other debilitating or life-threatening conditions, including diabetes and cancer. It's so dangerous to the arterial lining that it's worse than having high LDL cholesterol. And if you already have plaque, which acts as kindling for a heart attack or stroke, inflammation is what lights the match.

In the next chapter, you'll learn which simple blood and urine tests can detect this fiery process, including the recently discovered inflammatory marker we call "the joker." You need to find out if you have this dangerous wild card in the deck because it not only predicts future risk for CAD in healthy people—regardless of your risk factors—but it also predicts future cardiovascular events and whether they're likely to be fatal.

Although healthcare providers rarely order this very inexpensive blood test, the results can be lifesaving. As it turned out, Superman was one of the millions of Americans under assault by this cunning cardiovascular archvillain, and discovering the nemesis he faced was extremely important to guiding personalized treatment. Another of the tests in our "fire panel" revealed that Camille Zaleski's doctors had prescribed ineffective treatment after her heart attack—putting her at extreme risk for another event. And if you've ever been tempted to fib to your doctor about your health habits, you'll also want to know about the lifestyle lie detector test.

7

How Hot Are Your Arteries?

"A mighty flame follows a tiny spark."

—Dante Alighieri, ca. 1265–1321

Camille Zaleski and Juli Townsend were overwhelmed with fear and anxiety when they left the hospital after their heart attacks. Ratcheting up the fear factor even further for Camille was the realization that during her hospital discharge, doctors were already preparing her for the next heart attack—by warning her to remember her symptoms and call 911 if they occurred again—instead of telling her how to prevent it. And she was haunted by a scary statistic she'd read in a patient brochure: Nearly 25 percent of women (and 18 percent of men) die within one year after their first heart attack.

Also aware that women are far less likely than men to receive appropriate treatment after a heart attack, Camille worried that standard care wouldn't be good enough to save her life. Although the hospital doctors had prescribed an antianxiety drug (along with aspirin, a blood-thinning drug, and a statin), Camille was so frightened that she couldn't sleep, fearing that a heart attack might kill her during the night.

At home, Juli felt dangerously unprotected without doctors, nurses, and high-tech monitoring equipment watching over her 24/7, as they did in the ICU. She checked herself constantly for even the slightest symptom that might herald the onset of yet another attack. Very understandably, as she stressed over every tiny tinge and ache, she also feared that the hospital doctors had prescribed the wrong treatment. After all, she'd been mistakenly put on antibiotics—at the same hospital—when her first heart attack was misdiagnosed as bacterial pneumonia.

After the second heart attack, five days later, the doctors prescribed aspirin, a beta blocker, and a high-dose statin. Taking a cholesterol-lowering drug didn't make sense to Juli, since the hospital's healthcare providers had repeatedly told her that her cholesterol levels were "beautiful, like a teenager's." Remember, the only explanation she'd been given when she questioned the need for a statin was, "This is what we do after a heart attack," making it sound like she was getting one-size-fits-all medical care that wasn't appropriate for her case. When Juli developed a side effect—a skin rash—several days after starting the statin, she stopped taking the pills, believing they were unnecessary or even harmful.

Juli didn't realize that she was making a very dangerous mistake. No doubt she wouldn't have been so quick to quit statin therapy had she been aware of a frightening 2008 study of nearly 10,000 heart attack survivors. Those who discontinued statin therapy after the heart attack were 88 percent more likely to die during the following year than were patients who took the medication as directed by their healthcare providers. The researchers also found that halting other therapies, such as aspirin or beta blockers, was not linked to increased mortality in the study participants.

The Root of All Diseases?

Because Juli's doctors failed to provide proper patient education—or didn't know the answers to her questions—she thought she was being treated for a problem she didn't have: high cholesterol. In reality, statins can be a valuable part of an overall treatment and prevention plan after a heart attack or ischemic stroke, because they also combat another cardiovascular villain that's far more dangerous than high cholesterol: chronic inflammation, a key player in the plaque ruptures that lead to heart attacks and strokes.

For some patients with inflamed plaque, statins can actually be lifesaving, even if they *don't* have high cholesterol, as the landmark 2008 JUPITER trial dramatically revealed. In the study, more than 17,000 apparently healthy people with normal cholesterol, but high levels of C-reactive protein (an inflammatory biomarker discussed later in this chapter), were randomly assigned to either receive a statin or a placebo. In the group treated with the statin, risk for fatal and nonfatal cardiovascular events fell by nearly half over the next 1.9 years, compared to people who received a placebo.

Merely lowering cholesterol, on the other hand, may not be enough to prevent heart attacks and strokes. At the time of her seemingly inexplicable stroke, Lauralee Nygaard had been taking statins for a year and had been told shortly before the event that her cholesterol levels looked great. The plaque in her arteries remained inflamed, however, because she had untreated gum disease. As discussed in Part One of this book, plaque plus inflammation equals heart attack and stroke risk, even if you have optimal cholesterol levels (like Juli) and lack other traditional cardiovascular risk factors.

Chronic low-grade inflammation in the blood vessel lining is also powerfully linked with risk for developing coronary artery disease in the first place. People with very high levels of one of the inflammatory biomarkers discussed in this chapter are *nine times* more likely to develop blockages in their arteries than people with the lowest levels, greatly multiplying their threat of suffering a heart attack or stroke. An explosion of scientific studies has linked inflammation to many chronic diseases, from Alzheimer's to CVD, diabetes, autoimmune disorders, and even certain forms of cancer.

Some scientists have even hypothesized that chronic low-grade, systemic inflammation—fueled by such disorders as obesity or a large waistline, smoking, stress, poor diet, lack of exercise, insulin resistance, and periodontal disease—might be at the root of most or all chronic diseases, as a sort of "unified field" theory to explain why these lifestyle-linked maladies like vascular disease have reached epidemic levels in Western nations, while remaining relatively rare in developing countries.

Researchers also theorized that fire in the arterial wall was one of the missing puzzle pieces that explained the apparent mystery of why many people with normal or even optimal cholesterol levels suffer heart attacks and strokes, while other people with extremely high cholesterol never develop atherosclerosis. Until recently, however, there was no hard proof that inflammation causes coronary artery disease. For years, scientists hotly debated a chicken-and-egg question: Does fire in the arterial wall *cause* plaque buildup—or is inflammation merely a *result* of diseased arteries?

Why Chronic Inflammation Is So Dangerous

In 2012, two groundbreaking genetic studies published in *The Lancet* offered the strongest evidence to date that inflammation causes coronary heart disease (CHD). These studies were the first to demonstrate a cause-and-effect relationship between a specific inflammatory biomarker called interleukin-6 (IL-6) and the creation of the cat in the gutter—a discovery that could lay the foundation for revolutionary new strategies to treat and prevent the leading killer of Americans.

The first study analyzed genetic data and biomarkers from more than 200,000 participants in 82 earlier studies, focusing on people with a common variant of the IL-6R gene that reduces the body's inflammatory response. Specifically, these people have a smaller-than-usual number of receptors for interleukin 6 (IL-6), a cytokine (signaling molecule) involved in the first step of the inflammatory response.

For example, if you stepped on a rusty nail, cells in the affected area would mobilize immune system troops to battle the invading bacteria by releasing signaling molecules, such as IL-6, as a call to arms, along with chemical attractants. These compounds summon the body's defenders to the affected area, launching an immune system response known as the inflammatory cascade. It involves more than 20 proteins that blast the invaders with toxins to kill them and an assortment of odd-looking white blood cell components that *Scientific American* aptly described as resembling a casting call for characters in the horror movie *Creepshow 2*. Increased blood flow to the affected area creates the familiar signs of redness and warmth around the wound as it starts to heal.

Chronic inflammation, however, harms rather than heals, because the immune system attack never stops. The result is akin to being shot by "friendly fire" during a war raging within the body, triggered by the disorders discussed in the previous section of this chapter. Tissue damage is a hallmark of chronic inflammation,

105

which has a variety of harmful effects on the endothelium: the lining of the blood vessels that we call the tennis court, because if it was removed from the body and flattened, it would cover six tennis courts. As discussed in Chapter Two, the endothelium serves as the "brains" of the arteries by helping regulate blood pressure and other functions. The damaging effects of chronic inflammation lead to endothelial dysfunction, undermining the tennis court's ability to serve as a smart barrier between blood and the arteries. Fire can also occur in the intima (the layer below the endothelium), a problem that can be detected with the PLA2 blood test discussed later in this chapter.

For a heart attack or stroke to occur, the tennis court has to fail at least *twice*. First, chronic inflammation causes adhesion molecules to bind to the endothelium so it becomes sticky, like flypaper. White blood cells (another immune system defender) produced during the relentless inflammatory cascade become trapped in the sticky areas and then penetrate the endothelium, which normally serves as a protective barrier between blood and the arterial wall. When LDL cholesterol floats by, the Pac-Man-like white blood cell components gobble it up, forming fatty streaks that ultimately turn into plaque.

The second failure occurs when the plaque itself becomes inflamed, which either causes the cat in the gutter to grow and become more dangerous, or leads to a plaque rupture, followed by the formation of a blood clot that may obstruct flow to the heart or brain. If that happens, the result can be either a silent heart attack or stroke, or full-blown life-threatening events.

People with the IL-6R gene variant, however, have fewer-than-normal IL-6 receptors: molecular switches that are normally activated when IL-6 rises. As a result, a much smaller inflammatory cascade occurs when these cytokines molecules are released. The study found that although people with this variation had high levels of IL-6 circulating in their blood—an abnormality that's usually linked to *increased* risk for CHD—they were *less likely* to develop plaque in their arteries than were people without the variant.

Yet people with the variant had the same rates of smoking, high blood pressure, obesity, high cholesterol, and diabetes as a control group of people without the variant, indicating that the anti-inflammatory properties of the gene variant, rather than differences in other risk factors, explained the reduced risk for CDH. Furthermore, those with the variant also had lower levels of other inflammatory markers linked to CHD risk, such as C-reactive protein and fibrinogen (a protein involved in blood clotting discussed later in this chapter), offering further evidence that the variant reduced inflammation.

In the second study, the researchers analyzed data from 40 earlier studies of nearly 135,000 people, and reported that people who inherited two copies of the gene variant had a 10 percent drop in CHD risk, compared to a 5 percent drop in those with one copy. The study findings also suggest that a medication that blocks IL-6 receptors (currently used to treat rheumatoid arthritis) might offer a new approach to CHD prevention that merits study in clinical trials to see if it's safe and effective for this purpose.

The Fire Panel: Simple Tests to Check for Inflammation

In Chapter One, we told you about the written guarantee that we offer to all our patients stating that if they have a heart attack or stroke while under our care, they'll receive a refund of 100 percent of the fees they paid during the year. The "Fire Panel" of six simple blood and urine tests discussed in this section of the chapter is the reason that we're able to make this guarantee, even though most of our patients have many risk factors for cardiovascular events or have already suffered one or more heart attacks or strokes.

Just as firefighters have various ways to tell if a hidden blaze is raging inside the walls of a building—such as feeling heat, smelling smoke, or seeing the lights go out if the wiring is burning—we use a combination of lab tests to check for arterial wall inflammation. These inexpensive tests (most of which are covered by insurance plans) can all be done in the same medical visit and are available clinically through leading laboratories, such as the Cleveland HeartLab. Each of them can help save your life by alerting your healthcare provider if there is a tiny spark—or mighty flame—in your arteries that could ignite a heart attack or stroke.

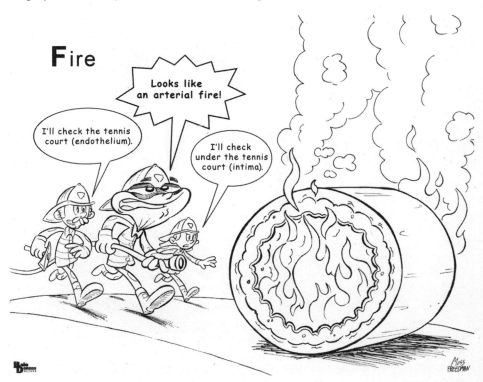

The Fire Panel serves four important purposes:

- Identifying people who are at risk for developing atherosclerosis, so their inflamed arteries can be treated *before* plaque develops (primary prevention).

- Determining if people who already have atherosclerosis have dangerously "hot" arteries, so they can be put on the right therapies to ward off a heart attack or stroke (secondary prevention).

- Evaluating patients like Juli and Camille, who have already survived one cardiovascular event, for fire in their arteries, so the blaze can be extinguished before they suffer another event (tertiary prevention). The two moms' lab results revealed that their diseased arteries were severely inflamed, indicating that without immediate changes in treatment, they were at very high risk for another heart attack.

Patient Identification

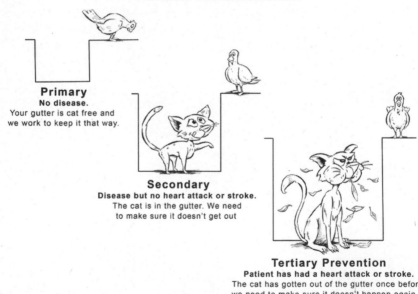

Primary
No disease.
Your gutter is cat free and
we work to keep it that way.

Secondary
Disease but no heart attack or stroke.
The cat is in the gutter. We need
to make sure it doesn't get out

Tertiary Prevention
Patient has had a heart attack or stroke.
The cat has gotten out of the gutter once before;
we need to make sure it doesn't happen again.

Ironically, Juli and Camille's intense fear and anxiety after their heart attacks may have worsened the fire in their arteries, a recent study suggests. British Heart Foundation researchers reported that patients who were the most terrified that they'd die after a severe cardiac event had the highest levels of inflammatory markers in their blood three weeks later, putting them at risk for worse long-term outcomes compared to patients who were the least fearful.

- Monitoring patients' response to treatments, to find out if the therapies that have been prescribed have successfully "cooled" inflammation in their arteries. In Superman's case, he initially responded to the treatments we prescribed. His cholesterol dropped to normal and the plaque in his neck arteries started to shrink.

But when we repeated the Fire Panel a year later, his inflammatory markers were significantly *worse*. The results were so alarming that we asked him to come to our office with his wife to discuss our findings. During the visit, we examined with cIMT and discovered that Superman had even *more* "kryptonite" in his neck arteries than he did during his initial visit. In other words, he was on the fast track to a heart attack or stroke.

We asked some probing questions and he admitted that he'd stopped taking one of the treatments we'd prescribed (niacin) because of a side effect: facial flushing. We explained that temporary redness in his face wouldn't kill him, but without treatment the severely inflamed plaque in his arteries erupt into a fatal heart attack. Superman quickly turned into a meek Clark Kent as his wife gave him a long, stern look, and then turned to us. "He'll take the niacin," she announced.

For Juli and Camille, our treatment and prevention plan for the two women included stress management to quell the anxiety that was fueling inflammation after their heart attacks. We also prescribed niacin, an Omega-3 supplement, and a different statin for Juli, at a lower dose that didn't cause any side effects. Changes in Camille's treatment included a diabetes drug, since her doctors had missed her prediabetes, and an ACE inhibitor, as well as following the diet-and-exercise plan presented in Part Three of this book. One year after her heart attack, she was 45 pounds thinner and so fit that she competed in a half-marathon.

The Fire Panel

This panel of tests should be repeated at least once a year even if the results are normal, since changes in your lifestyle (such as increased stress, less exercise, lack of sleep, a poor diet, or weight gain, particularly in the belly) or in your health (such as dental infection, developing an inflammatory disorder like rheumatoid arthritis, or the other red flags listed in Chapter Three) can trigger a flare-up of inflammation. If you're at increased risk for cardiovascular events, your healthcare provider may recommend having your inflammatory markers checked more frequently. We retest high-risk patients every three months, and medium-risk patients every six months.

If you have abnormal results on any of the six tests discussed in this section, it's extremely important to identify and treat *the root cause* of the inflammation. Ask your healthcare provider if the conditions that are sparking the fire in your arteries are being adequately addressed by your current treatment, since a rise in inflammatory biomarkers suggests that you may need different therapies or additions to your current prevention plan.

Also alert your dental care provider to your inflammation problem, since periodontal disease may be causing or contributing to the rise in your biomarkers. In Chapter Ten, we'll alert you to two saliva tests your dentist can use to evaluate your oral health more rigorously, and, in Chapter Fourteen, we'll cover the best treatments for periodontal disease—as well as what you can do to prevent this dangerous disorder, which can double or even triple your risk for a heart attack or stroke.

Typically, the first line of defense to extinguish fire in the arteries is lifestyle changes to combat the abnormalities that usually trigger inflammation, such as getting more exercise if you've slipped into a sedentary lifestyle, losing weight to combat insulin resistance and the toxic effects of belly fat, quitting smoking, managing stress, improving your oral health with optimal dental care, and eating a diet that's rich in antioxidants (found in many healthy foods, particularly fruits and vegetables) and fish (which has also been shown in studies to reduce inflammation in general and hs CRP in particular). You'll find detailed advice on the best diet to protect your heart in Chapter Twelve, including specific foods that help add years to your life.

Should these healthy changes not be enough, you may also need some of the medications and supplements discussed in Chapters Thirteen and Fourteen. Statins are one of the best medications to combat inflammation and also have recently been shown to have antioxidant properties. Niacin (vitamin B3) and fish oil can also be valuable treatments.

We recommend being checked with the six tests presented below at least once a year, or more often if you're at increased risk for cardiovascular events. We retest high-risk patients every three months. And the good news is that with the right treatment, elevated inflammatory biomarkers typically drop quickly, signaling that you're no longer on the fast track to a heart attack or stroke.

F2 Isoprostanes

What the Test Checks for:

We've nicknamed this blood test as the "Lifestyle Lie Detector" because it can reveal whether or not our patients are practicing heart-healthy habits. Recently, an executive we're treating claimed he'd been following all of our lifestyle recommendations to the letter, boasting that he'd quit smoking, hit the gym daily, ate a healthy diet high in fruits and vegetables, and made sure to get eight hour of sleep a night.

His abnormal level of F2 isoprostanes, however, suggested that he was lying—and when he was confronted with his test results, he confessed that he'd been staying up late every night to work on an important business project, had let his fitness slide, and was mainly eating junk food from the local greasy spoon. Overwhelmed with the stress of this project, he'd also been sneaking cigarettes. By the end of the visit, he was apologizing profusely for trying to deceive us. "I just can't get away with anything with you," he remarked, before vowing to mend his ways.

Because lifestyle is the most important therapy for heart attack and stroke prevention, this test helps motivate patients to actually practice healthy habits, rather than just pretending they do, in the hope of avoiding a lecture from their healthcare provider. The test isn't just a lifestyle lie detector, however: It also reveals how fast your body is aging—and if you might be on the fast track to a heart attack or stroke.

The test measures F2 isoprostanes, a biomarker of oxidative stress, an imbalance between formation of free radicals and protective antioxidant defenses. Increased oxidation puts you at risk for accelerated aging, cancer, and cardiovascular disease. One study found that people with the highest level of F2 isoprostanes were nine times more likely to have blockages in their coronary arteries than those with the lowest level.

Essentially, the goal of the test is to find out how fast your body is oxidizing, or breaking down. Although oxygen is essential for our survival, it also can be corrosive. When a freshly cut apple turns brown, a copper penny turns green, or a wrought-iron railing gets rusty, the culprit is oxidation, a reaction between oxygen molecules and substances they touch. As you may remember from high school chemistry, oxidation is the process of removing electrons from a molecule or atom.

Your body generates energy by burning fuel (compounds from digested food) with oxygen. One byproduct of normal metabolism—as well as smoking and other unhealthy habits—is formation of free radicals, highly unstable atoms or molecules that are missing one of their electrons. To achieve stability, they steal an electron from nearby molecules, leading to a domino-like chain reaction, in which the attacked molecules become free radicals and then rob their neighbors.

As a free radical chain rips through cells like a tornado, they can cause extensive injury to crucial components. If DNA, the cell's blueprint, is damaged, mutations that might lead to cancer could result, while damage to proteins, the cell's workhorses, can make the cells dysfunctional and more susceptible to disease. The F2 isoprostanes test measures a marker of free radical damage to lipids (blood fats like cholesterol).

The body also has antioxidant defenses to protect against free radical damage, however, including physical barriers to cage free radicals, enzymes to neutralize dangerously reactive forms of oxygen, antioxidants in our diet (found in fruits and vegetables, among other foods) that donate electrons and defuse free radical chain reactions, repair processes to fix damaged DNA, a garbage disposal system to sweep up these destructive scavengers, and other responses, such as programmed cell suicide if the damage is too extensive.

Therefore, the key to slowing down aging and protecting your cardiovascular health is achieving a balance between destructive oxidation and antioxidant defenses. Among the ways you can strengthen your antioxidant defenses—and reduce the rate at which your body is "rusting"—is by following healthy habits, including avoiding smoking, eating a Mediterranean-style diet that's high in fruits and vegetables and low in saturated fat, managing the stress in your life, and exercising regularly.

What the Results Mean:

A normal F2 isoprostanes level is less than 0.86 ng/L, while an optimal result is less than 0.25 ng/L. Although abnormal levels typically signal an unhealthy lifestyle that could cause premature aging, an important caveat is that some professional athletes or extremely amateur dedicated fitness buffs, may also have increased oxidation because of the extreme stress they're putting on their bodies.

With exercise, as with other healthy behaviors, it's crucial to find the sweet spot between doing too little and doing too much. A 2012 study published in *Mayo Clinic Proceedings* found that extreme endurance training may cause long-term heart damage in some marathoners, professional cyclists, and ultra-marathon runners, prompting the researchers to recommend moderate exercise or interval training (minibursts of high-intensity exercise that will be discussed later in the book) as healthier for the heart.

Fibrinogen

What the Test Checks for:

This blood test measures your level of fibrinogen, a sticky, fibrous protein produced by your liver. Fibrinogen helps stop bleeding by causing blood to clot. While fibrinogen's clotting effects can be lifesaving after an injury, abnormally high levels in the bloodstream can be dangerous, by contributing to the clotting cascade that leads to heart attacks and strokes. Fibrinogen is also a marker of inflammation, but other factors can boost levels, so this test shouldn't be used as the sole method of checking for fire in the arteries.

The higher your blood level of fibrinogen, the greater the risk of cardiovascular events. One large study called the EUROSTROKE project reported that "fibrinogen is a powerful predictor of stroke," including both fatal and nonfatal strokes, as well as first-time strokes, ischemic strokes, and hemorrhagic strokes (those caused by a torn or ruptured blood vessel). The researchers divided the study participants into four groups (quartiles) based on their levels of fibrinogen, and found that risk for stroke rose by nearly 50 percent for each quartile. People whose fibrinogen levels were in the highest quartile were nearly seven times more likely to suffer a hemorrhagic stroke than those in lowest quartile, and had double the risk of a fatal stroke.

In addition, higher levels of fibrinogen elevated stroke risk independently of such major cardiovascular risk factors as high blood pressure, diabetes, high cholesterol, and smoking. High blood pressure plus high fibrinogen, however, packed a double whammy, magnifying risk even more than high fibrinogen alone. That's probably because fibrinogen and its byproducts, such as fibrin, contribute to vascular disease by damaging the blood vessel lining, while high blood pressure further increases wear and tear that makes it easier for plaque to burrow inside. Plaque often contains large amounts of fibrin.

A large body of research has also established that elevated fibrinogen levels raise risk of coronary heart disease. In one study, researchers measured the fibrinogen levels of 2,126 people being treated in an outpatient preventative cardiology clinic, and divided then into four quartiles according to their test results. About half of the patients had coronary artery disease and on average, their fibrinogen levels were higher than patients who didn't have CAD. Among patients in the two highest quartiles, about 75 percent of the men and 50 percent of the women were diagnosed with CAD.

To show that elevated levels of fibrinogen weren't just an aftereffect of CAD, the researchers then tracked the patients (including 939 who were initially free of CAD) for an average of two years after their treatment. The researchers discovered that high fibrinogen was a strong, independent predictor of death from cardiovascular and other causes in both men and women, with the mortality rate in the highest quartile being seven times greater than in patients with the lowest fibrinogen levels.

High fibrinogen has also been linked to other diseases, including diabetes, cancer, and high blood pressure, and is frequently elevated in people with insulin-resistant conditions, such as metabolic syndrome. And for people with coronary artery disease, elevated fibrinogen increases the risk that a clot will form if plaque ruptures, setting the stage for a heart attack.

What the Results Mean:

The normal value is less than 500 mg/dL. In one study, having a fibrinogen level of 600 mg/dL was associated with a 200 percent increase in risk for cardiovascular events, compared to people whose fibrinogen level was normal.

High Sensitivity C-Reactive Protein (hs CRP)

What the Test Checks for:

This inexpensive blood test uses a technology called laser nephelometry to rapidly measure very small amounts of C-reactive protein (CRP) with high sensitivity (accuracy). CRP, a protein produced by the liver, rises in the bloodstream when there's inflammation throughout the body, which may indicate fire in the arteries that could ignite a heart attack or stroke.

The downside of the test, however, is that it's possible to have high levels of CRP *without* vascular disease, because infections, injuries, having a fever, or inflammatory disorders (such as rheumatoid arthritis) can also cause a spike in levels. Despite this limitation, large studies have consistently shown that abnormally high CRP levels can be a strong predictor of cardiovascular danger. In the Physicians Health Study, which tracked about 18,000 apparently healthy doctors, elevated levels of CRP were linked to triple the risk of heart attack, compared to doctors with normal levels of CRP.

The Harvard Women's Health Study reported that results of the hs CRP test were *more* accurate than cholesterol levels in predicting risk for cardiovascular events, while another study of women found that those with high levels of CRP were up to four times more likely to suffer a heart attack or stroke than were women with lower levels. Elevated CRP is even more dangerous if you also have a large waist, the leading sign of insulin resistance, which further magnifies heart attack and stroke risk.

In a joint scientific statement, the American Heart Association and the Centers for Disease Control and Prevention (CDC) recommended hs CRP as a more sensitive (accurate) test to predict risk for vascular disease, compared to traditional CRP tests that use less-sophisticated technology. Based on a systematic analysis of peer-reviewed studies examining the link between inflammatory markers and coronary heart disease and stroke, the AHA and CDC reported that:

- Hs CRP is a global indicator of risk for future cardiovascular events in people with no previous history of CVD.

- Hs CRP improves risk detection and treatment outcomes in such patients.

- In people who have already had vascular events, hs CRP can serve as an independent marker for risk of recurrent events, such as a heart attack or new blockages in someone who has undergone stenting or bypass surgery.

- Hs CRP is particularly beneficial for people with intermediate Framingham 10-year risk scores (10 to 20 percent) or LDL levels below 160 mg/dL.

What the Results Mean:

A score of under 1.0 mg/L is normal, while a score of 0.5 is optimal, since it's extremely unlikely that someone with that score has any inflammation in the arterial lining, meaning that short-term risk for cardiovascular events is very low. It's important to have the test repeated periodically, however, since even a slight elevation could be an early warning sign of increased heart attack or stroke risk.

Although it's comforting to have a normal or optimal level of CRP—indicating that the arterial lining is *not* inflamed—a high level, as discussed above, isn't conclusive evidence of heart attack, stroke, or CAD risk. Therefore, if your hs CRP results are abnormal, and there's no other apparent reason for inflammation, your healthcare provider will probably advise repeating the test a week later to confirm the results.

To find out if arterial wall inflammation is causing persistently elevated CRP, it's helpful to compare hs CRP results with those of the test described below, microalbumin/creatinine urine ratio (MACR). Since the two tests measure completely different biomarkers that may signal fire in the arteries, if both are elevated—as was the case with Superman and Juli—there's a very strong probability that blood vessel inflammation is the culprit.

Microalbumin/Creatinine Urine Ratio (MACR)

What the Test Checks for:

This test detects small amounts of albumin, a blood protein, in the urine. The term "microalbumin" refers to amounts of albumin that are too small to detect in urine dipstick test used for routine urinalysis during annual physicals. Having protein in the urine is abnormal, because albumin is a large molecule that circulates in blood and shouldn't spill from capillaries in the kidney into urine. Therefore, the test checks for a biomarker of endothelial dysfunction, as an indication of vascular disease. The urine ratio compares the amounts of microalbumin with those of creatinine (CR) a waste product produced by muscles.

Although this simple urine test costs just pennies, is covered by virtually all health plans, and provides valuable information about arterial wall health, healthcare providers rarely use it for this purpose, even though it's an extremely cost-effective way to check for evidence of arterial disease. Instead, MACR is most commonly performed to screen people with diabetes, high blood pressure, or kidney disorders for kidney damage.

The Framingham study found that MACR is an independent biomarker that predicts risk for cardiovascular events, while hs CRP and fibrinogen were not independent predictors in that study. Therefore, *an abnormal UACR is an important warning sign of cardiovascular danger, even if your hs CRP and fibrinogen levels are normal.* The researchers found that people with an elevated UACR had 20 percent higher rate of CV events, even when other risk factors were taken into account.

Another insight from research is that MACR is more accurate than the conventional albumin urine test often used in routine annual physicals because MACR takes into account how much water the patient has consumed and calculates the concentration of albumin in the urine accordingly.

What the Results Mean:

Very recently, new evidence from the large Framingham Offspring study shows that UACR results that have traditionally been considered "normal" can signal increased risk for cardiovascular events. Specifically, women whose MACR was above 7.5 and men with a ratio above 4 had nearly triple the risk for heart attacks, strokes and other cardiovascular events over six years of follow-up in that study. Therefore, ratios of 7.5 or lower for women and 4 or lower for men are optimal, rather than higher numbers that are still considered "normal" by standard care.

Based on the Framingham Offspring study results, Juli's UACR of 11 and Superman's ratio of 7.1 were quite alarming, since these numbers put them in the highest risk group for a heart attack or stroke. Yet practitioners of standard care would have patted them on the back and assured them the test results were perfectly "normal," had these healthcare providers even ordered this extremely valuable and cost-effective, but rarely used inflammatory biomarker test in the first place.

Lipoprotein-Associated Phospholipase A-2 (Lp-PLA2)

What the Test Checks for:

This blood test measures lipoprotein-associated phospholipase A-2 (Lp-PLA2), a blood vessel–specific enzyme that's mainly attached to LDL (bad) cholesterol.

Levels of Lp-LPA2 rise when arterial walls become inflamed, which may indicate that plaque is more likely to rupture, which could lead to a heart attack or stroke. The Lp-PLA2 test was FDA approved for coronary heart disease assessment in 2003 and ischemic stroke risk assessment in 2005.

This enzyme is now emerging not only as a biomarker of arterial wall inflammation, but also a direct *player* in the atherosclerotic disease process, with a recently published study suggesting that Lp-PLA2 plays a key role in cholesterol plaque formation and vulnerability (risk that the plaque may rupture explosively and trigger a heart attack or stroke). The researchers note that their findings support reducing Lp-PLA2 as a strategy for preventing CHD. Evidence-based guidelines from the American Heart Association and other groups also endorse the test as "reasonable" to screen symptom-free people who are at intermediate risk for heart disease or increased risk for stroke.

Unlike the UACR test, which evaluates the health of the endothelium (by checking if the blood vessel lining had become so dysfunctional that large molecules of albumin are spilling from the bloodstream in the kidneys into the urine), the Lp-PLA2 test is designed to answer a different, but extremely important question: How hot is it *under* your tennis court? In other words, is there fiery plaque hidden inside the artery wall that might erupt like a volcano?

What the Results Mean:

Lp-PLA2 values of less than 200 ng/mL are considered normal. In the Mayo Heart Study, 95 percent of patients with scores under this threshold did *not* have a heart attack or stroke in the next four years, even though they had coronary artery disease (CAD). The researchers also found that the higher Lp-PLA2 levels, the greater the risk for a first heart attack, stroke, or major CV event. Compared to patients with normal levels, those with scores of 200 to 266 ng/mL had a 70 percent higher risk of these events over the next four years, while a level of 267 or above more than doubled risk.

For Camille, whose UACR was in the optimal range, the Lp-LPA2 test sounded a potentially lifesaving alarm by revealing that several weeks after her heart attack, the plaque inside her arterial wall remained dangerously inflamed, even though her tennis court looked normal. Her score of 257 ng/dL meant that the treatments her doctors had prescribed weren't good enough to prevent another heart attack, because they'd failed to put the fire out.

To illustrate just how dire the young mom's risk would have been without changes in her treatment, in the KAROLA Heart Study, which looked specifically at people who had already experienced cardiac events, participants with this score were *2.3 times* more likely to suffer a recurrent event—or sudden cardiac death—over the next 4.5 years than those with lower scores. And the main clue that her arteries were still on fire was the Lp-PLA2 test results, since almost all of her other inflammatory biomarkers were in the normal range.

Myeloperoxidase (MPO)

What the Test Checks for:

This FDA-approved blood test measures myeloperoxidase, an enzyme that the immune system uses to fight infection. Normally, it's only found at elevated levels at the site of an infection. We call it "the joker" because if it's elevated throughout the body—as occurs in about two in fifty people, a similar distribution to the jokers in a deck of cards—all bets are off. Of all the inflammatory biomarkers, it's the worst: If this wild card, which appears to be genetically influenced, gets played, without the right treatment your game of life might be over.

One reason that MPO is so dangerous is that it produces numerous oxidants that make *all* cholesterol compounds more inflammatory. This includes HDL, the "good" cholesterol that normally helps clean the arteries, protecting against plaque buildup. If your blood levels of MPO are high, HDL goes rogue and joins the gang of inflammatory thugs. The joker also interacts with hydrogen peroxide in the bloodstream to produce hypochlorous acid (the active ingredient in bleach). Inside the blood vessels, this acid attack can eat holes in the tennis court, making it easier for cholesterol to penetrate and form plaque.

Another of MPO's nasty tricks is reducing the body's production of nitric oxide (NO), the best "food" to nourish the endothelium and protect its health. Lowering NO weakens the integrity of the tennis court, which can either promote atherosclerosis, or for people who already have plaque in their arteries, magnify the risk that the cat will leap out of the gutter and cause a heart attack or stroke. The joker also contributes to creating vulnerable plaques by making the normally protective fibrous cap that covers plaque more prone to rupture.

What the Results Mean:

The normal value is less than 420 pmol/L. Elevated MPO predicts future risk for coronary artery disease and cardiovascular events, including fatal heart attacks and strokes. In a recent study, people with high levels of the joker were 2.4 times more likely to die from heart disease over the next 13 years. Superman's level was a whopping 834 pmol/L,

Learning that he had extremely elevated levels of three out of the six inflammatory markers for which the Fire Panel checks was an important wake-up call, says the dad of two young sons. "Just looking at me, you would have thought I was in perfect health. My cholesterol had dropped to optimal levels and I felt really great, so I thought I could get away without taking the niacin. Seeing these incredibly abnormal numbers brought me back to reality.

"My goal is to be around to see my kids grow up and without these tests, I probably would have had a heart attack or stroke, based on what happened to my father," he adds. "Deciding to give the niacin another try was a no-brainer—and within three months, I was able to tolerate it well, without any flushing. Today, I have ideal numbers on all of the inflammatory tests, and am just as healthy on the inside as I look on the outside."

Action Step: Get an In-Depth Cholesterol Test

Did you know that up to one-third of heart attack victims have an inherited cholesterol problem that is not even routinely measured in the United States? What's more, this lipid menace boosts risk for having a heart attack or stroke at an unusually young age. We frequently see survivors of these events, including Juli and Camille, who have never been checked for this cholesterol factor. Yet it can be detected with a $20 blood test that also includes a comprehensive lipid profile that can better identify heart attack and stroke risk.

In the next chapter, you'll be surprised to learn that your LDL (bad) cholesterol level is *not* the most important number on the standard cholesterol test. Here's a startling secret your healthcare provider hasn't told you—or may not know: A simple math formula—using just two numbers from your cholesterol results—is such an accurate predictor of heart attack and stroke risk that life insurance companies have used it for years to rate their customers' risk. To find out *your* number, and what it reveals about your risk, go to the next page.

Sizing Up Cholesterol

"A cowardly cur barks more fiercely than it bites."

—Quintius Curtius Rufus, ancient Roman historian

When Jack Grayson woke up from the sedation he'd received for his angiogram, four grim-faced cardiologists were standing at the foot of his hospital bed. "They showed me a drawing and said that my coronary arteries looked terrible," says Jack, who served as Chairman of the Price Commission of the United States under President Nixon. Not only was one of his major coronary arteries 100 percent blocked, but three others, including the "widow-maker" artery (the left anterior descending artery) were at least 70 percent obstructed.

"The doctors had a debate about treatment—stents or bypass surgery—and decided that stents would be best," adds the Texas businessman. "They asked when I wanted to schedule the operation. I said, 'What are the other options?' I was told that they could try drugs or radiation therapy, but I'd be taking a lot of risks."

Jack declined any surgical procedure. A few months later he was exposed to our method at a presentation we gave in Houston. He decided then to become a patient and follow the Bale/Doneen Method. Jack realized that the angiogram did not explain why he had such terrible heart disease in the first place. Then 83, Jack had no obvious risk factors other than his age. A nonsmoker, he was exceptionally fit, with low (but healthy) blood pressure and excellent blood sugar, weight, BMI, and waist circumference numbers. He was anxious to plug into our method to uncover the reason for his disease.

Being told that he urgently needed surgery to "fix" his horrible and seemingly inexplicable disease left Jack with a sense of fear and futility. Since his extremely healthy lifestyle wasn't enough to protect him, there seemed to be nothing he or his cardiologists could do to prevent new blockages from forming in his already severely diseased arteries. Not did only Jack—a grandfather of two who enjoys skydiving—turn to us to save his life, but he also hoped we could help him achieve a remarkable ambition. "My goal is to live to 113, with a great quality of life," he told us.

With conventional treatment, however, it was questionable if Jack would have lived very long after his terrifying diagnosis. As you learned in Chapter Four, the trip to the operating room for stents or bypass surgery is rarely a one-time journey, because even procedures as extensive as quadruple bypass surgery only treat a few inches of the body's more than 60,000 miles of blood vessels. For someone Jack's age, repeated surgeries would have been very dangerous. Nor do these operations cure arterial disease, which continues to progress unless the root cause is identified and treated.

Like Joe Inderman and Dead Man Walking, Jack felt the first glimmer of hope when he learned that our science-based method is designed to find and treat the root cause of arterial disease, not just its symptoms, such as blockages. After we explained our written money-back guarantee and signed the document, Jack added his signature with a flourish. "Finally, someone was telling me that I wasn't going to die from a heart attack or stroke," he recalled during a recent interview.

The Dangerous Cholesterol Most Doctors Don't Check

Understandably, Jack assumed that his doctors had checked him for all cholesterol abnormalities that might explain why he had such horribly blocked arteries. After all, the blood test he'd received certainly sounded comprehensive: It's called a "lipid profile" or a "coronary risk panel." Since all of the blood fat numbers that were checked—his levels of total cholesterol, low-density lipoprotein (LDL), high-density lipoprotein (HDL), and triglycerides—were in the "optimal" range, he also assumed that his severe coronary artery disease wasn't caused by a cholesterol problem.

All of these assumptions were wrong, however. As you'll learn in this chapter, myths about cholesterol—the most demonized and misunderstood substance in both our bodies and our diet—abound. Among the most widespread, and harmful, of these misconceptions is the belief that doctors routinely test and treat patients for *all* forms of harmful cholesterol that raise heart attack and stroke risk. In reality, most healthcare providers don't check patients for a common-inherited cholesterol problem that's been shown, unequivocally, to actually *cause* heart attacks. We call this disorder the "mass murderer," because elevated levels of this cholesterol triples risk for heart attacks, according to three large studies involving nearly 45,000 participants. High levels of Lp(a), which is also known as "lipo (a)," also boost the threat of having heart attacks or strokes at young ages.

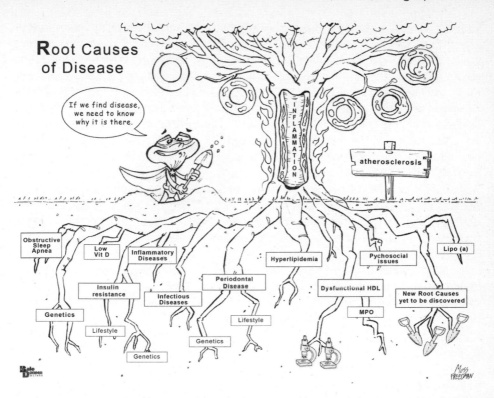

In June 2010, the European Atherosclerosis Society (EAS) issued a scientific statement recommending routine screening and treatment for this dangerous disorder, found in about 20 percent of the population, as an important "priority to reduce cardiovascular risk." Yet in the United States, it's *still* not the standard of care to treat—or even measure—this dangerous form of cholesterol, found in elevated levels in up to one-third of heart attack victims. At the Heart Attack & Stroke Prevention Center, we routinely see patients who have already suffered a heart attack or stroke—or even multiple events—and still haven't been tested or checked or treated for a cholesterol problem that's been proved to actually cause these catastrophes!

You're probably shocked and wonder what this dangerous cholesterol is. It's called lipoprotein (a), or Lp(a). Have *you* ever heard of it? Has your health provider ever measured your Lp(a) levels? If the answer is no, consider this: Being left in the dark about this important cholesterol test nearly cost Juli, Camille, Lauralee, and Jack their lives. Had their healthcare providers ordered this blood test, it would have revealed that all four of these patients had high levels of Lp(a), solving the apparent medical mystery of why they had developed such severe coronary artery disease despite a lack of traditional risk factors.

Instead of recommending Jack undergo potentially risky—and costly—heart surgery at age 83, his healthcare providers could have treated him with a simple vitamin pill and other over-the-counter supplements discussed in Chapter Twelve. These inexpensive therapies might also have prevented the three young moms' life-threatening cardiovascular events, had their Lp(a) problem been detected through the routine screening advised by EAS and treated *before* it triggered Lauralee's stroke and Camille's and Juli's heart attacks.

Incredibly, even after Juli had suffered *two* heart attacks at age 37, her Lp(a) levels still weren't checked. Instead, she was assured that her cholesterol levels were "beautiful, like a teenager's"—at least according to the standard lipid test most doctors use. Lauralee's stroke, also at age 37, was deemed "medically inexplicable" since she'd been on statin therapy for an entire year prior to the event. Because the statin had successfully reduced her previously high LDL levels to the normal range, she believed, mistakenly, her cholesterol issue had been solved. Actually, the medication was only treating *half* of her cholesterol problem because unlike high LDL, elevated Lp(a) does *not* respond to statin therapy or lifestyle modification.

Currently, scientists don't know why elevated Lp(a) is so hazardous. Linked to genes on chromosome 6, this condition appears to be a genetic "misfire" in the path of evolution. It's thought be a variant of the gene that makes plasminogen (a protein involved in blood clotting) since Lp(a) and plasminogen have almost identical sequences of amino acids. Lp(a) is only found in Old World monkeys, hedgehogs, and humans.

Although the link between elevated Lp(a) levels and increased risk for cardiovascular events was first discovered in the 1970s, Lp(a) wasn't known to cause heart attacks and strokes until 2009, when three conclusive genetic studies, involving hundreds of thousands of patients, were published in *JAMA (Journal of the American Medical Association)* and *New England Journal of Medicine.* Some experts used to argue that elevated Lp(a) wasn't known to be dangerous for African Americans, but a 2011 study established that this cholesterol *is* a risk factor for that group, while the prevalence in other ethnic groups is still under investigation. This important epidemiological research will be key to understanding demographic differences in rates of CVD.

Everyone, regardless of ethnicity, should be checked for Lp(a), using a simple blood test that can be performed at the same time as the conventional cholesterol test healthcare providers typically use or the advanced lipid profile discussed later in this chapter. Lp(a) testing used to be extremely expensive when it was first introduced about 15 years ago, then costing about $1,000, but recent technological breakthroughs have now slashed the cost to about $20.

Since levels are mainly determined by genetic factors—not lifestyle—if your Lp(a) is normal, then there's no need to have it checked again, since your genes don't change. If your Lp(a) level is abnormally high, several inexpensive supplements discussed in Chapter Twelve can potentially lower it. For example, taking niacin (vitamin B3) can reduce levels by up to 40 percent, according to the European Atherosclerosis Society. There's also some evidence that lowering LDL helps counteract much of the cardiovascular risk associated with elevated Lp(a). Several over-the-counter supplements discussed in Chapter Twelve have also shown some effectiveness in reducing Lp(a).

Uncovering the main reason for Jack's disease gave him comfort and hope. Not only did he feel better once the "why" was explained, but diagnosing his Lp(a) problem meant there were simple steps he could take to ward off heart attacks and strokes—without the risks of undergoing stent or bypass surgery. Now 90, he takes niacin every day, watches his LDL, and continues to enjoy an active lifestyle. He's an avid skydiver and travels the world without fear of a heart attack or stroke. He recently had an exhilarating adventure with his sons and grandkids, gliding through California treetops on a zip line swing 50 feet above the ground with boyish glee. And Jack remains determined to reach his 113th birthday—or beyond—while enjoying life to the fullest along the way.

A Surprising Cholesterol Number That Predicts Heart Attack Risk

Life insurance companies know a secret that most doctors never tell patients: When it comes to calculating your risk for a fatal heart attack, the *least* important cholesterol number is your level of LDL, the notorious "bad" cholesterol that has long been vilified as public enemy number one by the medical profession. In fact, life insurance companies don't even look at LDL levels, because large studies have shown that it's the *worst* predictor of heart attack risk.

Instead, life insurance companies use a simple formula, based on two numbers that should be in everyone's medical record, to rate heart attack risk: They divide your total cholesterol by the level of HDL (good) cholesterol. The result, called total-cholesterol-to-HDL ratio (TC/HDL ratio), was found to be the *best* predictor of heart attack risk in the long-term Women's Health Study.

Life insurance firms stand to lose millions of dollars if they rate somebody's risk improperly. So they've been quick to grasp the predictive value of TC/HDL ratio. For decades, it's been the main cholesterol number their actuaries look at, while healthcare providers continue to place huge importance on LDL, as opposed to superior indicators of risk like TC/HDL. Most doctors don't educate patients about the importance of TC/HDL ratio, even though this number is often included in the lab report.

If your TC/HDL ratio doesn't appear on your cholesterol test results, doing the math yourself is very simple. For example, if your total cholesterol is 180 mg/dL and your HDL is 60 mg/dL, you'd divide 180 by 60 to get your TC/HDL ratio of three. While life insurers consider people with a ratio of 5 or lower to be "preferred best" insurance risks (the category of customers who qualify for the lowest premiums because they're deemed healthiest), research shows that having an even lower number is much safer. In the Women's Health Study, for example, the mean TC/HDL ratio in women who suffered cardiovascular events, such as heart attacks and strokes, during 11 years of follow-up was 4.7, compared to a ratio of 3.9 in women who didn't have events.

Based on scientific evidence from multiple studies, we consider a TC/HDL ratio of 3.5 a desirable target and a number below 3 to be optimal. People with a ratio below 3 and no inflammation in their arteries enjoy vastly superior protection against heart attacks and strokes and are also less likely to develop arterial disease at all, compared to people with higher numbers.

Debunking The "Cholesterol Hoax" and Other Lipid Myths

Research shows that of all of the cholesterol villains—LDL, very low density lipoprotein (VLDL), intermediate low density lipoprotein (IDL), and that mass murderer Lp(a)—LDL is arguably the wimp of the gang of four: the "cowardly cur" whose bark is worse than its bite. Yet standard cardiology guidelines emphasize the value of reducing LDL as a primary goal in heart attack and stroke prevention, while ignoring superior predictors of risk, such as TC/HDL ratio.

None of the hundreds of cholesterol studies conducted to date have ever shown that LDL causes heart attacks. This unscientific belief remains so ingrained in medical thinking, however, that it's been termed "the great cholesterol hoax." *Again, we emphasize that the key player in both the development of coronary artery disease and the plaque ruptures that lead to heart attacks and strokes is inflammation. If your arteries aren't hot, you are unlikely to suffer these calamities, even if your cholesterol levels are extremely high or you have cholesterol plaques in your arteries.*

Here's a look at 15 common misconceptions about lipids that can harm patients—and the facts you need to protect your cardiovascular health.

Myth #1: Cholesterol is inherently evil.

Fact: You couldn't survive without cholesterol, since this waxy substance produced by the liver plays many essential roles in our body, from waterproofing cell membranes to helping produce vitamin D, bile acids that help you digest fat, and many types of hormones, including the sex hormones testosterone, estrogen, and progesterone. It also helps form synapses, the circuitry through which nerve cells communicate.

Cholesterol is ferried through your body by molecular "submarines" known as lipoproteins, such as lipoprotein (a), low-density lipoprotein (LDL), and high-density lipoprotein (HDL). LDL transports cholesterol from the liver to cells where it's needed, while HDL carries cholesterol back to the liver, where most of it is secreted in bile used to break down food. Both LDL and HDL are crucial for our bodies to function, so in the proper ratio, both are actually "good."

Myth #2: The conventional cholesterol test accurately measures LDL.

Fact: One little-known drawback of the traditional lipid test is that it doesn't directly measure LDL. Instead, it tallies total cholesterol, HDL, and triglycerides, then uses a mathematical formula to calculate LDL. This formula can be unreliable, however, particularly if your triglycerides are high, sometimes creating a false sense of security.

Advanced lipid tests directly measure LDL for a more accurate reading, using a variety of technologies. One commonly used test (NMR LipoProfile) gauges size by analyzing the magnetic properties of LDL particles. Another test called VAP (Vertical Auto Profile) sorts particles by spinning them in a high-speed centrifuge, since the big ones are more buoyant.

For the most accurate cholesterol test results, both the standard test and the advanced lipid profile should be performed in the morning after an overnight fast. Fat from a meal can artificially boost your lipid levels, particularly of triglycerides, on the test.

Myth #3: HDL cholesterol is always "good."

Fact: Although HDL is often hyped as "good" cholesterol, people with seemingly healthy levels may not be getting as much protection as they think. Having a lot of small, dense HDL particles can actually raise the threat of a heart attack or stroke, while a predominance of bigger, more buoyant particles can lower it. Both the quality and quantity of your HDL particles are important to cardiovascular risk, because the bigger particles are better at grabbing harmful cholesterol and dumping it into the liver for disposal.

Myth #4: Eggs clog up your arteries.

Fact: Because cholesterol has been so demonized by both the medical establishment and the media, many people view foods that contain this nutrient as practically poisonous. We've been bombarded with warnings that consuming foods that are high in cholesterol, such as hamburgers, steak, lobster, and liver, boost risk for atherosclerosis and heart attacks. Eggs have been particularly demonized as "a heart attack in a shell," because the yolk contains upwards of 200 mg of cholesterol, more than two-thirds of the American Heart Association's recommended daily limit of 300 mg per day.

The "lipid hypothesis"—the theory that there's a direct relationship between eating foods that are high in cholesterol, such as eggs, lobster, steak, and liver, and developing cardiovascular disease—has long been controversial, however. Recent research suggests that dietary cholesterol isn't nearly as dangerous as most people believe. One study found that when people ate three or more eggs per day, their level of LDL rose, as expected—but the surprise was that HDL also went up.

An even more interesting finding was that when people ate three or more eggs per day, their bodies produced larger LDL and HDL particles than when they ate no eggs. That's important for two reasons: Bigger LDL particles are less likely to invade the arterial wall and clump into plaque, while bigger, more robust HDL particles are better at ridding the bloodstream of harmful cholesterol. The researchers concluded that most people's bodies handle dietary cholesterol from eggs in a manner that's unlikely to harm the heart or blood vessels.

The biggest factor influencing cholesterol levels is actually heredity, not diet. Therefore, people who are watching their cholesterol can safely eat eggs in moderation. The biggest threat to our heart health is that most of us consume too much fattening food of all types and exercise too little, leading to expanding waistlines and increased risk for insulin resistance.

Myth #5: There are no visible symptoms of high cholesterol.

Fact: Some people with high cholesterol develop yellowish bumps called xanthomas that can occur on their eyelids, joints, hands, feet, or other parts of the body. The bumps can be tiny or as large as three inches in diameter. People with diabetes, certain cancers, or familial hypercholesterolemia (an inherited condition in which the liver is unable to remove cholesterol from the bloodstream, resulting in very high cholesterol levels) are more likely to have xanthomas, which are also more common in elderly people with high cholesterol. Research also shows that high cholesterol increases risk for kidney disease, Alzheimer's disease, and erectile dysfunction.

Most people with high cholesterol don't have any outward warning signs and feel fine. The only way to find out if your lipids are too high is to have them checked with a blood test at least every two years—or more often, if advised by your healthcare provider. It's also extremely important to have your Lp(a) levels checked at least once, as discussed earlier in this chapter.

Myth #6: Americans have the world's highest cholesterol levels.

Fact: Contrary to the stereotype that most of us are just a few Big Macs away from a heart attack because of sky-high lipid levels, in reality, the United States is solidly in the middle when it comes to cholesterol levels. U.S. men rank 83rd in the world in average total cholesterol and U.S. women 81st, according to the World Health Organization (WHO). For both sexes, the average is 197 mg/dL, slightly below the level the American Heart Association classifies as "borderline high" (200 to 239 mg/dL).

In Columbia, men average a whopping 244 mg/dL—a level that doubles heart-disease risk—while Israeli, Libyan, Norwegian, and Uruguayan women are in a four-way tie for the highest average with 232 mg/dL. Another WHO multicountry analysis found that mean serum cholesterol tends to be higher in young men in England, Germany, and Japan, compared to their counterparts in Scotland, Thailand, Jordan, Mexico, and the U.S.

Another surprise is research showing that cholesterol levels are dropping in the United States, despite the growing obesity epidemic. In the 1960s, about 33 percent of Americans ages 20 to 74 had high cholesterol (defined as above 240 mg/

dL) and the average was 222 mg/dL. From 2003 to 2006, only 16 percent of people in this age group had high cholesterol and during those years the average fell to 200.

Myth #7: You're protected against stroke if your cholesterol is low.

Fact: HDL levels are a strong independent predictor of ischemic stroke risk, even in people with low LDL, research shows. In fact, one major study found *no* link between stroke rates and either LDL or total cholesterol levels. Higher levels of good cholesterol are so beneficial for your brain that we call HDL "brain food." And raising HDL even slightly is a surprisingly effective way to ward off strokes. Researchers reported in a recent study that for each one mg/dL increase in HDL, stroke risk dropped by 1.9 percent.

To determine your ideal HDL number, divide your total cholesterol by three. Your HDL level should be higher than that. For example, if your total cholesterol is 210, your good cholesterol should be above 70 for the best defense against strokes and heart attacks.

Among the best ways to boost brain-protective good cholesterol are weight loss, improving your diet, and taking certain supplements, such as fish oil. Getting even one extra hour of moderate exercise per week can also increase HDL, a recent study found, working out several times a week is even better. If you smoke, here's yet another reason to snuff out the habit: quitting can boost HDL levels by up to 10 percent.

Myth #8: Food is heart-healthy if it has zero mg of cholesterol.

Fact: Some cholesterol-free foods are extremely unhealthy. Since the liver produces cholesterol, it's only found in animal-based foods, such as meat, eggs, or dairy products. Therefore, foods that don't come from animals can truthfully be labeled "cholesterol-free," even if they contain ingredients that can elevate cholesterol in the bloodstream, such as trans fats, which the Mayo Clinic calls "double trouble," because these foods boost bad cholesterol and lower good cholesterol.

Watch out for this misleading marketing ploy and check food labels to make sure the items you're buying are genuinely heart-healthy. The best foods for your heart are those that are low in sugar and saturated fat, but high in fiber. A recent study of nearly 400,000 people ages 50 and older found that a high-fiber diet reduced risk of death from cardiovascular causes by 59 percent during the nine-year study. Other research suggests that eating more fiber—and less red meat—would prevent about 45 percent of cancer cases in the United States.

Myth #9: Low cholesterol is always a sign of good health.

Fact: While the health risks of high blood levels of LDL cholesterol are commonly touted, most people don't know that low LDL has been linked to increased risk for certain disorders. For example, a 2012 study found that people who develop cancer typically have lower LDL levels during the 18 years prior to their diagnosis than people who don't get cancer. In the study, cancer patients were compared to a control group of cancer-free patients, matched by age, gender, smoking status, blood pressure, diabetes, and body mass index. None of the patients had taken statins.

Thirteen earlier randomized clinical trials evaluating statin therapy that included newly diagnosed cancer patients also reported a link between low LDL and a slightly higher rate of cancer (about one additional case per 1,000 patients), sparking medical debate about whether statins boost cancer risk. However, the 2012 study suggests that an as-yet-undetermined biological mechanism—not cholesterol-lowering drugs—appears to be the link between low LDL levels and cancer risk.

A recent study by French researchers found that older men with lower levels of LDL had nearly double the risk for developing clinical depression over the next seven years, while in older women low HDL was linked to increased depression risk. The researchers suggest that careful management of HDL and LDL levels, through a combination of diet and medication, may help prevent depression in the elderly, but that different treatments are needed according to the patient's gender. The study also found that in men, both LDL levels and genetic factors play a role in vulnerability to depression.

Myth #10: Children can't have high cholesterol.

Fact: Not only can kids develop high cholesterol, but in rare cases, they can even have heart attacks, as happened to a woman we know who suffered from familial hypercholesterolemia and had her first heart attack (of several) at age 16. In 2011, an expert panel convened by the National Heart, Lung, and Blood Institute (NHLBI) advised screening all American children for high cholesterol before age 11, a recommendation endorsed by the American Academy of Pediatrics (AAP).

Previously, the AAP and National Cholesterol Education Program had only advised cholesterol screening for children with a family history of high cholesterol or heart disease. A 2010 study, however, found that this approach missed about 36 percent of kids with elevated levels. The researchers evaluated health information on more than 20,000 fifth-grade students in West Virginia, 29 percent of whom had no red flags from family history, so they wouldn't have been checked under the government guidelines then in place.

The rationale for the NHLBI panel's guidelines is that kids with high cholesterol typically continue to have elevated lipids in adulthood, so it's preferable to detect and treat the condition early in life, typically through lifestyle changes such as a healthy diet and more exercise. The guidelines remain controversial, however, since other medical groups continue to recommend that screening start at age 20 or older.

Currently, one in five American children has abnormal cholesterol levels. However, a 2012 study by the Centers for Disease Control and Prevention offered heartening news, reporting that for the first time in nearly 20 years, kids' levels of harmful cholesterol have dropped, while the amount of good cholesterol has increased. These findings were surprising, since the childhood obesity rate remains high, but the researchers suggest that public health campaigns to reduce or eliminate trans fats in foods may explain the encouraging trend.

Myth #11: Everyone should strive for the same lipid levels.

Fact: Lipid levels, like other treatment goals, need to be individualized for each patient, depending on his or her other medical conditions and genes. For example, as discussed earlier in the chapter, studies suggest that people with an inherited Lp(a) problem can reduce their levels of this cholesterol by keeping their LDL numbers low. Similarly, diabetics and people who already have arterial disease need to set lower LDL targets than those of healthy people. In Chapter Eleven, we'll take a closer look at how to set optimal, personalized treatment goals for cholesterol and other cardiovascular risk factors.

Myth #12: If you have high cholesterol, you should be taking a statin.

Fact: Now the most widely prescribed drugs in the world, and taken by 30 million Americans, statins block a liver enzyme that helps produce cholesterol. The average person taking a statin will see his or her LDL levels drop by 20 to 60 percent in a month. These medications aren't inoculations against heart attacks and strokes, however, because it takes a lot more than just lowering LDL to prevent these events.

In addition, about seven million Americans who take a statin don't need their LDL lowered, because it's already normal. Instead, they are being treated for other heart attack and stroke risk factors. Less well-known benefits of these drugs are that they make blood less prone to clot and also reduce inflammation, which has recently been shown to cause heart attacks.

While statins are valuable for certain patients, particularly people who have already had a heart attack, these medications are also overhyped and oversold. In the United Kingdom, for example, low-dose statins are available over-the-counter, which could encourage irresponsible use of these drugs. There have even been proposals to add statins to drinking water or offer them at fast food restaurants to counteract the effects of fatty meals.

For most people with high cholesterol, lifestyle modification remains the most powerful—and best—treatment to lower it.

Myth #13: High LDL is the leading risk factor for heart attacks.

Fact: A recent study reported that a stunning 75 percent of nearly 137,000 men and women hospitalized for heart attacks had LDL levels within currently recommended targets, and nearly half had "optimal" levels. As a result, practitioners of standard care wouldn't have deemed the vast majority of these patients candidates for therapies that might have prevented their heart attacks. That's a horrifying example of how the LDL cholesterol hoax puts lives at risk because doctors continue to focus on a risk factor that's the *least* predictive of heart attack and stroke danger.

The study also found that levels of HDL have dropped in American heart attack patients over the past several years, probably because of rising rates of obesity, diabetes, and insulin resistance in the U.S. population. Nearly 55 percent of the patients studied had abnormally low levels of HDL, while only 2 percent had ideal levels of both LDL *and* HDL. The researchers concluded that current national guidelines do not effectively identify most patients who will suffer fatal or nonfatal heart attacks.

A particularly shocking finding was that nearly half of the heart attack patients studied had suffered a prior cardiovascular event, highlighting the urgent need for the comprehensive prevention plan presented in this book. It's extremely important to identify and manage disorders known to actually cause heart attacks and strokes, including inflammation, insulin resistance, and elevated Lp(a).

Myth #14: All LDL particles are equally dangerous.

Fact: The size of LDL particles matters. Some LDL particles are small and dense, making it easier for them to penetrate the arterial lining (if the endothelium is damaged by inflammation) and then form plaque. Other LDL particles are big and fluffy, so they tend to bounce off the artery wall. Think of the difference between bullets and beach balls. Compared to people with big, fluffy LDL particles, those who mainly have small, dense ones are up to three times more likely to have heart attacks. Magnifying the danger, people with small, dense LDL particles also have a higher number of particles, a factor that has also been shown to predict increased cardiovascular risk.

Because the conventional cholesterol test doesn't measure particle size or the number of LDL particles, the only way to check is with an advanced cholesterol lipid profile. This more comprehensive blood test, which costs about $80 and is usually covered by health plans, provides an in-depth analysis of both cholesterol quantity and quality by looking at cholesterol subtypes not included in the standard test.

It's not essential, however, for your healthcare provider to know your particle size or number. In fact, he or she can usually predict whether you have small, dense particles based on your levels of triglycerides and HDL, as measured by the conventional cholesterol test. The combination of high triglycerides and low HDL is usually associated with having small, dense LDL particles and a higher number of LDL particles.

Myth #15: High triglycerides trigger coronary heart disease.

Fact: Although triglycerides are the most common type of fat in the body, they don't cause arterial disease, because they don't penetrate the arterial wall and form plaque. Your body produces some triglycerides (formed from a single molecule of glycerol combined with three molecules of fatty acids), but most come from the food you eat. When you consume more calories than you burn, the extra calories are converted into triglycerides and stored in fat cells until they're needed for energy. In other words, when fat accumulates on your thighs or belly, that's where excess triglycerides end up.

For people who already have CAD, high triglycerides nearly triple heart attack risk, according to a Harvard-led study. This finding dovetails with another recent study showing that VLDL and IDL are both inflammatory to the artery and more than triple the threat of heart attack. Since VLDL and IDL comprise the cholesterol content of the lipoprotein "submarines" that transport triglycerides in the bloodstream, this study suggests that it's not triglycerides themselves that drive increased heart attack risk, but rather these two cholesterol villains, which are part of the gang of four discussed earlier in the chapter.

Having high triglycerides (even if cholesterol levels are normal), however, magnifies heart attack danger by nearly threefold, while *people with the highest ratio of triglycerides to HDL (TG/HDL ratio) had nearly 16 times the risk of heart attack than those with the lowest.* The study, published in *Circulation,* compared 340 heart attack patients to 340 of their age-matched healthy counterparts. The researchers concluded that TG/HDL ratio is "a strong predictor" of heart attack.

As you'll learn in the next chapter, a high TG/HDL ratio is one of the warning signs of insulin resistance, the root cause of 70 percent of heart attacks and nearly 100 percent of cases of type 2 diabetes. Although most doctors don't check for this extremely common disorder, even in patients who have already suffered a heart attack or stroke, insulin resistance is easy to detect with a simple, universally available blood test that's usually covered by health plans. It can sometimes be diagnosed without doing *any* lab tests, based on information that should be in everyone's medical record. If you're insulin resistant, simple lifestyle changes can dramatically reduce your risk for developing diabetes and can also ward off a heart attack or stroke.

In the next chapter, you may be surprised to discover which everyday habit puts you at very extreme risk for developing this extraordinarily common disorder, which affects about 150 million Americans. This habit can be *more* dangerous to your cardiovascular health than smoking—and can lead to a wide range of diseases, including CVD, type 2 diabetes, obesity, depression, and cancer. We'll tell you easy ways to protect yourself, including a health-boosting activity that only takes one minute and helps slim your waist, reduces triglycerides and inflammatory markers, and also lowers blood sugar.

Action Step: Get Your Blood Sugar Checked

More than 102 million Americans have diabetes or prediabetes, and 34 million of them don't know it, either because they haven't had their blood sugar measured or they were checked with unreliable tests. Like many of our patients, you may be shocked to discover how alarmingly inaccurate some diabetes screening tools can be: One widely used blood-sugar test misses up to 64 percent of patients with prediabetes and can even fail to detect full-blown diabetes.

As a result, these patients go undiagnosed while the disease silently damages their blood vessels, setting the stage for cardiovascular events. Not only are people with diabetes up to four times more likely to have heart attacks or strokes than nondiabetics, but diabetics typically suffer these calamities at a younger age. If you're middle-aged and have diabetes, some studies suggest that your risk for a heart attack or stroke is as high as that of a nondiabetic who has already had one. In addition, heart attacks and strokes are more likely to be fatal in people with diabetes.

In the next chapter, you'll find out which inexpensive blood-sugar test can reveal if you're insulin resistant. Most healthcare providers don't use it this way, depriving patients of extremely valuable information that can save lives. The good news is that with the right treatment, including healthy lifestyle changes, insulin resistance, prediabetes, and even the early stages of diabetes can often be reversed, powerfully reducing the risk for dangerous or even deadly complications, including a heart attack or stroke. Go to the next page to find out if you might be at risk—and what you should do right now to protect yourself.

The Hidden Cause of Most Heart Attacks

"Discover the root cause. Apply the proper remedy. That is the way of the wise."

—Sayings of Bhagavan Sri Sathya Sai Baba

Five years ago, Berend Friehe noticed a seemingly trivial symptom. Then 52, the farmer and pilot from Moses Lake, Washington, developed persistent tingling in his left hand and foot. "It was so slight that I almost ignored it, but finally decided to mention it to my family doctor during my next regular checkup."

The physician ordered a brain MRI, which revealed that Berend had experienced a transient ischemic attack (TIA), also known as a ministroke. "Hearing that the MRI found an injury to my brain scared the living daylights out me and I was disappointed in the way my family doctor handled it. I got the impression that he didn't have the time or knowledge to figure out how I could prevent a full-blown stroke in the future," recalls Berend. "He just said to take more Lipitor—two pills a day instead of the one I'd previously been taking for my high cholesterol."

Doubling up on a medication that hadn't prevented the ministroke didn't sound like good enough protection to the father of four children, then ages 16, 19, 22, and 25. Desperate to "fix" any problem that might have contributed to the event, Berend, who was a little overweight, with 215 pounds on his 6'1" frame, switched to a low-carb Atkins-type diet. "I was so scared and stressed that I had no appetite and rapidly lost 30 pounds."

Increasing the fear factor was his family history of dementia, a memory-robbing disorder often triggered by reduced blood flow to the brain because of a stroke or series of ministrokes. Without knowing why he'd had a TIA or how to prevent another more serious—or even fatal—brain attack, he became so anxious that he developed insomnia. Like Camille Zaleski, he was afraid to go sleep, not knowing if he'd wake up in the morning. "I was in a state of panic and kept thinking, ''Man, I'm doomed.''"

Can *You* Solve This Medical Mystery?

When we reviewed Berend's medical records during his first visit to our clinic, we spotted three clues that revealed one of the root causes of his ministroke: His triglycerides were high, his HDL was low, and he was taking medication for high blood pressure. Based on what you've read so far in this book, can you guess what diagnosis we made—before we'd done a single lab test? (Hint: You read about this dangerous cluster of heart attack and stroke risk factors in Chapter Four.)

If you guessed metabolic syndrome, congratulations! You've just made a diagnosis that many healthcare providers would have missed, despite the glaring red flags in Berend's medical records, because they don't check patients for this extremely common—and dangerous—disorder, which triples risk for a heart attack and quintuples it for type 2 diabetes. And if you also figured that by definition, Berend must also have insulin resistance, kudos on being a brilliant disease detective! You've just solved the medical mystery that had left this father of four so frightened that he couldn't sleep at night, believing himself to be "doomed."

Using the highly accurate two-hour oral glucose tolerance test (OGTT) discussed later in this chapter, we confirmed that Berend had insulin resistance (IR), the root cause of more than 70 percent of heart attacks, many strokes, and almost all cases of type 2 diabetes. IR delivers a devastating one-two punch to the cardiovascular system, because it's the leading cause of vascular blockages *and* of chronic inflammation, the "fire" in arteries that ignites cardiovascular events. What's more, IR speeds up the progression of arterial disease, research in both humans and animals shows. In a 2010 study of mice that were prone to atherosclerosis, those that were insulin resistant developed plaque deposits that were twice as big as those in animals without IR.

Discovering the root cause of Berend's disease opened the door to additional therapies. Like many people with IR, he had plaque buildup and high levels of inflammatory markers, the "fire" in the arteries that ignites heart attacks and strokes. That meant the medications he was taking weren't doing enough to protect him from another cardiovascular event. The good news, however, is that once insulin resistance is detected and correctly treated, it's usually curable—preventing both progression to type 2 diabetes and cardiovascular events such as TIAs (transient ischemic attacks), strokes, and heart attacks.

Berend was already on the right track by losing weight, since large studies show that even in people who are already prediabetic, losing as little as 5 to 7 percent of their body weight, plus exercising more, trims the risk of progressing to type 2 diabetes by up to 70 percent. We added several therapies described in Part Three of this book to Berend's treatment, including a diet-and-exercise plan tailored to his DNA, dietary supplements, and a diabetes drug that increases sensitivity to insulin. In just six months, his IR was successfully reversed.

The results have been amazing," says Berend. "I used to have hot arteries—the problem that kills people—and was headed for diabetes. Now my arteries are 'cold,' I no longer need a diabetes drug, and I can get on a treadmill and run like guys in their thirties or forties. I wish I'd found out about my insulin resistance *before* my arteries got so plugged up that I had a ministroke, but now that I'm making better choices about food and lifestyle—and my vascular disease is under control—I hope to have many years of quality life left."

Patients in Peril

It's very common for people to be diagnosed with diabetes right after they've suffered a cardiovascular event. Patients often chalk this double whammy up to bad luck, believing that they were inexplicably hit with two seemingly unrelated medical conditions at once. Others wonder if the heart attack somehow triggered their diabetes. We've even heard people say, "I went to the hospital with a heart attack (or a stroke) and caught diabetes while I was there."

Of course heart attack and stroke survivors don't "catch" diabetes at the hospital, since the disease isn't contagious. Nor does it strike suddenly. Insulin resistance is a continuum of increasing risk, often taking a decade or longer to generate a CV event or diabetes if it goes untreated. In a recent study of people treated in the emergency room for a heart attack, the researchers found that 20 percent of the patients were known diabetics. Of the remaining patients, blood tests revealed that 65 percent had abnormal blood-sugar levels, with about half of this group having previously undiagnosed diabetes, while the other half met criteria for prediabetes, an earlier stage of the disease.

The study findings—and the experiences of many of the patients you've met in this book—highlight a potentially deadly gap in our healthcare system: Medical providers aren't doing an adequate job of screening for insulin resistance, even though it affects about 150 million Americans, putting them at risk for two potentially fatal diseases—type 2 diabetes and coronary artery disease. Insulin resistance frequently goes undiagnosed *after* a heart attack or stroke, leaving survivors at high risk for recurrent events. As you learned earlier in this book, *one in three heart attacks and one in four strokes is a repeat event.* One major contributing factor for the alarming rate of recidivism of cardiovascular events is the failure to diagnose insulin resistance.

Very often, these life-threatening events could easily have been prevented if more healthcare providers followed "the way of the wise" advised by spiritual leader Bhagavan Sri Sathya Sai Baba: discovering the root cause of arterial disease and applying the proper remedy. Yet in our practice, we frequently see patients who feel just as "doomed" as Berend and Dead Man Walking did, simply because the highly treatable condition that was causing their vascular disease had been overlooked. Instead, they were left to live in terror of their next event.

Why does this happen when insulin resistance can easily be diagnosed with a simple blood test covered by almost all health plans? Our patients' stories illustrate the most common scenarios:

1. Not being informed about abnormal blood-sugar test results.
    Prior to our initial evaluation of new patients who consult us at the Heart Attack & Stroke Prevention Center, we comb through their previous medical

records for clues that they might have arterial disease or be at high risk for developing it. Frequently, we find lab reports indicating that a patient had abnormal results on one or more blood-sugar tests, but when we ask the person, "How long have you been prediabetic?" the response is often bewilderment, followed by anger because the patient's healthcare provider has never told him or her that anything was wrong.

One such patient was Joe Inderman, whom you met in Chapter Four. Although he had consulted several specialists—and underwent quadruple bypass surgery—none of his doctors picked up the root cause of his disease, even though it was clearly indicated in his medical records. Instead of being treated for the prediabetes that had been detected a few years earlier, he was told that his only hope for survival was getting a heart transplant, because according to the specialists he'd consulted—including two cardiologists—he'd exhausted all other treatment options.

We share our patients' anger that they were left in the dark about a highly treatable disorder that is known to silently damage blood vessels. A groundbreaking 1999 study published in the excellent medical journal *Lancet* was the first to report that this harm starts at the onset of insulin resistance— and continues to progress as long as this prediabetic disorder remains untreated. As soon as someone becomes resistant to his or her insulin, a cascade of dangerous events begins at the cellular level, affecting all of the body's arteries.

Because IR is fundamentally an inflammatory disorder, it injures the arterial lining, making it easier for white blood cells and cholesterol to pierce the "tennis court" and form plaque. Cholesterol issues are also much more complex in people with IR, who tend to have high triglycerides (TG) and low HDL levels. As you'll learn later in this chapter, your TG/HDL can actually be used to determine if you have insulin resistance or not. These cholesterol problems are not usually adequately treated with statin medications, which lower LD, while having little or no effect on HDL and TG.

Once disease develops, other biochemical changes further weaken the blood vessel lining, boosting the risk that the "cat in the gutter" will leap out and cause a heart attack or stroke. Multiplying the cardiovascular danger, people with IR also have blood that's more prone to form clots. That means that if a plaque rupture occurs, the resulting blood clot will typically be bigger and therefore more likely to trigger a more massive heart attack or stroke.

Despite the abundance of evidence of IR's extremely damaging effects on blood vessels, even today medical dictionaries typically ignore this devastating complication, perhaps explaining why some healthcare providers apparently don't consider prediabetes a huge threat to cardiovascular health or are too lazy to notify patients that they have it. Instead, IR is typically described solely as the problem that heralds the beginning of the long, silent march to type 2 diabetes, the form that affects 90 percent of diabetics.

Unlike type 1, an autoimmune disorder in which insulin production irrevocably halts because of antibodies that attack and destroy the insulin-producing beta cells in the pancreas, people with type 2 do produce insulin, but their body doesn't use it properly. Normally, this hormone helps cells in the body use glucose for energy. When people develop insulin resistance, their muscles, fat, and liver cells become insensitive to insulin, forcing the pancreas to crank out higher and higher amounts, trying to keep up with demand. Often people with IR have high levels of both insulin and glucose circulating in their bloodstream.

Think of this situation as a factory in which the workers are forced to toil longer and longer hours on the assembly line to meet ever-higher production quotas. Eventually, the workers grow so fatigued that they can no longer do their jobs and either collapse or go on strike, causing the assembly line to grind to a halt. Similarly, as insulin resistance worsens, the beta cells in the pancreas become exhausted and glucose (blood sugar) levels start to rise.

By the time someone with untreated insulin resistance crosses the line into type 2 diabetes, arterial damage and accelerated vascular aging have typically been occurring for at least 10 years—and in some cases for 20 or more years—explaining why diabetics are up to four times more likely to have heart attacks or strokes than nondiabetics. If you're middle-aged and have diabetes, some studies suggest that your risk for a heart attack or stroke is as high as that of a nondiabetic who has already had one.

In addition, heart attacks and strokes are more likely to be fatal in diabetics, and typically occur at a younger age. That's why early detection and treatment of IR is the best diabetes and CVD prevention strategy; it can also save your life! *As we've emphasized earlier in the book, whenever you get a medical test—including having your blood sugar measured—it's crucial to ask for your lab results and check them yourself.*

All too often, patients assume that no news is good news, when it may mean that your healthcare provider hasn't read the lab report or hasn't disclosed an abnormal result to you. Unfortunately, today's increasingly hectic healthcare environment, in which providers may be seeing several patients per hour, only increases the risk of such dangerous mistakes, even by doctors and nurse practitioners who are caring and well-intentioned. And if you don't understand your lab results, it's an excellent idea to schedule an appointment with your provider to go over the findings and treatment options.

2. Not being screened for high blood sugar at all.

Prior to her heart attack, Juli Townsend had never had her blood sugar measured. Don't blame her primary care provider, however, because she didn't have one. "I didn't go to doctors," says Juli, who thought it was safe to forgo physicals, because she considered herself to be in perfect health. In addition, Juli didn't want to incur the out-of-pocket cost of a medical visit and lab tests under her high-deductible health plan, believing the expense was unnecessary. After all, she looked and felt fine.

Besides, she was so busy juggling a full-time job and caring for her three-year-old daughter that she felt she didn't have time to get preventative care.

Yet the mom did take her daughter to the pediatrician for well-child care, recognizing that regular checkups are important to help kids stay healthy. It's very common for moms, who have been called the "chief medical officers" of their families, to put taking care of their own health last on their to-do list, while making sure that the rest of the family gets preventative care.

Tragically, many patients only seek help after they've had a heart attack or stroke—or develop obvious symptoms of type 2 diabetes, such as unusual thirst, frequent urination, blurred vision, numbness and tingling in the hands and feet, or recurring skin, gum, or bladder infections, warning signs that typically occur relatively late in the disease. Patients' not seeking screening is one reason that one-third of America's 26 million diabetics, and 87 million people with prediabetes, are currently undiagnosed.

While Juli didn't think she had any symptoms of disease, in reality there was a sign that she was at risk: even though her weight was normal, she had a large waist, the leading indicator of IR. As discussed earlier in the book, the size of your waist is a much stronger predictor of cardiovascular risk—and insulin resistance—than your overall weight or BMI. Had Juli known this, or had she consulted an alert healthcare provider who would take 30 seconds to measure her waist and followed with an OGTT, she would have discovered that she wasn't as healthy as she thought.

It's also important to recognize that both arterial disease and insulin resistance are silent, progressive diseases that may not cause *any* outward signs or symptoms until they become severe enough to trigger life-threatening events, such as the two heart attacks Juli suffered in a single week. That's why the only way to prevent these catastrophes is through early detection and treatment.

3. Not being adequately screened for insulin resistance, even after a cardiovascular event.

It should have been obvious that Camille Zaleski was at high risk for developing type 2 diabetes, since she had the classic risk factors found in medical textbooks. Ninety percent of people who develop this disease are overweight or obese, with a sedentary lifestyle. At the time of her heart attack, Camille was carrying 245 pounds on her 5'4" inch frame and rarely had time to exercise. She also had a family history of both diabetes and CVD, further magnifying the threat of high blood sugar.

Yet none of her healthcare providers had measured her blood sugar with the OGTT, even after her massive heart attack. Had they checked for a fatigued pancreas by challenging it with a load of sugar and then seeing what the sugar level was one or two hours later, they would have discovered that she was prediabetic. Instead, like Henry Nugent (aka "Dead Man Walking"), she was only checked with a far less sensitive test called the fasting plasma glucose (FPG) blood test, which is often used as part of the "metabolic panel" of blood tests typically performed during annual physicals or after patients have suffered cardiovascular events.

While the FPG test can usually identify people who are already diabetic, it's notoriously inaccurate at detecting insulin resistance, making this test a poor diagnostic tool for finding the condition. Here's why: In this test, blood is drawn after an overnight fast. A fasting blood sugar level of less than 100 mg/dL is considered normal, while 100 to 125 dg/dL is classified as prediabetes, and a level of 126 dg/dL or higher means you have diabetes.

If you're insulin resistant, however, your pancreas is working overtime to crank out increased amounts to overcome the resistance. As a result, when you haven't eaten for 10 or 12 hours, the higher level of insulin in your bloodstream—combined with lack of calories—will often result in a seemingly "normal" fasting sugar level. Because the pancreas isn't being challenged to put out extra insulin, as it is when you've ingested food, fasting blood sugar will frequently appear fine until you actually becomes diabetic, studies show.

Because Camille wasn't checked with the most sensitive test for IR, her doctors failed to discover that because she'd had untreated insulin resistance for so many years, she was prediabetic. Because the root cause of her heart attack was missed, she was sent home from the hospital with instructions to get ready for her next heart attack by remembering her symptoms and calling 911 if they occurred. No wonder she was so terrified that she couldn't sleep at night, fearing that she might not wake up in the morning!

Similarly, Dead Man Walking and Berend were understandably shocked when we diagnosed them with IR, based on their OGTT results, because they'd been told that their blood sugar was "normal" when it was evaluated with an unreliable three-month average test (hemoglobin A1c) or was simply measured in a fasting state (FBG). Henry was checked with the FPG, while Berend was checked the A1C test discussed in the next section.

Henry was extremely angry that he'd been handed a death sentence after a quadruple bypass operation, followed by stent placement in the same arteries six months later, had failed to halt his highly aggressive CVD. A panel of specialists convened by the hospital where he was being treated had reviewed all of his medical records—including his "normal" FPG results, before telling him that there was nothing further that could be done to save his life.

He'd told every doctor he'd ever consulted that his father who had died from CVD was a type 2 diabetic, intuitively suspecting that there was a link between his father's health problems and his own extremely aggressive CVD. Yet the root cause of his disease was still overlooked, simply because his doctors had used a normal fasting blood-sugar level as all the evidence needed to rule out IR.

4. Faulty medical guidelines for IR/prediabetes screening.

Henry, Camille, and Berend's physicians were *not* incompetent. They were simply following medical guidelines that consider all three blood tests—OGTT, FPG, and A1C—acceptable ways to screen people who are at risk for diabetes or prediabetes. Like most patients—and apparently many healthcare providers—Berend didn't know the A1C frequently yields misleading results, for diagnosing insulin resistance/prediabetes. This misconception for A1c probably stems from the American Diabetic Association's (ADA) advice to use A1c alone to diagnose prediabetes.

Unlike the FPG and OGTT tests, the A1C blood test doesn't require fasting before blood is drawn. Instead of measuring the patient's blood sugar level on the day of the test, it checks the average blood-sugar level for the previous three months, by measuring what percent of hemoglobin (a protein in red blood cells that carries oxygen) is coated with sugar.

But here's the problem: The A1C is has a 15 percent margin of error, and several studies have concluded that until the results reach a value of 6.5 percent (defined as the start of the diabetic range by the ADA), the test is *not* a reliable indicator of problematic blood sugar. Yet the ADA has recommended the use of AIC test to diagnose people "at risk for diabetes" (those with insulin resistance/prediabetes) when the value reaches a range of 5.7 to 6.4 percent.

In a study we presented in 2011 at the 4th International Congress on Prediabetes and Metabolic Syndrome in Spain, we found that of 527 patients who were checked with various blood-sugar tests, using the above A1C criteria alone would have missed 63 percent of those with IR/prediabetes.In addition, 27 percent of the patients that the A1C test classified as prediabetic actually had normal blood sugar when checked with the more accurate OGTT test.

A recent study published in *New England Journal of Medicine* also found that the ADA's "at risk" values for the AIC test were actually a poor predictor of future diabetes. The researchers measured the A1C levels of more than 11,000 healthy people, and then tracked them for an average of 14 years. Only those with A1C levels of 6.5 percent or greater were significantly more likely to be diagnosed with new onset diabetes during that time span. The A1C's alarmingly high error rate and poor predictive power are why we recommend against this using this test, or the FPG to make a diagnosis of IR/prediabetes.

This disorder is so dangerous that medicine needs to operate just the opposite of our judicial system. People with known CVD must be considered guilty of IR until proven innocent by the OGTT. A normal A1C and or fasting blood sugar do not prove innocence!

In the next section of this chapter, you'll find a detailed list of warning signs that you might have IR or be at risk for developing it. If you have any of them, ask your healthcare provider to measure your fasting blood sugar and if it is normal, to measure it one and two hours after having you drink a specified amount of sugar (the oral glucose tolerance test—OGTT).

If the results are normal, then we recommend having the test repeated every three to five years, or sooner if advised by your doctor or nurse practitioner. It's also crucial to be rechecked if you have major changes in your health, such as being diagnosed with cardiovascular disease, or your blood sugar was previously measured with the often-faulty FPG or A1c tests discussed above.

Watch Out for These Warning Signs!

Since insulin resistance doesn't cause any noticeable symptoms, many people aren't diagnosed until they develop diabetes. There are several tip-offs, however, that you may have IR or be at risk for developing it. One important clue is your lipid levels, which can be another way to diagnose IR. Surprisingly, people with IR usually don't have high levels of bad cholesterol, which is why statins usually aren't helpful. Instead, the numbers to look at are your triglycerides and HDL levels, since studies show that TG/HDL ratio can actually be used to *diagnose* insulin resistance.

The numbers that can signal the IR condition, however, vary by ethnicity, The IR diagnostic cut points for the TG/HDL ratio are: > 3.5 in Caucasians, > 3.0 in Hispanics, and > 2.0 in African Americans. (Cut points for other ethnicities have not yet been established.) To calculate your ratio, simply divide your triglycerides level by your HDL level. For example, if your triglycerides are 200 and your HDL is 50, your ratio is 4 (too high). It's also important to realize that even if your TG/HDL ratio is normal, you could still have insulin resistance. In other words, the ratio is only significant if it's abnormal.

Another way to diagnose insulin resistance is to find out if you have metabolic syndrome, the "three-strikes-and-you're out cluster" of abnormalities we described in Chapter Four: a large waist, high blood pressure, elevated blood sugar, low HDL cholesterol, and high triglycerides. If you have any three (or more) of these factors, you have metabolic syndrome—also known as "insulin resistance syndrome" because almost everyone who has it is insulin resistant. If you have these factors—or any of the other warning signs of insulin resistance discussed in this section—it's essential to work with your healthcare provider to achieve optimal control of all of these issues to reduce your cardiovascular risk. In Chapter Eleven, you'll find detailed guidance on setting optimal treatment goals.

You'll know if your healthcare provider is attuned to the dangerous cluster of heart attack and stroke risk factors that comprise metabolic syndrome if he or she measures your waist. Incredibly, even though waist circumference has been considered a "vital sign"—on par with blood pressure and pulse—for years, many providers still don't check this simple measurement, which would have revealed that all of the patients discussed in this chapter had the number-one warning sign of IR: a waist measurement greater than 40 inches for a man and 35 inches for a woman.

Optimal vs. Standard of Care

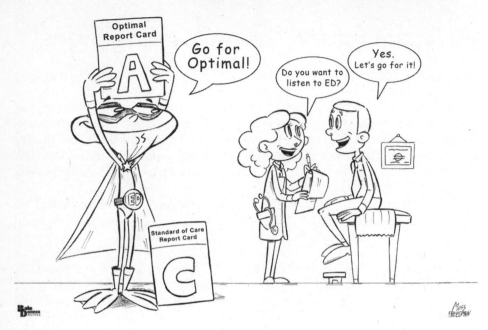

Other indications that you may be insulin resistant include:

- Having a heart attack or stroke. About 7 out 10 people who suffer these events will harbor IR—and as you learned in this chapter, many of them go undiagnosed. Therefore, we recommend that anyone who has suffered a cardiovascular event—including a heart attack, stroke, ministroke (also called a transient ischemic attack or TIA), bypass operation, or other procedures to treated blockages, such as stent placement or a balloon angioplasty without stenting—be considered "guilty" of insulin resistance, unless proven innocent by the two-hour oral glucose tolerance test described in the next section of this chapter.

- High blood pressure. One of the ways that IR harms vascular health is by robbing the blood vessel lining of its most important nutrient: nitric oxide (NO), a gas that acts as a chemical messenger within and between cells. (Nitric oxide shouldn't be confused with a similarly named compound: nitrous oxide, the anesthetic known as "laughing gas.") Nitric oxide causes blood vessels to relax and widen, increasing blood flow, while the low levels of NO associated with insulin resistance cause arteries to become narrower, a key reason that people with insulin resistance are more likely to develop high blood pressure.

- Your lipid levels, Surprisingly, people with IR usually don't have high levels of bad cholesterol (LDL-C). As mentioned earlier they tend to have high TG and low HDL levels. IR also usually causes a preponderance of small, dense LDL particles (the cholesterol "bullets" that are most likely to penetrate the endothelium and form plaque), even if your overall LDL level is normal. The whole gang of lipid villains (apoB) may be elevated in people with IR subjects. The "advanced" cholesterol tests described in the previous chapter can shed additional light on the potential for underlying IR.

- A history of gestational diabetes (high blood sugar during pregnancy) or pre-eclampsia (high blood pressure, swelling, sudden weight gain, and protein in the urine during pregnancy).

- Polycystic ovary syndrome (PCOS), a common hormonal disorder in women of reproductive age that causes the ovaries to become enlarged, with many small cysts. Brothers of women with PCOS are also at increase risk for insulin resistance. PCOS typically causes such symptoms as infrequent or prolonged periods, excessive hair on the face and body because of elevated levels of male hormones, adult acne, and weight gain.

- Erectile dysfunction. Because insulin resistance lowers production of nitric oxide (the gas that helps blood vessels expand), one consequence can be reduced blood flow to the penis, causing a man to be unable to achieve or sustain a sufficient erection for sex.

- Ananthosis nigricans, a skin condition marked by thick, dark, velvet-like patches in the armpits, neck, groin, or other body creases that's common in people with IR or diabetes, particularly those of Mexican American, African American, or East Indian ancestry.

- Periodontal disease. There seems to be a two-way link: Periodontal disease worsens insulin resistance, and having IR raises the threat of developing gum disease, too.

- Sleep deficiency. A recent study reported that people who sleep fewer than six hours a night are three times more likely to develop prediabetes, while a number of studies link skimping on slumber to significantly higher risk for both insulin resistance and diabetes.

- Your age. Because type 2 diabetes is more common in middle-aged and older people, the American Diabetes Association advises screening for everyone age 40 or older, or at a younger age, if advised by your healthcare provider because of such risk factors as obesity or family history.

- A family history of diabetes *or* cardiovascular disease. Not only is a family history of diabetes a powerful predictor of risk for insulin resistance, but having relatives who developed CVD, particularly at young age, can also be a warning sign, given that IR is the root cause of most heart attacks and ischemic strokes. Because this prediabetic condition often goes undiagnosed and untreated, sadly many people with IR perish from cardiovascular events before their blood sugar level reaches the diabetic level. Therefore, a family history of cardiovascular events indicates increased risk for insulin resistance, even if none of your relatives have been diagnosed with diabetes or IR.

- Abnormal A1C or fasting plasma glucose test results. Although these tests aren't very reliable because they may result in false alarms (mistakenly abnormal results in people who are actually healthy)—or more important, miss IR/prediabetes—an abnormal result on *any* blood-sugar test demands further investigation, using the more accurate two-hour oral glucose tolerance test described in the next section of this chapter. And if you don't know what your blood sugar results are, ask your healthcare provider for a copy of your lab report, which will indicate if the numbers are abnormal or not.

Insist on the Best Blood-Sugar Test

If you have any of the red flags or risk factors listed above, the best way to find out if you have insulin resistance, prediabetes, or diabetes, is with the two-hour oral glucose tolerance test, in which you challenge your pancreas by drinking a sugary liquid containing 75 grams of glucose after an overnight fast. Blood samples measuring glucose are drawn at one and two hours after consumption of the drink containing sugar. It is important to look at the fasting level prior to drinking the liquid as some people will actually discover their level is already in the diabetic range. Obviously, those individuals should not proceed with the test.

When you are insulin resistant, the beta cells in the pancreas become fatigued over time. When sugar levels are generally low, such as in a fasting state, the pancreas even when 'fatigued' can still produce enough insulin to keep the blood level "normal." When there is a sudden surge in the blood sugar after drinking a sugary beverage, however, these fatigued cells cannot crank out enough insulin to keep the sugar levels down one or two hours later. Therefore, insulin resistance that may not show up when you're in a fasting state (as in the FPG test) is revealed when the pancreas is challenged by processing the glucose drink used in the OGTT.

Historically, the ADA has defined an OGTT two-hour sugar level of less 140 mg/dL or lower as "normal," a level of 140 to 200 mg/dL as marking prediabetes, and a level above 200 mg/dL as diagnostic of diabetes. Recent research shows, however, that the danger zone for IR actually starts well before 140 mg/dL. In fact, Dr. Frank DeFronzo, a world expert in diabetes has published excellent data in peer-reviewed journals indicating that once the two-hour sugar reaches 120mg/dL or higher, at least 60 percent of the beta cells are fatigued. Once 90 percent are fatigued (also known as beta cell function loss), you are diabetic.

Dr. Defranco has also shown that once the one-hour sugar levels are greater than 125 mg/dL the person should be considered prediabetic. If the one-hour goes above 150mg/dL, that person is 13 times more likely than the average person to progress to diabetes in the next seven to eight years. Anyone who is prediabetic should be considered insulin resistant. If you have IR/prediabetes, the OGTT also provides an objective measurement to follow in tracking your response to treatment. The test can be repeated in a year to see if you have moved toward or away from diabetes. In other words, have you lost more beta cell function or gotten some of it back?

Some people are reluctant to spend about three hours in a lab to get this test. Consider this: In the same amount of time that you'd spend at the movies—probably swigging soda or another sweet drink—you can learn if you have a potentially life-threatening disease that may still be curable. A common misconception, even among some healthcare providers, is that once diabetes starts, the disease is irreversible because the beta cells have died. If the disease is caught and treated soon enough, however, it's sometimes possible to "cure" type 2 diabetes.

In our practice, we've seen a number of cases in which type 2 diabetics who were diagnosed and treated early (usually within one to two years of the onset of their disease) recovered enough beta cell function to ultimately achieve normal blood-sugar levels without medication. For some people diagnosed even in the initial stages, however, type 2 can't always be cured and, after a few years, it's almost always irreversible.

However, early detection and treatment of insulin resistance—prior to type 2 diabetes—always provides an opportunity to avoid the many hazards of diabetes, which include lower limb amputations, blindness, nerve damage, and high risk for cardiovascular disease, which strikes two out of three diabetics during their lifetime. Getting the OGTT is a crucial part of your heart attack and stroke prevention plan. Finding out you're insulin resistant alerts your healthcare provider to the need for additional therapies, such as those that helped Berend escape the "doom" he feared, allowing him to look forward to a long and healthy future.

The Number-One Habit That's Jeopardizing Your Health

If you're perched in a chair—or sprawled on the couch—as you read this chapter, you may have a disease that's rapidly becoming one of the most common—and dangerous—health threats to Americans, according to several recent studies. An estimated 50 million adults in the United States suffer from "sitting disease," a new medical label for an epidemic of deadly disorders linked to an overly sedentary lifestyle, from obesity to diabetes, coronary artery disease, some forms of cancer, and early death.

Some experts are calling sitting "the new smoking," because of the health toll our increasingly inactive lifestyles are taking on our health. Incredibly, surveys show that average adults now spend 90 percent of their leisure hours parked on a chair—usually after long hours at a desk during the workday. In fact, all this rump-resting and its associated maladies has even spawned a new field of scientific research called "inactivity physiology," devoted to studies of all the ways that too much sitting is making us sick.

What can you do to protect yourself? Simply standing up more could lengthen your life, according to a study of more than 222,000 adults aged 45 or older. The researchers found that people who sat for 11 or more hours a day had a 40 percent higher risk of dying in the next three years—regardless of how much they exercised the rest of the time—compared to those who spent fewer than four hours sitting, even when such factors as weight, activity level, and overall health were taken into consideration.

Another recent study found that too much time watching TV can actually be fatal, with those who spent four or more hours a day in front of a screen (usually glued to the tube, but also playing video games or surfing the Web) had double the risk for a major cardiovascular event causing hospitalization, death, or both—further evidence that unplugging the TV is one of the easiest and healthiest ways to avoid insulin resistance, which is strongly linked to both obesity and sedentary habits.

The more often you get up and move, the greater the benefits to both your cardiovascular system and your waistline. Researchers recently reported that even among people who spent much of the day sitting, those who took the most activity breaks—even ones as brief as one minute at a time—had, on average, thinner waists (by nearly two inches), lower levels of the inflammatory marker C-reactive protein, triglycerides, and blood sugar than those who rose from their chair least often.

In other words, even short breaks from sitting help combat several of the adverse effects of insulin resistance. Working out for 30 minutes a day at least five days a week has an even more powerful effect: It's been proved to prevent prediabetes from progressing to diabetes 60 percent of the time and has similarly dramatic benefits for preventing metabolic syndrome.

One excellent way to motivate yourself to get your feet moving is to clip on a pedometer. People who do so take up to 2,500 additional steps doing the day, according to a review of earlier research by researchers at Stanford University of School of Medicine. They analyzed 26 studies involving nearly 3,000 people, most of whom were overweight and inactive at the start of the study.

One takeaway from the new research is that simply going to the gym regularly may not be enough to counteract the effects of spending the rest of your waking hours slumped in a chair. Therefore, to trim your risk for both insulin resistance and metabolic syndrome, it's essential to rise up against sitting disease, by making simple changes throughout the day, such as by doing things the hard way. For example, an intriguing study by scientists at the Mayo Clinic found that "non-exercise activity thermogenesis" (NEAT) can often explain the difference between which people are overweight and which ones are slim.

Thinner people torch more calories thorough the day through such habits as standing and pacing during phone calls, parking at the far end of the lot when they go to stores or work, taking the stairs instead of the elevator, and even fidgeting while they're seated. On average, people with higher levels of NEAT activities burned about 100 more calories than those with the lower amounts, even when their levels of conventional exercise were about the same, the researchers reported.

Watch Out for This New Dental Danger

As this book goes to press, we have breaking news to report about another hidden cause of heart attacks. A recent study published by Dr. Tanja Pessi and colleagues in the American Heart Association journal *Circulation* demonstrates that endodontic disease (tooth decay) is also a significant player in driving heart attack risk.

In the study, 101 people who were in the throes of a heart attack were evaluated. The research team removed the culprit blood clots (those that were causing the heart attack) and used DNA analysis to look for oral pathogens. They also collected arterial blood samples from each patient to do the same analysis. The researchers discovered that the concentration of oral germs was 16 times greater in the clot than in the arterial blood, indicating that the pathogens came from the underlying plaque deposit that had ruptured through the artery wall. The DNA analysis also showed that 75 percent of the clots had oral pathogens that cause dental cavities and 35 percent of the clots contained bacteria that causes periodontal disease.

Another startling discovery: the team performed oral panoramic X-ray imaging on 30 of the patients and discovered that 50 percent of them had infected teeth. These patients were 13 times more likely to have DNA of pathogens that cause dental cavities in the culprit blood clot responsible for their heart attack. The researchers then examined nine of the clots with an electron microscope and found fragments of oral bacteria in 100 percent of the clots and in three of the clots, the germs were still whole.

These findings suggest that 50 percent of heart attacks may be triggered by an infection in the mouth. This study seems to match our clinical observations. More than a decade ago, we were shocked when a patient we were managing suffered a heart attack. He was treated with a stent and while still in the hospital, mentioned that one of his teeth had been bothering him for about a month. When he was examined by a dentist, the infection turned out to be so severe that the tooth was extracted at the hospital.

It's also possible to have a severe dental infection without any obvious symptoms. After Pessi's study was published, a 61-year-old man consulted us a few months after suffering a heart attack. To his knowledge, he had no dental infections and he had no discomfort, bleeding gums, loose teeth, or obvious periodontal problems. Because of Pessi's study, we referred him to a dentist with expertise in oral medicine. The dentist called to tell us that not only did the patient have gum disease, but he also had three severely abscessed teeth that needed immediate extraction. One dental abscess was so large that it had actually spread to his sinus cavity. After the horribly infected teeth were removed and the gum disease treatment, the inflammation in the patient's arteries was extinguished.

Right after this case, we saw a 54-year-old gentlemen after he had suffered a heart attack requiring a triple coronary bypass surgery, followed by another event requiring a stent seven weeks later. He made an appointment to be evaluated with the Bale/Doneen Method, but told us that it would be more than a month before he could fly in for his appointment. Again, in light of this study by Dr. Pessi, we immediately referred him to a dentist, who report that the man has gum disease. When we asked about dental cavities, the dentist replied that he actually hadn't checked for that because the patient had no complaints and he didn't see any signs of cavities.

We told the dentist about Dr. Pessi's study and recommended that he ask the patient to return for sophisticated imaging looking for infected teeth. The dentist called back in a few days, asking us if we possessed a crystal ball. He did find a severe abscess in the lower left second molar. The tooth was so diseased that the patient was immediately referred to an oral surgeon for extraction. Lab tests done prior to the dental care demonstrated significant arterial inflammation. The same tests repeated a few weeks after his oral care showed the "fire" was out.

From Dr. Pessi's study—and our own experiences—it appears the oral systemic connection is actually even more important than we realized. We now believe that any patient who suffers a heart attack deserves an immediate referral to an oral medicine specialist: a dentist who can evaluate the person with the DNA testing for periodontal disease discussed in Chapter Ten and cone beam 3-D radiography to check for asymptomatic infected teeth. Our goal is that medicine and dentistry join hands to optimize the health and wellness of the arterial system. Optimal dental care is crucial to save lives and prevent heart attacks and ischemic stroke.

Although good oral health is critical in maintaining arterial wellness, you may be surprised to discover in the next chapter that some supposedly healthy lifestyle habits that are often recommended to lower cardiovascular risk—including moderate alcohol consumption—can actually be dangerous for people with certain genotypes. Your DNA may also reveal that your true risk for heart attack and stroke is higher than you think, even if you *don't* have a family history of cardiovascular events, and influence your response to certain commonly prescribed therapies, including statins and even aspirin.

Action Step:
Personalize Your Prevention Plan

Millions of Americans unknowingly carry common genetic variations that can boost their cardiovascular risk. DNA, however, doesn't have to be destiny. Knowing what's in your genes can actually save your life by alerting you to potential risks and helping your healthcare provider choose the most effective personalized therapies to manage any threats lurking in your DNA.

These blood and saliva tests used to cost thousands of dollars. Now it's possible to have a comprehensive assessment for less than the price of a mammogram or colonoscopy, putting potentially lifesaving information within the reach of most Americans. And unlike most medical tests, genetic testing only needs to be done once, since your DNA doesn't change.

If you're a parent, you can also use this knowledge to protect yourself and your children from future cardiovascular risks, as Berend and his wife, Carla, did. Through tests performed at our clinic, the couple discovered that they both had genetic variations that have a powerful influence on how the body breaks down nutrients, making common foods that are healthy for most people the wrong choices for them—and for their four kids, then ages 16 to 25.

In addition, Carla, who consulted us about her high cholesterol, turned out to have inflamed plaque in her arteries. Finding out her genotype enabled her to get personalized treatment, including specific dietary changes tailored to her DNA, to prevent a heart attack or stroke. In the next chapter, you'll discover how your genetic information can guide you—and your family—to the most heart-protective lifestyle. You'll also learn smart, simple steps to safeguard your health, including a strategy that can help lengthen your life no matter what is written in your DNA.

10 Decoding Your DNA

"The rapid pace of advancement in genetic technology offers great promise in its potential to transform patient care."

—American Heart Association 2012 policy statement, "Genetics and Cardiovascular Disease"

Four years ago, Katharina Friehe seemed to have it all. Then 25, she had just landed her dream job, working for an international nonprofit that helps entrepreneurs in developing countries build thriving businesses. And after work, the beautiful blonde loved to party. Nearly every night she could be found at a bar, with a drink in one hand and a cigarette in the other, regaling her friends with tales of her travels to exotic countries.

"I went from a background in corporate public accounting where I'd stare at the cubicle walls and fantasize about a career that took me to faraway places, to actually being a business adventurer, having amazing, once-in-a-lifetime experiences in countries like South Africa," says the young CPA. "Frankly, life doesn't get more exciting than that."

During her travels, she received troubling news. Her father, Berend, had suddenly lost a lot of weight and seemed anxious about his health. "When I told my parents that I was coming home for a visit, they said there was something they wanted to tell me. I immediately started imagining worst-case scenarios: I was afraid that my dad had cancer," she recalls.

Instead, she was stunned—and frightened—to learn that both of her parents had a disease that kills nearly twice as many Americans as all forms of cancer combined: atherosclerosis. Then came another shocker: Katharina's parents were worried about *her* health. "They'd found out that they had a genetic factor that put them at higher risk for heart attacks and strokes, so they wanted me to be checked out in case I was at risk too."

When Katharina was evaluated at the Heart Attack & Stroke Prevention Center, she was horrified by her test results. "At 25, I had the arteries of a 55-year-old woman. It was incredibly shocking to find out that my arteries were older than my mom's age! And even though I don't have a weight issue, I was prediabetic," says the 5'9", 150-pound blonde. "Learning that I was on the verge of diabetes scared me the most, even more than a heart attack, since it was hard to believe that I could be at risk for one at my age."

Like both of her parents, she also carried a variant of the Apo E gene that not only boosts lifetime risk for cardiovascular events, but also affects how the body metabolizes alcohol and food. "I heard that I couldn't smoke, drink, or eat cheese—all the things I loved to do socially," adds Katharina. "At first, I was very angry about having that genotype and thought, 'This stinks! I'm a healthy, slim blonde girl and at my age, I should be enjoying life instead of worrying about old people's diseases.'"

These days, however, Katharina has a totally different perspective. "It took me a couple of years to say that I'm thankful I know my genetics," she says. "This knowledge is very powerful and I can use it to protect myself. Just knowing that I'm at risk reminds me to watch what I eat, even if I'm not consciously thinking [about] my genetics. And since I only smoked when I was out with friends, quitting wasn't such a big deal as I'd expected."

Katharina still goes to lots of parties, but has cut back on booze and bar snacks. "I can have a glass or two of wine on special occasions, as long as I don't define four nights a week as occasions," she says. "When I see my friends drinking, smoking, or pigging out on high-fat foods, I think, 'Do you have a genotype that might let you get away with that, or are you a walking time bomb because you have a genotype like mine—and don't know it?'"

A New Era in Preventive Medicine

More than 50 percent of Americans carry one or more gene variants (also known as polymorphisms) that dramatically increase risk for heart attacks and strokes. Until 2007, DNA tests to check for cardiovascular threats were extremely expensive and only offered in research studies. In November of that year, deCODEme Genetics launched the world's first direct-to-consumer genetic health scan, amid headlines hailing this technology as "the innovation of the year."

Our patient Jack Grayson was the first person who received the then-highly controversial test, which involved purchasing a test kit, swabbing his cheek to collect DNA, and sending the saliva sample to the company to be scanned for markers for various disorders and conditions, from CVD to diabetes, some forms of cancer, Alzheimer's disease, and even obesity.

"When deCODEme mapped my genotype, I found out that I had a 27 percent risk of dying from heart disease," says Jack, who was *not* frightened by his genetic results. Instead, his only regret is that this type of testing wasn't available decades earlier—*before* he developed a 100 percent blockage in a major coronary artery, along with such severe obstructions in two other arteries that he was deemed a candidate for an emergency triple-bypass operation.

"The sooner you find out about a potential problem, the easier it to prevent it," says the Texas businessman, who runs a private-sector nonprofit organization to help American business, healthcare, and educational enterprises improve productivity and remain globally competitive. "It's like manufacturing cars: instead of having to issue recalls to repair defects after they occur, you want to work on prevention at the front end, so the vehicles don't break down in the first place."

Like many of our other patients, Jack was excited about the potential to use genetic insights to protect his own health and that of his family. In fact, he ordered cheek-swab kits for his four sons, so that they could make smart lifestyle choices and receive preventative care for any health threats that were detected in their DNA. For example, one of his sons was identified as being at risk for celiac disease, an autoimmune disorder that makes the body unable to tolerate gluten. When his son switched to a gluten-free diet, a skin condition that had plagued the young man for years finally cleared up.

Jack credits another genetic discovery with actually saving his life. As discussed in an earlier chapter, a simple blood test that we ordered as part of his evaluation detected a previously undiagnosed, inherited cholesterol problem—elevated levels of lipoprotein (a)—as the root cause of his highly aggressive arterial disease. Treatment with an inexpensive vitamin and other simple steps allowed him to avoid potentially risky—and very costly—triple-bypass surgery. Through genetic knowledge coupled with a personalized prevention plan, the 90-year-old grandfather is now optimistic that he'll attain his goal of living to 113—or beyond.

Jack had to shell out thousands of dollars for the cheek-swab kits he purchased online from a company based in Iceland in 2007. Since then the price has plummeted, thanks to technological breakthroughs such as high-throughput next-generation gene sequencing. DeCODE Genetics remains involved in cutting-edge genetic research and offers its resources to consumer-focused genetic testing companies, but no longer offers direct-to-consumer testing itself. Several American genetic diagnostics labs have developed specific tests for four genes now known to be powerful predictors of lifetime cardiovascular risk: 9P21 (the "heart attack gene"), and variants of the apolipoprotein E (Apo E), KIF6, and interleukin-1 (IL-1) genes. These four blood or saliva tests, which we recommend for all of our patients, cost about $100 per gene for the 9P21, Apo E, and KIF6 tests, and $200 for the Il-1 test, putting this potentially lifesaving genetic knowledge within the reach of most Americans. Since genetics is among the fastest-growing fields of medicine, we anticipate that further scientific study will ultimately validate additional tests as clinically useful in medical practice.

If you have diabetes, you'll also want to know about another recently developed test, described later in this chapter, that checks for a variant of the haptoglobin gene that boosts heart attack danger in diabetics as much as smoking. This gene influences the amount of iron in your blood, which can harm heart health in several ways that we'll discuss in this chapter. If you have this genotype, however, the good news is that an inexpensive supplement sold over-the-counter in every drugstore can almost entirely eliminate the added cardiovascular menace that this variant would otherwise pose.

Surprisingly, the same supplement that can be potentially lifesaving for diabetics with this haptoglobin genotype appears to be hazardous for everyone else. In fact, studies suggest that this supplement *raises* risk for heart attacks and even early death in people *without* this polymorphism. That's a powerful example of one of the biggest benefits of DNA testing: *actionable* insights, backed by the latest science, which you and your medical provider can use to protect your health. You'll also learn how your genotype can influence your response to medications and even nutrients in your diet—and which easy actions to take if you have any of the potentially harmful genetic mutations described in this chapter.

Should You Get Genetic Testing?

Although much remains to be discovered about genes that elevate cardiovascular risk, the genetic knowledge we already have is starting to transform patient care—and "represents a great opportunity to improve human health," the American Heart Association (AHA) reports in a 2012 policy statement supporting use of genetic tests in medical practice. With the ever-accelerating pace of new discoveries about DNA and vascular disease, the AHA now recommends that *all* health professionals be trained in genetics and genomics.

Because genetic testing for lifetime cardiovascular risk is rapidly evolving, most patients—and many healthcare providers—aren't familiar with the tests that are now available or the explosion of scientific studies demonstrating their enormous potential to transform patient care. Here's a look at some common questions and concerns you may have about decoding your DNA.

- If I have the heart attack gene, do I really want to know?

   A widespread misconception is that genetic testing for heart attack risk is akin to opening the Pandora's box of Greek mythology that unleashed horrifying diseases and misery, without arming carriers of high-risk genes, such as 9P21, with any weapons to protect themselves. Recently, we read about a 40-year-old man, Jimmy Daniel, who was so worried that he might keel over with a heart attack while playing golf that he carried a portable defibrillator on his golf cart, so his caddie could try to jumpstart his heart should he go into sudden cardiac arrest on the links.

   One of Jimmy's motives for this extraordinary precaution was his terrifying family history: His father had died from a heart attack, while his mother has survived two heart attacks, one of which was treated with triple-bypass surgery. His sister has suffered two strokes, and nine other members of his extended family had heart disease.

   To Jimmy, this meant, "I was in the crosshairs. Nothing I can do about my DNA. I was a heart attack waiting to happen," he told *Golf Digest* magazine. Believing doom was written in his genes, he hoped to save the lives of others by combining his favorite sport with a mission: He embarked on an effort to set a new Guinness World Record for playing the most rounds of golf in one year, with his portable defibrillator at the ready, as part of a campaign to convince golf courses to have these devices available to treat victims of sudden cardiac arrest (SCA).

This condition, which kills up to 450,000 Americans a year, occurs when the heart's electrical rhythms suddenly become so chaotic that the heart can no longer pump blood. Without immediate medical treatment, such as a shock from a defibrillator, SCA is so lethal that 95 percent of its victims die before they reach the hospital.

It's understandable why Jimmy considered himself at risk. SCA almost exclusively strikes people with coronary artery disease, sometimes during or after a heart attack. The best defense, however, isn't having someone fire up a defibrillator after cardiac disaster occurs—it's protecting yourself with a personalized prevention plan, tailored to your DNA, to keep your heart healthy.

As you'll learn in this chapter, cardiovascular events are *not* inevitable, even for people with high-risk genes. While it's very common for people to assume, as Jimmy did, that there's nothing they can do about their DNA, in reality, genetic testing offers powerful, *actionable* insights to guide medical and lifestyle decision-making. By harnessing this knowledge to turn around their health, patients like David Bobbett and Camille have successfully overcome arterial disease, even though both of them are homozygous for the 9P21 gene (the riskiest genotype).

There's a growing recognition that every patient shouldn't be treated according to the average results of large studies. Instead, treatment needs to be personalized according to the patient's genetics to provide an optimal prevention plan. With easy lifestyle changes and optimal care, no one, regardless of family history or genotype, needs to feel like "a heart attack waiting to happen." If you know what risks are spelled out in your DNA, you can fight them with scientifically proven strategies tailored to your genes.

- If I have a dangerous gene, will my insurance rates go up?

  Surveys show that only 16 percent of Americans know that this type of genetic discrimination has been illegal since November 2010. Hailed as "the first major new civil rights bill of the twenty-first century," the Genetic Information Nondiscrimination Act (GINA) bars health plans from using genetic information—whether from your genetic test results or family history—for underwriting purposes (such as denying you coverage or hiking your premiums).

  In addition, under this law, employers aren't allowed to base hiring, firing, or promotion decisions on your genetic profile, or that of your family members. Not only does GINA guard against genetic bias in the workplace, but it also limits employers' and health plans' access to your genetic data. The law does have some loopholes, however, in that it contains no provision to prevent underwriters at life insurance, long-term care insurance, or disability insurance carriers from basing their decisions on your family history or genetic test results. Also, its provisions don't apply to companies with fewer than 15 employees.

  While these gaps in GINA urgently need to be fixed, research shows that contrary to what most people think, documented cases of genetic bias are actually extremely rare. In addition, there are no laws to prevent plans or employers from discriminating against people with other risks for developing arterial disease, such as high blood pressure. Yet to date, we've never encountered a patient with concerns about having his or her blood pressure checked.

In our opinion, while there is a slight risk that your genetic profile might be used against you by some insurers, the benefits of finding out if your genes predispose you to a heart attack or stroke—and taking action today to avoid these potentially fatal events—far outweigh the very remote possibility that you might face higher life or disability insurance premiums down the road.

And you might even have the opposite experience: One of our patients recently qualified for the *lowest* available rate for 10-year term life insurance, despite having both high blood pressure and genetic risks for CVD, because his insurance carrier was impressed by the comprehensive treatment and preventative care he was receiving at our clinic. In fact, his premiums were cut by nearly 50 percent!

- Is there any need for genetic testing if I have no family history of heart disease?

Research, as well as the experiences of our patients, shows that family history alone can be a poor predictor of heart attack or stroke risk for a variety of reasons. Because arterial disease typically develops silently, it often goes undetected for decades until it becomes severe enough to trigger a cardiovascular event. As a result, you may think you have no family history of CVD when, in reality, one or more of your relatives may have undiagnosed disease. It's also possible to carry genes that predispose you to a heart attack or stroke even if you have *no* affected relatives.

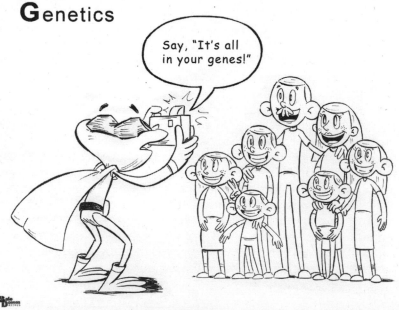

Genetics

Say, "It's all in your genes!"

Juli Townsend is a case in point. When she suffered two heart attacks at age 37, she was particularly shocked—and scared—because she had no known family history of coronary heart disease, nor did she have any of the traditional risk factors. A month after her heart attack, however, her seemingly healthy father suffered an ischemic stroke, indicating that he also had disease in his arteries, but didn't know it until the cat leapt out of the gutter, an all-too-common scenario, as we've emphasized in this book.

Along with having a parent with undiagnosed arterial disease, Juli also turned out to have the same inherited cholesterol problem that Jack did: elevated levels of lipoprotein (a). As you learned in Chapter Eight, this frequently undiagnosed disorder, which we call "the mass murderer," has not only been shown to *cause* heart attacks, but also triples the risk of having one, often at an early age.

Therefore, Juli's apparent lack of a family history of vascular disease was deceptive, since her genes actually did put her at high risk. Although a simple blood test could have identified the young, physically fit mom's true danger prior to her heart attack, she hadn't gotten a checkup for several years, mistakenly assuming that no health threats lurked in her family tree.

There are several other ways that family history can be misleading. For example, many people have faulty or incomplete information. A survey sponsored by the Centers for Disease Control and Prevention found that while almost everyone polled agreed that family history was important, fewer than one-third of respondents had ever inquired about their family members' health data. In the Framingham Heart Study, only 28 percent of participants correctly reported that they had a family history of early onset heart disease.

The AHA points out that to be accurate, family history relies on an unbroken chain of events: First, a relative with potentially harmful genes must develop CVD, which may not occur if that person practices an excellent lifestyle or dies from other causes. Next, the family member must be accurately diagnosed with arterial disease, which is frequently missed until it become so severe that it triggers a heart attack or stroke. Then, other family members must correctly recall the relative's diagnosis and communicate it to their healthcare provider.

This chain of events happens so infrequently that a recent study found that out of six common conditions that run in families, CVD was the disorder that patients are *least likely* to report to their doctor. Some patients are unaware of inherited cardiovascular threats because they're adopted, come from small families, or don't keep in touch with their relatives, so may not learn about cardiovascular events. All of these factors explain why people with no family history of CVD can benefit from opening the book on their DNA through testing.

The AHA reports that genetic tests can result in up to 70 percent of patients being reclassified as having higher risk for heart attacks than their risk factors, including family history, would suggest. By more accurately pinpointing which people are in danger, the AHA's expert committee concluded, genetic tests can improve clinical management of any threats that are identified, such as more-aggressive treatment of cholesterol issues in patients with genes that make them more susceptible to heart attacks.

- Can I order these tests on my own?

Unlike the saliva-swab test kits that Jack purchased from deCODEme (or other panels for an array of diseases and conditions offered by other companies, such as 23andme), the genetic tests we recommend in the next section of this chapter are *not* marketed directly to consumers. Instead, your healthcare provider must order the tests from a genetic diagnostics laboratory, such as Celera, which offers genotype tests for the KIF6, 9P21, and Apo E genes discussed in the next section of this chapter or ARUP Laboratories (an enterprise of the University of Utah), which has recently introduced the haptoglobin genotype test.

The Interleukin-1 gene test, which identifies people with a heightened inflammatory response that magnifies risk for cardiovascular disease *and* periodontal disease (which in turn, multiples heart attack and stroke risk) is available through dentists, who can order the test through a genetics diagnostics lab. Should any cardiovascular threats be discovered, it's crucial to discuss a personalized prevention plan to manage and mitigate these risks. If the IL-1 test identifies you as being at increased risk for arterial disease and periodontal disease, your dental and medical providers should work together to address these risks, using a team approach designed to optimize both your oral and arterial health with appropriate individualized medical and dental therapies.

Because many healthcare providers have not yet received the training in genetics and genomics that the AHA recommends, it's possible that your medical and dental providers are not familiar with these tests. If that's the case, the genetic diagnostic labs that market these tests provide extensive information for clinicians and patients on their websites, including scientific evidence from peer-reviewed medical journals. We suggest printing out the materials on each test and showing them to your medical or dental provider. Usually genetic testing is not covered by health plans unless you have a family history of cardiovascular disease. This trend is starting to change, however, with some insurance carriers now recognizing the value of genetic testing and supporting this type of health evaluation.

Wondering if you should get a health panel for other diseases and conditions? Although genetic tests from direct-to-consumer companies are not part of the Bale/Doneen Method, if our patients wish to get this testing on their own, we'll review the results with them. Our experience, however, is that patients often receive such an abundance of data on myriad diseases and conditions—some of which may not be actionable in terms of specific steps to protect their health—that the test results may end up being filed away, instead of guiding heart-smart treatment and lifestyle choices. It's also crucial to realize that although these tests include genetic data on heart disease risk, the direct-to-consumer health scans currently on the market don't check for all of the high-risk genes discussed below.

Do You Have the Heart Attack Gene?

Genetic testing is a rapidly evolving field, so we anticipate that additional tests will become available in the future, both directly to patients and through their healthcare providers for an even more comprehensive cardiovascular threat assessment. *Currently, we recommend that all patients get the 9P21, Apo E, KIF6, and IL-1 genotype tests described in this section. We only recommend having your haptoglobin genotype checked if you're diabetic, since there's no known link between this genotype and cardiovascular risk in nondiabetic patients.*

9P21 Genotype: Identifies Carriers of the Heart Attack Gene

This blood or saliva test checks for the 9P21 gene, often called "the heart attack gene," because it's an independent predictor of cardiovascular event risk even when such factors as family history, diabetes, high blood pressure, elevated levels of the inflammatory marker C-reactive protein, and obesity are taken into account. About 25 percent of Caucasians and Asians are *homozygous* for 9P21, meaning that they have inherited the gene from both their mother and father. Studies link this genetic profile to a:

- 102 percent rise in risk for suffering a heart attack or developing heart disease at an early age, compared to noncarriers of the gene.
- 56 percent overall increase in lifetime heart attack and heart disease risk.
- Much higher risk for severe coronary artery disease (CAD), affecting multiple arteries, both at a young age or over a lifetime.
- 74 percent jump in risk for aortic abdominal aneurysm, a weak, ballooning area in the heart's largest blood vessel that's often fatal if it ruptures.
- 400 percent increase in risk for CAD—and double the risk of death in the next 10 years—in people with poorly controlled diabetes, compared to diabetic noncarriers with poor glycemic control.

About 50 percent of Caucasians and Asians are *heterozygous* for 9P21. Since they only carry one copy of the gene (inherited from one parent), studies calculate that they have half the risk of each of the outcomes above. The frequency of this gene in African Americans and other populations has not yet been determined.

As we emphasize to our patients, DNA does not have to be destiny. About half of Americans carry at least one copy of the heart attack gene, yet by managing their risks with proved prevention strategies and optimizing their lifestyle, they can still avoid a heart attack. If you carry the 9P21 gene, we recommend the following eight steps. Steps two through eight are also the key to heart attack and stroke prevention even if you're not a carrier of the 9P21 gene.

1. At age 40, get an abdominal aortic aneurysm (AAA) scan. (This ultrasound test is described more fully in Chapter Six.) If the results are normal, have the test repeated every five years, while abnormal results will require more frequent follow-up, as advised by your healthcare provider, to see if the aneurysm is growing. Typically only large aneurysms require treatment to prevent rupture. Ruptured AAA kills about 30,000 Americans a year.

2. Avoid smoking. Not only is smoking the leading risk factor for heart attacks and strokes, but it also greatly increases the threat of developing an aneurysm. Other contributing factors include obesity, diabetes, high cholesterol, high blood pressure, and genes.

3. Exercise at least 22 minutes daily. A recent study found that this amount of exercise, which can even include a brisk walk, reduces cardiovascular risk by 14 percent, while working out 44 minutes daily lowers risk by 20 percent.

4. Keep your blood pressure under control. About one in three adults have high blood pressure, but many of them don't know it. This silent killer ranks as the leading risk factor for stroke and a major contributor to heart disease, heart failure, and kidney disease. In the next chapter, you'll find out how to set and achieve optimal goals for your blood pressure and other cardiovascular risks.

5. Maintain healthy cholesterol levels. Genetic factors, such as elevated levels of Lp(a), may make it necessary to set more-aggressive targets for lowering your LDL than are typically advised by standard care. As you learned in Chapter Eight, it's also important to pay attention to your total-cholesterol-to-HDL ratio—the best predictor of heart attack risk in the Women's Health Study—and your ratio of triglycerides (TG) to HDL. In the next chapter, you'll find a list of all of the optimal treatment targets we recommend, plus tips on how to achieve them.

6. Maintain optimal blood-sugar levels, following the advice in Chapter Nine and Part Three of this book.

7. Keep your weight down and eat a diet based on your DNA, as discussed in the material below on the Apo E genotype test.

Apo E Genotype: Predicts Heart Disease and the Best Diet to Avoid It

This blood or saliva test analyzes your Apolipoprotein E (Apo E) genotype, which influences lifetime risk for coronary heart disease and Alzheimer's disease, as well as how your body metabolizes nutrients in your diet, including fats and carbs, a topic we'll explore more fully in Chapter Twelve. As the Friehe family discovered, certain Apo E genotypes make common foods that are healthy for people with other Apo E genotypes potentially harmful.

The Apo E gene has three variants (E2, E3, and E4), resulting in six possible genotypes: Apo E 2/2, Apo E 2/3, Apo E 2/4, Apo E 3/3, Apo E 3/4, and Apo E 4/4. A few insights from research:

- The Apo E 2/2 and 2/3 genotypes, which occur in 11 percent of the population, are associated with the lowest risk for CVD. If you have one of these genotypes, your best bet for disease prevention is a moderate-fat diet containing about 35 percent fat from heart-healthy sources, such as omega-3 rich oily fish or olive oil.

- People with the Apo E 2/4 and 3/3 genotypes, which are found in 64 percent of the population, have intermediate cardiovascular disease risk and benefit from the conventional Mediterranean-style diet that's typically advised to protect heart health. This diet should contain about 25 percent fat.

- About 25 percent of people, including Berend, Carla, and Katharina Friehe, have the Apo E 3/4 or 4/4 genotypes, which are linked to the highest lifetime risk for CVD. This group can trim the threat by following a very low-fat diet (no more than 20 percent fat) and limiting or avoiding alcohol consumption. The Apo E gene also has an impact on exercise on the magnitude of the cholesterol surge that occurs after a meal. In a recent study in which people with various Apo E genotypes exercised then ate 500 calories of food 30 minutes later, those with the Apo E 2/3 genotype had the smallest rise in lipid levels. People with the Apo E 3/3 genotype also benefited from exercising before the meal, but to a lesser extent, while people with Apo E 3/4 didn't have any change in their cholesterol surge. (The study didn't include people with 2/4 or 4/4 genotypes.) Of course, exercise is extremely important for everyone, regardless of Apo E genotype, but this study shows that it has an additional benefit for those with the 2/3 and 3/3 genotypes.

- Berend, who has the 4/4 genotype, is right to be concerned about Alzheimer's disease (which affects his mom), since several studies have found increased risk for dementia in carriers of this Apo E genotype. The memory-robbing disorder also occurs in people with other genotypes, however, while many people with the 4/4 genotype never develop Alzheimer's disease (AD).

- Regardless of your Apo E genotype, regular exercise—for both your body and your brain—are extremely important to keep your wits sharp as you age. While there is no surefire way to prevent AD, which strikes one in eight adults over age 65, evidence is mounting that a diet that's high in antioxidant-rich colorful fruits and vegetables (such as blueberries, cherries, and beets), whole grains, and fish benefits the brain.

- Columbia University Medical Center also reported that elderly adults who exercise vigorously at least 1.3 hours a week were 33 percent less likely to develop AD, compared to couch potatoes of the same age. In that study, seniors who combined hiking, jogging, or biking with a Mediterranean-style diet whittled their AD risk by more than 60 percent during the 5.5-year study.

- Studies also show that the most mentally active people also have a lower rate of AD. One study of older nuns and priests found that those who devoted the most time to such activities as going to museums, doing crossword puzzles, reading the newspaper, and even listening to the radio had a 47 lower rate of AD. Other brain boosters include taking courses at a community college, learning a foreign language, playing bridge or video games, and surfing the Web.

- Get-togethers with friends and neighbors can have a surprising payoff, Harvard researchers found. In a study of people in their fifties and sixties, those who were the most socially connected had half the rate of memory impairment during the six-year study as those who were socially isolated. Good ways to stay socially engaged include volunteer work, travel, and joining a club or community group.

- Controlling cholesterol is especially important for people with the Apo E 4/4 genotype. Research shows that middle-aged adults with total cholesterol levels of 240 mg/dL or higher were 60 percent more likely to develop AD decades later, while people with readings of 200 to 239 had a 52 percent jump in risk.

KIF6 Genotype: Predicts Statin Response and Heart Attack Risk

This blood or saliva test checks for a variant of the KIF6 (Kinesin family member 6) gene. The KIF6 gene's job is to make a protein that transports other substances, such as protein complexes, within cells. Which version of the gene you carry influences both your risk for a heart attack and whether you'll get any benefit from the statins most likely to be prescribed for heart attack prevention.

Here's scary news: if you're on Lipitor (atoravastin)—the most commonly prescribed statin—or Pravachol (pravastatin)—as your sole therapy, there's a 40 percent chance that you're getting *no* cardiovascular protection at all, even if your cholesterol numbers look great. Three large randomized clinical trials found that these drugs *only* reduce the risk for heart attacks, strokes, and mortality from cardiovascular causes in the 60 percent of Americans who have the KIF6 variant.

These statins had no effect on rates of these events in the 40 percent of patients who didn't carry the variant.

Thirty million Americans take statins, which rank among the most-widely prescribed drugs in the world. If you have high cholesterol or coronary artery disease, you're probably on a statin. Since these cholesterol-lowering medications also combat the inflammation that drives heart attacks, almost all patients who have suffered cardiovascular events are put on a statin to help prevent recurrence. It's essential to find out your KIF6 status so you can get the most-effective treatment.

Because Lipitor and Pravachol are so commonly prescribed—usually without checking the patient's KIF6 status—we wonder if ineffective treatment explains why 33 percent of heart attacks and 25 percent of strokes occur in people who have already survived one or more of these events. To get the best protection from these events, it's essential to learn your KIF6 status so your healthcare provider can tailor your treatment to your DNA.

In addition, women should be aware that in a very large clinical trial, taking Lipitor actually *raised* women's heart attack risk by 10 percent while reducing risk by 42 percent in men. While the researchers concluded that the increased risk in women was not statistically significant, because the study included fewer women than men, the findings suggest that Lipitor may not be an effective treatment choice for women.

There's controversy about the effect of the KIF6 variant on lifetime CVD danger. In five large studies, untreated carriers of the variant were at up to 55 percent higher risk for heart attacks, strokes, or death from cardiovascular causes, compared to untreated participants without the variant. In two clinical trials, carrying the variant had a bigger impact on raising heart disease risk than being older than age 55, abnormal levels of LDL or HDL cholesterol, or high blood pressure. Only smoking and diabetes trumped the KIF6 mutation for boosting disease risk.

Interleukin 1 (IL-1) Genotype: Escalates the Body's Inflammatory Response

This cheek-swab saliva test checks for two genes, interleukin-1A (IL-1A) and interleukin-1B (IL-1B), that regulate the interleukin-1 family of cytokines: chemical messengers that are involved in immune system and inflammatory responses. These variants are linked to heightened response to inflammation, the immune system's defense against injuries and infections. Since these genes are among the first to be activated during the body's inflammatory response, they ignite a chain reaction in which other inflammatory chemicals are released at higher-than-normal levels to escalate and sustain the blaze. As a result, carriers of these genes have a more-intense acute response to any type of inflammation and are also more prone to chronic inflammation.

To visualize the effect of these genes, imagine two forests, one in an area with normal rainfall and the other in a region parched by drought. Think about what would happen if kids were wandering in the woods, playing with matches: In one forest, there might be a small blaze that soon ran out of fuel, while in the other, the result could be an inferno that raged out of control. Similarly, carriers of these genes have a more-intense acute response to any type of inflammation and are also more prone to chronic inflammation.

Since inflammation is known to trigger atherosclerosis, it's not surprising that carrying genes that intensify this fiery process boosts risk for developing earlier and more severe CVD. In fact, if you have these two IL-1 variants, your lifetime cardiovascular disease risk equals that of a smoker. In one study of people who underwent a test to diagnose the cause of chest pain, those with the Il-1 genotype were nearly four times more likely to have coronary artery disease (CAD) than noncarriers, while another study of patients with chest pain found that IL-1 carriers and smokers were at the highest risk for being diagnosed with clogged arteries, with double the danger of those who had high cholesterol.

The reason IL-1 variants are so strongly linked to severe CAD is that they pack a one-two punch. Not only are carriers far more predisposed to develop chronically inflamed blood vessel linings, making it easier for LDL to invade and form plaque, but people with this genotype are also nearly four times more likely to develop periodontal disease (PD). The good news, however, is that finding out if you're a carrier allows you to take charge of your cardiovascular health by taking the right steps to prevent chronic inflammation. We recommend following the firefighting tactics in Part Three of this book, which counteract several factors that contribute to inflammation, with science-backed strategies to quit smoking, manage stress, lose weight, improve sleep, and personalize your diet and exercise program.

Since studies show that IL-1 carriers have higher loads of dangerous bacteria in their mouth—and increased risk for gum disease—if you have this genotype, it's also crucial to see your dental provider every three months, for optimal oral care.

There is now a sophisticated diagnostic tool to detect gum disease: Two companies, OralDNA and Hain Diagnostics, offer salivary DNA tests that identify the concentration of bacteria in the mouth that are known to be associated with cardiovascular risk. These tests use high-tech DNA analysis, a more reliable technology than traditional culturing techniques. Studies are now demonstrating that it's the burden of these germs that drives CV risk, as opposed to simply making a clinical diagnosis of periodontal disease through a traditional dental exam. The advances in testing are improving diagnosis of PD.

Do You Need an Oral Disease Detective?

Wesley Robinson used to be one of our most baffling cases. At each follow-up visit, despite aggressive treatment with lifestyle changes and medications, the 6'1" Texan, whom we'd nicknamed Superman because of his brawny build and six-pack abs, *still* had the cardiovascular equivalent of kryptonite in his arteries: inflamed plaque. And no matter what we tried, his disease kept getting worse. It looked as if Wesley, 44, might be headed for the same fate as his father, who was disabled by a stroke at age 55, and then suffered a heart attack at 58—or his grandfather, who had died from a heart attack at 60.

At one point, as you read in Chapter Seven, we thought we'd solved the mystery. When we summoned Superman and his worried wife, Kelly, to our office to discuss his alarming lab results, he admitted that he'd quit taking one of the medications we'd prescribed (niacin) because of a minor side effect. After we pointed out that Wesley could live with a slight medication side effect, but might not survive a heart attack or stroke, Kelly fixed Superman with a gimlet gaze and announced, "He'll take the niacin."

Wesley did resume treatment—and achieved excellent cholesterol levels. At first, his inflamed arteries appeared to cool down, but then his inflammatory markers started to rise again, despite his compliance with niacin treatment. The continuing inflammation indicated that he was still on the fast track to a heart attack or stroke. Knowing that Superman had a family history of severe periodontal disease—in fact, his father had lost all of his teeth at age 35—we always suspected that PD might play a role in Wesley's disease.

When he was queried about this possibility, however, we were always reassured that his dental checkups were fine. In addition, at the time, we were not using the two tests discussed in this chapter: the IL-1 genotype test and MyPerioPath. When we later became of aware of the availability of these tests, we incorporated them into the Bale/Doneen Method. Because several of Wesley's inflammatory markers remained elevated, we recommended that he undergo these oral health evaluations.

Superman's wife, Kelly, a dentist, questioned the need for testing. "I was skeptical, because although there were a few areas in his mouth that could be better, there was nothing to make me think that he had active periodontal disease," says Kelly. "Overall, his gums looked healthy, so I was shocked when the MyPerioPath test came back positive for periodontal disease, showing that my husband had very high levels of three types of bacteria."

Superman also turned out to be a carrier of the IL-1 gene, explaining why he was so prone to both inflammation and oral infections. His MyPerioPath results included recommendations from the diagnostics lab about which antibiotics might be helpful, as well as his levels of 11 pathogens (disease-causing bacteria) that cause gum disease and boost risk for tooth loss. Kelly decided to try treating her husband with antibacterial mouthwashes, improved oral care, including twice-a-daily brushing and flossing, and thorough professional dental cleanings every three months.

"We were amazed at how quickly his inflammatory markers fell once the bacterial load in his mouth was under control," says Kelly, who was extremely relieved when a cIMT scan confirmed that her husband was no longer on the fast track to a heart attack or stroke. "I was very skeptical about this testing, since his mouth looked pretty healthy, but the results have made me a believer."

Should you get salivary DNA testing to check for dangerous oral bacteria? We recommend this screening test if you have persistently high inflammatory markers, a history of clinically diagnosed PD, or have suffered a cardiovascular event. If none of these factors apply, we recommend that you get regular dental care, according to the schedule advised by your dental provider. This should include screening for PD, which involves taking painless measurements of pocket depths with a periodontal probe. *If you have any pockets in your gums measuring 3 mm or greater, then you have periodontal disease and need the treatments discussed in Chapter Fourteen to protect both your oral and cardiovascular health.*

Haptoglobin Genotype: Predicts Cardiovascular Danger in Diabetics

Although this blood test, which checks for variants of the haptoglobin (Hg) gene, costs more (about $400) and is harder to get than the other genetic tests discussed in this chapter, it provides valuable information if you have diabetes. Not only can you find out if you have an Hp gene variant that raises the lifetime threat of CVD as much as smoking does, but also if you do have this high-risk genotype, research suggests that you can almost entirely eliminate this increased risk by taking an inexpensive over-the-counter supplement.

The Hg gene regulates haptoglobin, a protein produced by the liver that binds to hemoglobin, a substance produced when red blood cells die. If hemoglobin isn't bound quickly, it will release iron, which can harm arterial health in several ways. For example, the iron will oxidize LDL cholesterol, making LDL more harmful to your arteries. When Hg binds to hemoglobin, white blood cells can quickly clear this damaging substance from the bloodstream, neutralizing these threats. In diabetics, hemoglobin will also attach to HDL, negating many of its protective properties. It just so happens that a particular genetic variant of Hg known as 2-2 does not bind well with hemoglobin, but what does get bound to it sticks to HDL extremely well! Therefore, Hg 2-2 packs a dual punch of bad news!

Hp production is genetically controlled and varies by genotype. The Hg gene has two alleles, called Hg1 and Hg2. Since you inherit one allele from each parent, the three possible combinations are Hg 1-1 (low risk), Hg 2-1 (intermediate risk), and Hg 2-2 (high risk). If you have the 2-2 genotype, your lifetime risk for CVD is triple that of a diabetic with the 2-1 genotype, and five times higher than that of a diabetic with the 1-1 genotype. About 16 percent of people carry the Hg 1-1 genotype, 48 percent carry Hg 2-1, and 36 percent carry Hg 2-2.

Researchers have demonstrated, however, that type 2 diabetics with the Hg 2-2 genotype can counteract almost all the increased risk by taking 400 i.u. of the antioxidant vitamin E daily. While you may wonder if all diabetics should pop a daily vitamin E pill—and skip the gene test—studies show that unless you're a diabetic with this specific Hg gene variant, taking vitamin E not only has no cardiovascular benefits, but it can be downright dangerous for the heart. Since vitamin E usually *raises* risk for heart attacks and even early death, the *only* people who could benefit from taking it are diabetics with the Hg genotype.

This actionable insight is why we recommend that all type 2 diabetics get this genotype test. It doesn't just identify diabetics at greatly increased risk for CVD: the test results also reveal which patients might benefit from an inexpensive over-the-counter supplement that everyone else should avoid. Before taking any dietary supplement, however, discuss the potential risks and benefits with your health-care provider and whether this therapy would be an appropriate part of your overall treatment and prevention plan.

Action Step: Set Optimal Treatment Goals

Even if potential cardiovascular threats are spelled out in your DNA, setting—and achieving—optimal goals for both lifestyle and medical management of conditions that elevate heart attack and stroke risk provides powerful protection, as a 2012 study published in *New England Journal of Medicine* demonstrates. The researchers, who analyzed health records covering 50 years for more than 250,000 Caucasian and African American adults, found that 45-year-old men who avoid smoking and maintain optimal blood pressure, blood-sugar, and cholesterol levels, had only a 1.4 percent risk of having a heart attack or stroke during their lifetime, or of dying from cardiovascular causes—compared to a nearly 50 percent risk for men with two or more of these factors.

"Just even one small increase in risk, from all optimal risk factors to one that isn't optimal, such as slightly elevated cholesterol or blood pressure, significantly bumps up a person's lifetime risk," reported the study authors. They also found that for a 45-year-old nonsmoking woman with optimal blood pressure, cholesterol, and blood sugar, lifetime heart attack or stroke risk was 4 percent, compared to 31 percent in women with two or more of the factors the study looked at.

In the next chapter, you'll discover what your optimal treatment goals should be and why some of the targets set by practitioners of standard care may not be good enough to protect you from a heart attack or stroke. You'll also learn which dangerous disorder affects 87 million Americans—and remains out of control in most of them—even though most people with this condition consult a doctor at least twice a year *and* take medication that's supposed to solve their problem.

Part **Three**

Your Action

Plan

Setting Optimal Treatment Goals

"Don't bunt. Aim out of the ballpark."

—David Ogilvy

Although Darren Liens, 39, was almost obsessive about healthy eating, exercised strenuously every day, and had the ripped musculature of a NFL player, he used to think he was "leading a doomed existence." His belief that he was destined to die young, no matter what he did, stemmed from a harrowing tragedy that occurred when he was 22.

When Darren was growing up, he literally looked up to his tall, muscular father, Craig, a beloved small town football coach, whose powerful physique was the envy of the entire middle school team. "Guys would look at my dad's biceps and say, 'I wish I had "guns" like Coach Liens,'" recalls Darren, who worked out with weights as a teen and felt very proud when he achieved a build that was almost identical to his father's.

After graduating from the University of Michigan, where he was a star defensive back on the varsity football team, Darren moved back home and became very close to his dad. Almost every afternoon that year, father and son went hunting or fishing. One crisp November afternoon, before grabbing their rifles and heading off to hunt deer, the pair sat on the front porch of the family home, eating a snack.

"My dad had been raking leaves and I noticed that he looked very sweaty for such cool weather," recalls the insurance adjuster from Chandler, Arizona. "He started grumbling a little about his back aching. Since it wasn't like him to complain about anything, I made an awful joke that I've regretted ever since. I said, 'Well, you're not having a heart attack, are you?'"

"Absolutely not," retorted Craig, as he walked into the house. A minute later, the 46-year-old coach collapsed on the floor. After a few convulsions, his body went rigid and his face turned bright red. Darren called 911 and frantically began mouth-to-mouth resuscitation. "I wasn't trained in CPR and did things incorrectly.

It probably took five minutes for the ambulance to come but it seemed like forever. The whole way to the hospital, I kept saying, 'Come on, Dad!'"

At the hospital, Darren watched emergency physicians work on his father. "They were trying to jumpstart him like a motor that wouldn't turn over. They shocked him with paddles over and over. Each time, they'd get a heartbeat or two, then his heart would flat-line. After 25 minutes, his face was deep purple, nearly black. The doctors were about to give up, but they decided to shock him one more time—and got his heart going."

Craig was put on a ventilator and rushed to a major medical center. After being treated with a stent, the coach remained in a coma while Darren, other family members, and friends kept a vigil at his bedside, praying for his recovery "Everyone was ecstatic because his heart had started beating again," says Darren. "We took turns sitting in his ICU room, holding his hand and talking to him, hoping he'd wake up soon."

That never happened. "During subsequent days, we found out that because he'd gone without oxygen for so long after the heart attack, he had no brain activity. My mother was beside herself, and our pastor asked if I knew what my father's wishes would have been in this situation."

Darren's mind flashed back to an eerie conversation. "Crazy as it sounds, a month earlier, while my dad and I were hunting, he looked at me and said, completely out of the blue, 'If something ever happens to me, I don't want to be on life support.' It was as if he'd had a premonition. At the time, I didn't know what he meant, so I just said, 'OK,' never imaging that at age 22, I'd actually be faced with the decision to pull the plug on my father."

Seventeen years later, Darren still cries when he remembers what happened next. After being taken off the ventilator, the big, muscular football coach survived another 23 days, with his family at his bedside, until his slow, raspy breaths finally ceased. "Even though I knew this is what my father wanted, and doctors were telling me he was brain dead, every time I hear about someone coming out of a coma, I get choked up, wondering if I deprived him of that chance," says the insurance adjuster.

Hundreds of friends—and students—packed the high school gym for Coach Liens's funeral. "Some of the kids—and even the adults—were so grief-stricken that they actually threw themselves on my dad's casket," recalls Darren. To spare his girlfriend, Alicia, similar anguish, he suggested they break off their relationship. "I told her that I could pass away at 46 and she might be better off with someone who would live longer."

Alicia said she'd stand by him—and help him fight any genetic dangers he might face. The following year, she supported Darren through another terrifying crisis when his 49-year-old uncle needed emergency quadruple bypass surgery. "Alicia had a background in cardiac rehabilitation and after we got married, she told me that I needed to be proactive about my health, so I didn't have a fatal heart attack at 46, like my dad, or need quadruple-bypass surgery at 49, like my uncle."

Standard Care May Not Be Good Enough to Prevent a Heart Attack

When Darren, then 33, consulted us six years ago, he was frightened and frustrated. Like our patient Dead Man Walking, the young insurance adjuster was convinced that he was leading a "doomed existence." Darren actually dreaded his birthday, feeling each year that he was moving closer to his "expiration date" of 46. Even looking in the mirror added to his anxiety, he said recently. "Physically, I'm a carbon copy of my father, so I could see that I had inherited his genes."

Before being evaluated at our clinic, Darren had gone to several physicians for help, all of whom had checked for two risk factors: high cholesterol and high blood pressure. And after each exam, says the six-foot-tall, 195-pound Arizonan, "Everybody told me, 'You're in great shape, just continue what you're already doing.' One doctor said that at 136/88, my blood pressure was a little high, but it was nothing to worry about, because I was at the high end of the range accepted as normal. He said I was too young to worry about heart problems, but if I was still concerned after I turned 40, to come back for a cardiology work-up then."

According to the cardiovascular guidelines used in standard care, Darren was worrying needlessly—and didn't need any treatment—because his lipid levels and blood pressure were already within accepted targets. What most patients don't realize is that the medical practice guidelines are similar to a city's building code—a minimum safety standard. Just as top-quality construction companies may exceed the building code to make homes and offices even stronger and safer from fires, earthquakes, and other catastrophes than is legally required in some cases, the Bale/Doneen Method sets higher standards for treatment and prevention than those of certain practice guidelines widely used in standard care.

Some of the treatment goals in this chapter may surprise—or even shock—you, because they are dramatically different from those most healthcare providers use to guide treatment decisions. To help personalize your prevention plan, this chapter includes a checklist of all the numbers you need to know, including optimal vital signs, lipid levels, inflammatory markers, and the lab results you want if your healthcare provider orders the inexpensive "happy heart" blood test discussed later in this chapter.

In Darren's case, if we practiced standard care, we would have patted this brawny young man on the back, assured him that he was in excellent health, and told him to keep up the good work. Had we done that, here's what we would have missed:

- A blood pressure disorder that puts one in three adults at increased risk for heart attacks and strokes—and actually doubles the danger of death from cardiovascular causes, yet often goes untreated. In fact, as you'll learn in the next section of this chapter, there's a very good chance that you are one of the nearly 70 million Americans with this dangerous disorder. If so, you've probably been told that your blood pressure is "normal," or that it's "a little high, but nothing to worry about," as Darren was told.

- An inherited cholesterol problem. Had Darren's healthcare providers used the advanced cholesterol test, instead of the basic lipid profile, they would have discovered that he had high levels of lipoprotein (a), the inherited cholesterol issue that we call the "mass murderer" because it triples heart attack risk. Elevated levels of this cholesterol have also been shown to actually *cause* heart attacks and strokes, often at an unusually young age.

- Fire in the arteries. Darren had a very high blood level of the blood-vessel enzyme Lp-PLA2, signaling that his artery walls were severely inflamed. This enzyme, which is mainly produced by white blood cells in the wall of the artery, reacts with the LDL (bad) cholesterol that has penetrated into the same space within the artery. The substances produced by this interaction play a key role in both plaque formation and vulnerability (the risk that plaque may rupture explosively and trigger a heart attack or stroke).

- An inflammation gene. Darren was also a carrier of the interleukin-1 gene, which we'll discuss in detail in Chapter Fourteen. This gene greatly magnifies the inflammatory response that drives arterial disease and cardiovascular-event risk. The IL-1 gene also boosts the threat of developing gum disease, which is now known to be a strong, independent risk factor for CVD. Further testing also revealed that Darren harbored high levels of a harmful bacterium in his mouth, compounding the danger to both his teeth and his arteries.

- Genetic risks. In addition to being clobbered by inherited cholesterol and inflammatory issues, Darren also turned out to be a carrier of the 9P21 "heart attack gene" *and* the KIF6 gene. In addition, the low-fat diet he was following, while healthy for some people, was completely wrong for his ApoE genotype. In other words, he had a perfect storm of cardiovascular perils brewing because of his DNA.

- Accelerated arterial aging. Despite his brawny physique and athletic lifestyle, at age 33, Darren had an arterial age of 45 on his cIMT test. Just as he had feared, he was on the fast track to heart disease and his arteries were showing signs of damage. The good news, however, was that the scan didn't detect any plaque in his carotid arteries. With so many cardiovascular threats working against him, however, Darren needed aggressive prevention to help him remain disease-free.

As you'll learn in this chapter, the best way to avoid a heart attack or stroke is tailored treatment to and prevention goals for your unique risk profile, and then work with your healthcare provider to achieve these objectives. For example, Darren's LDL (bad) cholesterol level of 106 mg/dL would be considered excellent, according to the American Heart Association. That LDL level, however, is *not* optimal for patients who have elevated levels of lipoprotein (a) as Darren does. Research shows that patients with this inherited cholesterol disorder need to keep their bad cholesterol even lower to head off a heart attack, with the optimal level for these patients being less than 70 mg/dL.

To help Darren attain this LDL goal, we prescribed a statin. Since these medications also combat inflammation, this therapy was doubly beneficial in his case, by also helping to extinguish the fire raging in his arteries. He also takes niacin (vitamin B3) daily—the most effective treatment to reduce Lp(a) levels—and has switched to a low-carbohydrate diet that includes a glass or two of wine or beer a day, an eating plan that's ideal for his genotype. And he's on medication that has successfully reduced his blood pressure to less than 120/80 (the healthiest range).

These days, says Darren, now 39, "I finally have a peace about me, right in my spirit, because I no longer dread getting closer to the age when my father passed away. I've been given a roadmap that says, 'Here are the problems that could kill you—and here's how to prevent them.' When I'm running or hiking with my wife, or spending time with my family, I feel like a weight has been lifted from my shoulders, now that I have a path to enjoying a long and healthy future."

Avoiding a Silent Killer

The world's leading cause of death and disability is also the most preventable: high blood pressure is an assassin that attacks stealthily, giving few hints that it's on the prowl, as it wreaks slow mayhem on your blood vessels and vital organs, including your heart, brain, and kidneys. Sixty-seven million Americans—about one in three adults—have hypertension, blood pressure in which the top number (systolic pressure) is 140 millimeters of mercury (mm hG) or greater *or* the bottom number (diastolic pressure) is 90 mm hG or greater. Having even one number within this range counts as high blood pressure, even if the other number is lower. For example, if your blood pressure is 140/85, you have hypertension.

Most people with hypertension take medication *and* have seen a doctor at least twice in the past year, yet their condition *still* isn't controlled, according to an alarming September, 2012 report from the Centers for Disease Control and Prevention (CDC). The report underscores the most profound—and deadly—failure of standard care, given that high blood pressure is the leading risk factor for stroke and a major contributor to heart disease, conditions that collectively kill nearly 1,000 Americans a day. What's more, uncontrolled hypertension greatly magnifies the danger of developing heart failure, metabolic syndrome, aortic aneurysm, and kidney disease, and can also lead to blindness and memory loss.

This scary situation prompted an urgent call to action by CDC director Thomas R. Frieden, MD, MPH, who told healthcare providers in September 2012, "We have to roll up our sleeves and make blood pressure control a priority every day, with every patient, at every doctor's visit. With increased focus and collaboration among patients, healthcare providers, and healthcare systems, we can help 10 million Americans' blood pressure come into control in the next five years."

Why are practitioners of standard care doing such a dismal job of fighting this silent killer? It's hardly news that uncontrolled high blood pressure is lethal: In the late nineteenth century, life insurance and mortgage companies were the first to realize that the higher a customer's blood pressure, the greater the person's risk of dying early. Since then, numerous epidemiological and treatment studies have documented that the threat of heart disease, stroke, and heart failure all soar in tandem with increasing blood pressure numbers.

Three major problems explain why high blood pressure ranks as the most common uncontrolled chronic disorder in the United States (and most other nations):

1. Lack of early detection and treatment.

   If you had a precancerous growth, wouldn't you want it removed *before* it turned into cancer? While you'd think healthcare providers would be equally proactive about catching elevated blood pressure in the early stages, unfortunately that's not the case. Although normal blood pressure is defined as a reading below 120/80, current medical guidelines say that any measurement below 140/90 is acceptable.

   These guidelines mean that a huge group of people not even mentioned in the CDC report are ignored: the nearly 70 million Americans with prehypertension, defined as systolic pressure between 120 and 139 *or* diastolic pressure between 80 and 89. Having one number in the prehypertensive range, and the other in the normal range, still counts as prehypertension. If you have this extremely common disorder, you've probably been told that your blood pressure is fine. Or, as occurred with Darren, your healthcare provider may have advised you that your blood pressure is "a little high," but still in the "normal" range.

   As a result of this medical neglect, most people with prehypertension assume that there's nothing to worry about—and therefore no need for such proven blood-pressure lowering treatments as weight loss, dietary and lifestyle changes, and, if necessary, medication. But is that really true? Let's look at some excellent scientific research published in leading medical journals:

   - In 2002, a major study reported that when blood pressure rises from 115/75 to 135/85, the risk of dying from CVD doubles.

   - In 2005, a study demonstrated that over a 10-year period, people with blood pressure in the prehypertensive range had more than triple the risk of suffering a heart attack, compared to those with normal blood pressure (below 120/80).

   - A 2005 study of more than 250,000 people, conducted by Kaiser Permanente, found that over a 20-year period, those with slight elevations in blood pressure had nearly double the threat of developing end-stage kidney disease, compared to people without prehypertension.

   - Although many people think that elevated blood pressure is mainly a threat to middle-aged or older people, a 2007 study of 2,000 young adults found that one-third of them had prehypertension, and that the increased force of blood pounding through their heart had already caused significant structural damage.

- Global data indicates that in 2008, prehypertension was the culprit in the majority of cardiovascular events around the world, while a 2011 study reported that prehypertension boosts risk for stroke by 55 percent.

- A recent global study found that *in most countries more than 80 percent of adults have blood pressure levels that put them in danger of developing CVD. The majority of this at-risk group have blood pressure below 140/90.*

- Evidence from a 2012 study tells us that if you have a cardiac calcium score between 100 and 399 (an indication of coronary artery disease), coupled with prehypertension, your risk for having a heart attack or stroke triples over the next seven years. The same study found that the combination of prehypertension and a cardiac calcium score of 400 or greater multiples heart attack and stroke risk by up to eightfold!

2. Dangerously unscientific guidelines.

By now, you're probably wondering why cardiology guidelines still say that this perilous blood pressure is okay, given such powerful scientific evidence, compiled over more than a decade, about its many dangers. To us, delaying treatment until people with prehypertension progress to full-blown high blood pressure makes about as much sense as waiting until people with coronary artery disease keel over with a heart attack to treat their disease.

There are a number of explanations for this appalling medical neglect, with many of them elucidated in a 2009 study published in *Journal of the American Medical Association (JAMA)*. Researchers funded by the government's Agency for Healthcare Quality and Research analyzed 53 medical practice guidelines issued by the American College of Cardiology (ACC) and the American Heart Association (AHA) encompassing 7,192 recommendations on 22 cardiovascular issues, and found that:

- Of those guidelines that included the level of scientific evidence supporting the recommendations, only a median of 11 percent were based on level A evidence (recommendations based on evidence from multiple randomized clinical trials—the gold standard of scientific research).

- Forty-eight percent of the recommendations were based on level C evidence (the lowest level of evidence, drawn from case studies, the standard of care, or merely the opinions of experts).

- More than 50 percent of recommendations in most current AHA/ACC guidelines are based solely on level C evidence. For some cardiovascular diseases, up to 70 percent of recommendations to healthcare providers are based on mere expert opinion.

- The number of recommendations with *no* conclusive scientific evidence is growing—yet these are guidelines that most healthcare providers rely on when they make decisions about cardiovascular care! The researchers say that the findings "highlight deficiencies" and warn that "clinicians need [to] exercise caution" about following the increasing number of medical guidelines that lack scientific support.

- It's also common for excellent science to be published a decade or two prior to being included in guidelines, because the recommendations are updated so infrequently.

As you've already seen with blood sugar and cholesterol testing, many medical guidelines are not optimal. But now that you've been empowered with the knowledge that even slight elevations in blood pressure can be hazardous, you'll understand why it's imperative to demand treatment if your blood pressure is 120/80 or above, even if your healthcare provider says there's no cause for concern. As you'll learn in the next chapter, an improved lifestyle—such as losing weight, exercising more, and eating the right diet—can often significantly reduce blood pressure. If these measures aren't enough, there are other effective therapies, such as the medications and supplements discussed in Chapter Thirteen.

The wonderful news is that these treatments greatly reduce cardiovascular risk. In 2006, a large study reported that when people with prehypertension were treated with medication and medical advice about lifestyle modification, their risk of progressing to full-blown hypertension fell dramatically. Recently, an analysis of health data from more than 250,000 people found that treating prehypertension can prevent lifelong disability—or fatalities—by reducing stroke risk by up to 70 percent. That finding is not surprising, given that high blood pressure is the number one risk for stroke, according to several large studies, and ranks as the fourth leading cause of heart attacks.

3. Failing to identify and treat the root causes of high blood pressure.

Since AHA/ACC guidelines and many government public health campaigns *do* emphasize the extreme importance of treating hypertension, why does it remain the most common uncontrolled chronic condition in the U.S. and much of the world? In a 2010 review article we wrote about this issue, published in *Journal of the National Medical Association,* we pointed to the problem of "therapeutic inertia," a provider's failure to increase therapy or try different treatments when blood pressure targets are not met. For example, a retrospective study found that medication adjustments were only made for 13 percent of patients with uncontrolled hypertension. Yet just reducing "therapeutic inertia" by as little as 20 percent would have improved blood pressure control for 46 to 66 percent of the patients studied, the researchers calculated, underscoring the need for healthcare providers to work harder on fine-tuning treatment, rather than giving up in despair if the first medication they try isn't effective.

A major reason that providers often find hypertension tricky to treat, even if they *are* willing to prescribe additional therapies, is that all too often, doctors don't look for the root cause of high blood pressure. Just as many heart attack and stroke survivors are told that their event was a medical mystery that was impossible to predict or prevent, people with high blood pressure are frequently left to believe that their condition defies medical explanation.

Actually, high blood pressure is frequently triggered by the same disorder that causes 70 percent of heart attacks: insulin resistance. An even more surprising—and often overlooked—culprit is obstructive sleep apnea (OSA), a disorder marked by bouts of interrupted breathing during sleep. The frequent, sudden drops in blood oxygen levels that result from this condition strain the cardiovascular system, raising risk for elevated blood pressure. And the more severe OSA is, the higher the threat of developing hypertension and other cardiovascular complications. Sleep apnea boosts risk for stroke, irregular heartbeats (atrial fibrillation), congestive heart failure, and sudden cardiac death.

We recently had two patients, whose blood pressure remained stubbornly high despite an entire year of treatment with several medications and other therapies. Since both had normal blood sugar levels (when measured with the two-hour oral glucose tolerance test discussed in Chapter Nine), we questioned the patients about OSA symptoms, such as loud snoring, waking up at night for no apparent reason, persistent daytime drowsiness despite adequate rest, and morning headache or sore throat.

Both patients denied having these symptoms, so we also questioned their spouses. People with OSA are often unaware of their loud snoring—the leading warning sign of this frequently undiagnosed disorder. Although the spouses were adamant that OSA couldn't possibly be the problem, we decided to refer the patients, who lived in different states, to sleep labs near their homes for an overnight sleep study. After the first patient spent the night in the sleep lab, hooked up to monitors, we received an early morning call from an alarmed sleep specialist, who told us that the patient had one of the worst cases of OSA the specialist had even seen.

A week later, we received an identical early morning call from the other sleep lab. Despite the severity of our patients' OSA, both were successfully treated with CPAP (continuous positive airway pressure) machines, which blow pressured air into a patient's nose and mouth during sleep, to keep the airway open. This treatment is often the best solution to obstructive sleep apnea, a disorder that causes the airway to collapse during sleep, resulting in interrupting breathing, often followed by a loud, rattling snore when breathing resumes. Once our patients' OSA was treated, we were finally able to get their blood pressure under control.

OSA is as common as type 2 diabetes, affecting about 18 million Americans, 90 percent of whom are undiagnosed. It's more common in men, people who are overweight and those who are older than 40. It can strike at any age, however, even during childhood. If untreated, not only can it lead to cardiovascular issues, including impotence in men, but it also raises risk for car crashes. In our opinion, it makes sense to discuss a sleep study with your healthcare provider if you have high blood pressure that doesn't respond to medication—or if you have any of the symptoms of OSA.

While achieving optimal blood pressure goals isn't always easy, doing so has huge health benefits. If prehypertension is so treacherous to cardiovascular health, what do you think uncontrolled hypertension does? As we're sure you've guessed, it's even more dangerous! The same study showing that going from 115/75 to 135/85 doubles the risk of dying from CVD also reported that going up to 155/95 quadrupled the risk, while a level of 175/105 multiplied risk by eightfold (compared to blood pressure of 115/75). Mixing high blood pressure with other disorders that raise heart attack and stroke risk only escalates the peril. For example, if you're diabetic, having hypertension triples the threat of cardiovascular events.

Again, the good news is that getting effective treatment significantly reduces the threat of serious complications. Research shows that if hypertension is under control, the risk for developing kidney disease falls by as much as 30 percent. A study involving nearly 500,000 people demonstrated that for each 10 mm hG drop in blood pressure, heart attack risk plummeted by 50 percent. Lowering blood pressure has been shown to protect against cognitive decline and to lower stroke rates by 40 percent in diabetics at high risk for cardiovascular events.

And it's never too late to reap the powerful benefits of blood pressure reduction. In fact, in a trial with nearly 4,000 people aged 80 or older, the benefits of hypertensive therapy was so great, compared to taking a placebo, that the trial had to be halted early, since it would have been inhumane to continue *not* treating the placebo group! Bottom line: The scientific evidence is unequivocal—achieving optimal blood pressure is one of the very best ways to enhance cardiovascular wellness.

Is Your Heart Happy?

We've all pondered the question of how "happy" our heart is from the emotional standpoint—and a positive answer is refreshing and good for our psychological well-being. But most people don't know that it's also important to find out if their heart is happy from the physical standpoint as well. That's right—there's a simple blood test that can literally quantify exactly how "happy" your heart is.

When the heart is under stress or struggling to function properly, it puts out extra amounts of a neurohormone called B-type naturetic peptide (BNP). Essentially SOS messages that the heart is in distress, naturetic peptides cause the body to excrete more fluid, lessening the amount the heart has to pump each time it beats. These peptides also cause arteries to dilate, lessening the force the heart must generate to circulate blood. Both effects reduce a struggling heart's workload.

B-type naturetic peptide is easy to measure with a rapid, inexpensive blood test known as NT-proBNP. When the level of this cardiac distress marker is below

125 pg/mL, there is a 98 percent chance your heart is very happy! Any test in medicine that can give you those types of odds is phenomenal.

How worried should you be if the level is above that? If that's the case, then there is about a 33 percent chance your heart is not totally happy and experiencing what we call dysfunction. While there is still a decent chance that you are okay if the level of this marker is elevated, the odds that there might be a problem are high enough that your healthcare provider may advise additional tests to evaluate your heart health, such as an echocardiogram (EKG).

It's also noteworthy that the heart-happy test was one of only two tests in the huge Framingham study that accurately predicted heart attack and stroke danger after the researchers made rigorous adjustments for every risk factor they could think of. (The other test was the microalbumin-creatinine urine ratio discussed later in this chapter.) It is extremely difficult for a lab result to qualify as an "independent predictor" of cardiovascular risk. We hope you request the NT-proBNP test and that your heart is happy!

Optimal Goals Checklist

What's the optimal blood pressure? Like other cardiovascular goals in the checklist below, your blood pressure target needs to be personalized according to your overall health and other medical conditions. The heart muscle is nourished mainly by diastolic pressure pushing nutrients and oxygen through the coronary arteries. Therefore some patients with very narrowed channels in their coronary arteries need a higher diastolic pressure (the lower number) to squeeze the blood through. If a patient sets a goal to reduce the pressure to 75 mmHg or less, he or she may not be able to adequately perfuse the heart muscle with blood, which might lead to a heart attack.

Similarly, some people with significant chronic kidney disease, which can result in narrowing of arteries feeding the kidney, may also be in trouble if their pressure is lowered too much. Each patient needs to be followed closely when they are receiving BP treatment and appropriate lab tests should be followed to make sure the pressure is not reduced too much. In a healthy population, scientific data would suggest that we'd be better off with a blood pressure just above the point where we might pass out. Some trials, however, have set very low blood-pressure goals for people who are not healthy, such as diabetics. Tragically, some participants in the "aggressive" treatment arm of these studies did very poorly and some even died.

In this type of study, everyone in a certain arm of the study is treated the same. No two people, however, are exactly alike. Excellent outcomes require personalizing care—not standardizing the same care for everyone! In the checklist below, you'll find the optimal treatment and prevention goals we recommend for the cardiovascular health metrics and tests discussed in this book. As discussed in Part Two, some of the numbers in your medical records can actually be used to diagnose disorders, including insulin resistance and metabolic syndrome, without doing *any* lab tests.

It's important to discuss your treatment and prevention goals with your healthcare provider, individualize them according to your overall health and any medical conditions you may have, and then be carefully monitored with periodic medical exams and tests as you strive to improve your cardiovascular health.

Optimal Vital Signs

- Body Mass Index (BMI)

  Goal: Less than 25

- Blood Pressure

  Goal: Less than 115/75, unless you have obstructive coronary disease or chronic kidney disease. If you have either of these disorders, discuss your blood pressure target with your healthcare provider.

- Waist Circumference

  Goal for Caucasians, African Americans and Hispanics: Less than 40 inches for men, less than 35 inches for women.

  Goal for Asians: Less than 35 inches for men, less than 31 inches for women

  Goal for Japanese: Less than 34 inches for men, less than 31 inches for women.

- Pulse

  Goal: Less than 75 beats per minute

Optimal Vascular Imaging Test Results

These tests to check for arterial disease are covered in detail in Chapter Six, including pros and cons, what's involved, what the results mean, and which patients should have these tests.

- Carotid Intima-Media Thickness (cIMT). This "ultrasound of the neck" checks for abnormal thickness of the carotid artery walls and plaque (disease). The results also include a calculation of your "arterial age."

  Goals: No areas of thickness greater or equal than 1.3 mm (plaque). If you do have plaque, the next two chapters of this book will alert you to the best therapies to treat—or possibly even reverse—your disease. Your arterial age is optimal if it's no more than five years "older" than your chronological age (a range that's within the normal margin of error for well-trained technicians).

The "younger" your arteries are, compared to your chronological age, the better.

- Coronary Calcium Score. This CT scan checks for calcium in the coronary artery walls, a strong predictor of heart attack risk.

  Goal: No calcium (score of zero). If you do have calcified plaque, then it's crucial to work with your healthcare provider to set optimal goals to halt the progression of your disease and prevent a heart attack or stroke. In the next chapter, you'll find some surprising—and fun—ways to improve your life-style, while Chapter Thirteen looks at medications and supplements that may be prescribed.

- Ankle/Brachial Index (ABI). This test is used to diagnose peripheral artery disease, a circulatory problem that results when plaque buildup reduces blood flow to the extremities, usually the legs.

  Goal: The normal range is between 0.9 and 1.4.

- Abdominal Aortic Aneurysm. This scan checks for weak, ballooning areas in the heart's largest artery and can also detect calcified plaque in the aorta.

  Goal: An aortic diameter of 3 cm and no arterial calcifications.

- Carotid Duplex Scan. Unlike cIMT, which directly checks the arterial wall for plaque, the carotid duplex looks for indirect signs of disease, such as block-ages, by measuring blood flow through the neck arteries.

  Goal: Results are expressed as percentages defined by each lab, with lower numbers representing the normal range (the optimal goal) and higher ones being increasingly abnormal.

Optimal Lipid Levels

Cholesterol tests and common misconceptions about lipids are explored in detail in Chapter Eight. As discussed in that chapter, we recommend calculating your ratios of total cholesterol to HDL (TC/HDL) and triglycerides to HDL (TG/HDL), the two lipid values that have proven to be *the most* predictive of cardiovascular risk in large studies. As you also learned in our cholesterol chapter, an abnormal TG/HDL ratio can actually be used to diagnose insulin resistance.

While the basic cholesterol profile most healthcare providers use only mea-sures total cholesterol, HDL, LDL, and triglycerides, the advanced cholesterol test discussed in Chapter Eight also checks levels of lipoprotein (a), the "mass mur-derer" that triples heart attack risk, and measures apolipoprotein B (Apo B), a conglomeration of all of the cholesterol bad guys. Recent research shows that Apo B levels are a better indicator of cardiovascular risk than LDL levels alone.

- TC/HDL ratio (Total cholesterol level divided by your HDL level)

  Goal: Less than 3.0 mg/dL

- TG/HDL (Triglycerides level divided by your HDL level)

  Goal: Less than 3.5 mg/dL if you're Caucasian

     Less than 2.0 mg/dL if you're African American

     Less than 3.0 mg/dL if you are Hispanic

- Lipoprotein (a)

  Goal: Normal range, as defined by the medical lab performing the test.

- LDL (bad) Cholesterol

  Goal: Most patients benefit from a goal of less 130 mg/dL. However, if you have plaque in your arteries (anywhere in your body—not just the coronary arteries), elevated levels of Lp(a), or are at increased risk for CVD due to genes, family history, or other factors, your healthcare provider may advise a goal of less than 70 mg/dL.

- Apolipoprotein B (Apo B)

  Goal: Less than 60 mg/dL

Optimal Levels of Inflammatory Markers

This "fire panel" of blood and urine tests, discussed in Chapter Seven, check how "hot" your arteries are, to evaluate heart attack and stroke risk.

- F2 Isoprostanes. This "lifestyle lie detector" blood test reveals if you're practicing heart-healthy habits and how fast your body is aging.

  Goal: Less than 0.25 ng/L

- High-Sensitive C-Reactive Protein (hs CRP). This blood test checks levels of a protein that rises when there's inflammation throughout the body.

  Goal: Less than 0.5mg/L

- Microalbumin/Creatinine Urine Ratio (MACR). As you learned in this chapter, this urine test, which costs just pennies, is one of just two biomarker tests that independently predicted risk for cardiovascular events in the very large Framingham study.

  Goal: Less than 4.4 for men and less than 7.5 for women

- Fibrinogen. This blood test measures levels of a sticky protein that causes blood to clot.

  Goal: Normal range, as defined by the medical lab performing the test.

- Lipoprotein-Associated Phospholipase A-2 (Lp-PLA2). This blood test measures levels of a blood-vessel specific enzyme that's mainly attached to bad cholesterol. In Darren's case, his Lp-PLA2 levels were extremely abnormal at 253 ng/mL during his initial evaluation, indicating high risk for developing plaque.

  Goal: Less than 180 ng/mL

- Myeloperoxidase (MPO). This blood test checks levels of an immune-system enzyme we call "the joker." Of all the inflammatory biomarkers, this one is the worst, since it's a wild card that makes all types of cholesterol (including HDL, the normal "good cholesterol") more inflammatory.

  Goal: Less than 420 pmol/L

Optimal Blood Sugar

As discussed in Chapter Nine, we recommend using the two-hour oral glucose tolerance test to check for insulin resistance and diabetes. Because your health-care provider may have used one of the two other commonly performed blood-sugar tests described in that chapter, however, we've included the optimal values for all three tests.

- Fasting Blood-Sugar Test

  Goal: Less than 100 mg/dL

- Hemoglobin A1C Test

  Goal: Less than 5.5 percent

- Oral Glucose Tolerance Test – with 75 g glucose

  Goal: One-hour blood sugar: Less than 125 mg/dL

  Two-hour blood sugar: Less than 120 mg/dL

Optimal Liver Function

Elevated levels of liver enzymes in your blood indicate that cells in your liver are dying more rapidly than they should be. While there are several reasons why this may be happening—including liver diseases like hepatitis and chronic alcohol abuse—elevated liver enzymes can also be a red flag that you've developed insulin resistance, and therefore could be headed for type 2 diabetes if your blood-sugar disorder goes untreated.

Therefore, if you have abnormal results on this lab test, which is widely used in routine medical checkups, we recommend that you ask your healthcare provider to check your blood sugar, using the two-hour oral glucose tolerance test. Another common culprit for elevated liver enzymes is medication side effects, particularly from cholesterol-lowering drugs called statins, which act on a liver enzyme. If you are taking this type of medication, your doctor or nurse practitioner is likely to advise periodic lab tests to check your liver enzyme levels.

> Goals: For the liver enzyme alanine aminotransferase (ALT), the optimal blood levels are less than 20 u/L for women and less than 34 u/L for men. For the liver enzyme gamma-glutamyl transferase (GGT), the optimal blood levels are less than 21 u/L for women and less than 47 u/L for men.

Optimal Kidney Function

Studies show that the worse the kidney function, the greater the risk for heart attack and stroke. This may be related to both conditions having common causes, such as insulin resistance and high blood pressure. The most common blood test used to evaluate kidney function is *serum creatinine,* which is usually included in the routine blood tests performed during annual physicals. In general, the lower the creatinine level, the better your kidneys are functioning.

Based on your creatinine level—and a complicated formula that factors in your age and gender—the lab can then calculate what is called an *estimated glomerular filtration rate* (eGFR). In simple terms, this number tells you how well your kidneys are working.

If you have lost a lot of muscle tissue due to aging or a disability, creatinine is not an accurate estimation of kidney function. Creatinine is derived from muscle tissue, so if there is not much muscle to generate creatinine the levels will be low even if the kidneys are not working well. In this circumstance, a test called cystatin C will provide a much better estimation of kidney function since its production has nothing to do with the muscles.

> Goals: Creatinine level: less than 1.2 mg/dL
>
> Cystatin C level: less than 0.89 mg/L
>
> Glomerular filtration rate: greater than 60 ml/min (estimated)

Optimal Thyroid Function

Thirteen million Americans, many of who are undiagnosed, have low levels of thyroid hormones. While you probably know that this problem can cause fatigue, weight gain, dry skin, forgetfulness, and heavier periods in women, you may be surprised that low levels of thyroid hormones also boost cardiovascular risk: one study reported that people with low thyroid had more than double the risk for a cardiovascular event over the next 2.5 years than those with normal thyroid. Another, much larger study, in which participants were tracked for 35 years, found that hypothyroidism increased risk for fatal heart attacks by 50 percent.

Since symptoms of thyroid dysfunction can be subtle, the only way to tell if the body's "master gland" is working properly is with a blood test to check levels of thyroid stimulating hormone (TSH) and the thyroid hormones T3 and T4. Although this simple, inexpensive test isn't always included in annual physicals, most experts advise being tested at age 35, even if you don't have any obvious warning signs of a thyroid disorder.

Goal: At this time, the optimal number for TSH is a moving target, since a growing number of specialists are viewing numbers that were previously deemed normal to be indicative of hypothyroidism. We recommend that you review your lab report and if any of the numbers are abnormal or even "borderline," discuss them with your healthcare provider. Thyroid dysfunction is highly treatable.

Optimal Heart Function

- NT-ProBNP Blood Test, the "heart-happy" test, described earlier in this chapter.

  Goal: Less than 125 pg/mL

- Electrocardiogram (EKG). For this exam, you're hooked up to electrodes that record the heart's electrical activity. EKGs are used to check for many heart problems, including heart attacks, irregular beats (arrhythmias), and heart failure.

  Goal: Normal Sinus Rhythm

Action Step: Follow a Diet Guided by Your DNA

In the next chapter, you'll find out which heart-protective diet is best for your genotype, and some remarkably effective, science-backed strategies to help you slim down without feeling deprived. If you have high cholesterol or genetic risks for cardiovascular disease, you'll be intrigued by the very surprising story of a patient who managed to overcome the most dangerous heart-attack risk factor of all—without taking pills.

Chapter 12

A Diet-and-Exercise Plan Based on Your DNA

"Let food be thy medicine."

—Hippocrates

Three years ago, Patrick Boub was in the best shape of his life. Then 39, he'd become an avid cyclist who was proud of his ability to beat much younger men in bike races. The 5'10", 150-pound CPA from Walla Walla, Washington, trained hard, averaging 150 miles per week on his bike, and began running every day.

Fueling his determination to achieve peak fitness was his alarming family history: one of his uncles had had a heart attack at age 50 and several relatives, including his mother, had required bypass surgery or other heart procedures to treat severely blocked coronary arteries. Patrick also had another major risk factor for coronary artery disease—high cholesterol—but treatment with a statin drug had successfully lowered his LDL into the normal range.

As Patrick intensified his training, he began to experience bouts of extreme leg pain and cramps. When the problem grew so excruciating that he was unable to run or bike at all—and his skin suddenly turned yellow—he consulted his family doctor. Blood tests showed that the CPA had developed rhabdomyolysis, a disorder in which breakdown of muscle fibers causes a protein called myoglobin to build up in the blood—a problem that often causes kidney damage. Among the causes of this very rare, but dangerous condition are severe exertion, such as marathon running, and side effects of certain drugs, particularly cholesterol-lowering medications (statins).

"The doctor said that I needed to stop exercising and quit statin therapy immediately, because my blood tests showed that I was at risk for going into kidney failure," recalls Patrick. "I was devastated. I didn't want to give up running and biking—exercise is my life—and was scared that without a statin, I'd die of a heart attack." Over the next year, his kidney function returned to normal and he was able to resume biking. Persistent problems with leg pain and cramping, however, continued to make running impossible. And he was particularly alarmed to see his cholesterol numbers become increasingly abnormal at each medical checkup.

An Optimal Lifestyle Is More Powerful Than Medicine or Surgery

When Patrick consulted us two years ago, the then-40-year-old dad had an extremely abnormal total cholesterol-to-HDL ratio, the strongest predictor of cardiovascular risk. His TC/HDL ratio of nearly 5.0 was linked to "moderately high" danger of developing heart disease in the next decade in the large Framingham Heart Study. (As you'll recall from Chapter Ten, the optimal ratio is below 3.0.)

Patrick was a carrier of the 9P21 "heart attack gene." Compounding the danger, at age 40 he had the arteries of a 70-year-old man, along with elevated levels of the inflammatory marker Lp-PLA2. In other words, his arteries were on fire—and he was on the fast track to heart disease. The wonderful news, however, was that both his cIMT scan and his coronary calcium score found no plaque in his arteries. Therefore, we urgently needed to get his cholesterol under control, before he developed the "cat in the gutter."

What made Patrick's case particularly challenging was that he had adverse reactions to every cholesterol-lowering medication we tried, including a very low dosage of a different statin, combined with niacin (vitamin B3). Instead, despite his complex cholesterol issues *and* a family history of early heart attacks, we had to manage this patient at high risk for developing arterial disease solely through helping him achieve an optimal lifestyle, tailored to his genes and medical conditions.

While you may think that lifestyle changes sound like a puny defense against a gang of cardiovascular thugs, in reality, as you'll learn in this chapter, a heart-healthy lifestyle is by far the best—and most powerful—weapon in your treatment and prevention arsenal. Published data show that lifestyle modification saves many more lives than any medicine ever invented or high-tech heart procedures, such as stents. Here are just a few compelling findings from recent studies:

- When adults age 70 or old followed an ideal lifestyle that included a Mediterranean diet, moderate physical activity, moderate alcohol consumption, and no tobacco use, their risk of dying from cardiovascular causes in the next decade dropped by 73 percent.

- These four lifestyle factors—plus having a body mass index of 25 or less—reduced ischemic stroke risk by 80 percent in a study of more than 110,000 initially healthy people. Not only did another study of more than 71,000 women produce identical results, but those researchers also reported that an unhealthy lifestyle was the culprit in at least 50 percent of strokes.

- While a number of large studies show that on average, moderate alcohol use (one drink per day for women, two for men) can be beneficial to the heart, it can also be hazardous to some people because of genetic factors, addiction issues or medical factors, as we'll discuss more fully in the next section of this chapter. In addition, consuming even one alcoholic beverage a day raises cancer risk in women, particularly for breast cancer. Research shows that an optimal lifestyle that *doesn't* include alcohol also save lives. For example, a major study found that people with five or more of the American Heart Association's "Seven Essentials for Heart Health" (not smoking, a heart-healthy diet, regular exercise, a BMI of 25 or lower, blood pressure below 120/80, total cholesterol below 200, and fasting blood glucose below 100 mg/dL), reduced their risk for death from cardiovascular causes by 88 percent!

- In patients who had already had a coronary event, following a medically advised diet and exercise plan trimmed risk for heart attack, stroke, and death in the next six months by 54 percent. Quitting smoking cut risk by 26 percent. Conversely, patients who made *none* of these lifestyle improvements had nearly quadruple the danger of dying in six months.

In this chapter and the next, you'll discover that achieving an optimal lifestyle that's personalized according to your genes, medical conditions, and health risks can be a lot simpler—and more pleasurable—than you might imagine. Some of the easy actions we recommend may surprise or even delight you. Among our "prescriptions" for better heart health are a daily "dose" of dark chocolate, taking frequent vacations, unwinding with a relaxing massage, listening to music, and making love, which literally does your heart good.

You'll also discover the easiest ways to exercise—and add years to your life without the expense of joining a gym, the most effective strategies to quit smoking, including two highly successful tactics that you probably haven't tried before, and simple, proved ways to shed unwanted pounds and keep them off for good, even if you've struggled with weight loss in the past.

Benefits of an Eating Plan Guided by Your Genes

Hundreds of diets offer a similar prescription for cardiovascular wellness, from anti-inflammatory eating plans to the Zone diet. In what might be called the low-fat vs. low-carb wars, the two rival weight-loss approaches have battled it out for years in medical journals, with some studies showing that cutting down on carbs seems better at getting the pounds off, and others finding that trimming fat appears more effective.

A recent study comparing the two strategies had intriguing results: Women were randomly assigned to one of four popular diets: the low-carb Atkins diet, the low-carb Zone diet, the super low-fat Ornish diet, or the low-fat LEARN diet. While the women lost slightly more weight, on average, on the Atkins diet, there was a puzzling range of results among those on each eating plan. Some women lost 30 or more pounds, while others *gained* 10 pounds. The contradictory findings highlight the frustration many dieters feel when no matter how hard they try, they just can't get the pounds off.

What the researchers proved, unintentionally, was that the one size-fits-all approach doesn't work. Similarly, studies of various dietary approaches intended to reduce cardiovascular risk—such as eating a Mediterranean-style diet, drinking moderate amounts of alcohol, or taking fish oil—reveal striking individual differences in response. That's not news to the American Heart Association, which has advised doctors that, "There needs to be an emphasis for focusing on gene influence to dietary factors." In another statement on nutrition, the AHA also noted, "Healthcare providers need to consider that genetics and metabolic differences may limit the potential for generalized dietary recommendations."

What's the best way to personalize your eating plan for optimal cardiovascular health? As you learned in Chapter Ten, the Apo E gene on chromosome 19 powerfully influences both your risk for developing chronic diseases—including arterial disease, insulin resistance and even memory-robbing disorders like vascular dementia—and which foods are likely to be most effective in combating those risks. Specifically, this gene plays a key role in how your body metabolizes the "Big Three" food types: carbohydrates, proteins, and fats.

The "Apo" in Apo E is short for "apolipoprotein." This family of proteins, each of which is named after a letter of the alphabet, serve as molecular submarines to ferry fats, such as cholesterol, through the bloodstream. The Apo E gene serves as a blueprint that tells the body how to manufacture Apo E, a key player in cholesterol metabolism. In its Scientific Conference proceedings on preventive nutrition, the AHA supported using genotype tests (e.g., the Apo E gene) to predict individual responses to dietary treatment options.

Following a diet based on your specific Apo E genotype fights the leading risk factor for heart attack and a major risk factor for ischemic stroke: abnormal lipid levels. Studies show that eating the right diet for your Apo E genotype can help boost heart-protective HDL cholesterol and trims levels of triglycerides, LDL (bad) cholesterol, *and* extremely bad cholesterol: small, dense LDL particles. People with a preponderance of small, dense particles have triple the heart attack risk—even if their LDL level is within normal limits—compared to people who mainly have large, buoyant LDL particles.

Are You Eating the Right Foods for Your Apo E Genotype?

Because many people haven't had the Apo E genotype blood or saliva test we recommend in Chapter Ten, we frequently see patients who are eating the worst possible diet for their genotype—or are unknowingly avoiding the very foods that are most likely to protect their heart health. For example, Patrick was so terrified that consuming even a trace of fat would cause his increasingly abnormal cholesterol numbers to get even worse that he'd put himself on an extremely restrictive, ultra-low-fat diet. Instead of enjoying family dinners with his wife and kids, he was racked by worry that just about anything he ate might be hazardous to his heart.

Actually, as DNA testing revealed, Patrick was *not* eating the optimal diet to protect his cardiovascular health. As it turned out, he had the Apo E 3/3 genotype—the most common genotype. People with this genotype, which is linked to intermediate lifetime risk for cardiovascular disease, benefit most from the conventional Mediterranean-style diet that's typically recommended for cardiovascular wellness. Based on foods traditionally consumed in countries that border the Mediterranean Sea, this way of eating emphasizes plant-based foods, such as fresh fruits and vegetables, nuts, whole grains, legumes, olive oil, herbs, and spices, along with moderate amounts of cheese, yogurt, fish, and wine.

Understandably, Patrick was a little skeptical when we told him that eating *more* fat (in the form of healthy oils) would help solve his LDL problem. He was even more surprised when we also advised him to add even more fat, with a daily dose of fish oil, an over-the-counter supplement that has been shown to improve levels of HDL, triglycerides, and small, dense LDL in people with all Apo E genotypes. And he was downright dumbfounded by our recommendation that he start eating small amounts of dark chocolate every day.

The highly restrictive ultra-low-fat diet he'd previously been following clearly wasn't improving his cholesterol numbers, however, so he was willing to give the new eating plan a try, along with making the heart-healthy lifestyle changes discussed in the next chapter. We emphasized that he should continue to limit or avoid saturated fat (the kind in fast food), which is extremely unhealthy for all Apo E genotypes—and to focus only on increasing heart-healthy oils.

Little by little, Patrick's lipid levels began to improve and his inflammatory markers fell. Much to his amazement, says the now-42-year-old CPA, "I was able to fight high cholesterol without a pill, when I thought that without a statin, I was headed for a heart attack." These days, he adds, "I have total confidence that I'm on the right track to better health, because all of my numbers look terrific." Patrick's total cholesterol-to-HDL ratio is now optimal at 3.0 and his arterial age had dropped from 70 to a number that's close to his chronological age.

The main reason that a conventional Mediterranean-style diet has been found to reduce risk for heart attacks and strokes as well as memory-robbing disorders like Alzheimer's disease—despite containing about 25 percent fat—is that it contains the ideal balance of fats, carbs, and protein for people with the Apo E 3/3 genotype, which is found in 62 percent of the population, and for those with the Apo E 2/4 genotype, found in 2 percent of the population. In other words, since about two-thirds of participants in these studies have a genetic make-up that responds favorably to the balance of fats, carbs, and protein in a conventional Mediterranean diet, it's not surprising that on average, people who follow it have excellent health outcomes in large studies.

There's a one in three chance, however, that you have a genotype that does *not* benefit from this specific balance of fats, carbs, and proteins. Or you may even be harmed by some components of the traditional Mediterranean diet, as was the case with Katharina Friehe, the hard-partying young CPA you met in Chapter Ten, who was eating too much cheese (and other high-fat foods) and drinking too much alcohol for her high-risk Apo E genotype—and was further escalating the danger by smoking. As a result, at age 25, she already had the arteries of a 55-year-old woman. In fact, her arteries were "older" than her mom was!

Katharina's dad, Berend, is another case in point. He assumed that the low-carb, high-protein Atkins-style diet he had adopted after suffering a transient ischemic attack (also called a ministroke) would lower his risk for the two problems he feared most: stroke and dementia. Actually, the best dietary bet for people with his Apo E 4/4 genotype, which confers the highest cardiovascular risk of all of the Apo E genotypes, is following exactly the opposite approach: a diet that's low in fat (containing 20 percent fat from healthy oils) and high in complex carbs, such as fruits, vegetables, and whole grains.

How Your Apo E Genotype Affects Your Health

As you learned in Chapter Ten, the Apo E gene has three variants: Apo E 2, Apo E 3, and Apo E 4. Since genes come in pairs, one inherited from each of your parents, there are six possible combinations: Apo E 2/2, Apo E 2/3, Apo E 3/3, Apo E 2/4, Apo E 3/4, and Apo E 4/4. These combinations are usually grouped as follows: You're considered an Apo E 2 if you have the Apo E 2/2 or Apo E 2/3 genotype; an Apo E 3 if you have the Apo E 3/3 or Apo E 2/4 genotype; or Apo E 4 if you have the Apo E 3/4 or 4/4 genotype. For example, if you inherited an Apo E 3 gene from each of your parents, as Patrick did, you'd have the Apo E 3 genotype, found in 64 percent of the population. This genotype is linked to intermediate lifetime risk for cardiovascular disease and is considered to have a "neutral" effect on how your body metabolizes fat.

The Apo E 2 and Apo E 4 genes have opposing effects on your lipid levels. The Apo E 2 gene slows down conversion of intermediate-density lipoprotein (a type of cholesterol particle) into LDL (bad) cholesterol. As a result, people with the Apo E 2 genotype, found in 11 percent of the population, tend to have lower total cholesterol on average than other genotypes—a key reason that these two genotypes are linked to the lowest lifetime risk for CVD. (See the table on page 195 for a summary of the health effects of each Apo E genotype in detail.)

Some people with the Apo E 2 genotype, however, have very high levels of triglycerides—and often receive dangerously faulty dietary advice for their genotype, since healthcare providers typically tell everybody with high triglycerides to cut down on fat. This seemingly healthy tactic actually puts people with this genotype in *increased* danger for suffering a heart attack. That's because, paradoxically, their levels of small, dense LDL particles (the extremely bad cholesterol that triples heart attack risk) *increase* if they follow a low-fat diet. Instead, research demonstrates that patients with these genotypes get the best cardiovascular benefit from cutting down on carbs, which helps reduce their level of LDL and the quantity of small, dense LDL particles.

If you have the Apo E 2 genotype, aim for about 35 percent fat in diet (from healthy oils). You're also likely to see improvements in both your LDL and HDL levels if you consume moderate amounts of alcohol (no more than one drink per day for women and two for men). Although it's often claimed that red wine is particularly good for the heart because it contains resveratrol, this is a myth. In fact, red wine only contains a miniscule amount of resveratrol and doesn't offer any greater cardiovascular benefit than do other forms of alcohol. All forms of alcohol have similar effects on LDL and HDL.

It's important to remember, however, that although moderate alcohol use may be good for your heart, it can also have health risks. For example, consuming even one alcoholic drink daily increases women's risk for breast cancer and may also raise risk for liver or rectal cancer. If you drink alcohol, discuss the potential risks and benefits with your healthcare provider. And if you don't normally drink alcohol, don't start. As you'll learn in this chapter and the next one, there are many other ways to keep your heart healthy.

The Apo E 4 genotype is associated with the highest lifetime risk for CVD and inhibits the ability of HDL (good) cholesterol to bind to LDL (bad) cholesterol. Like a vacuum cleaner, HDL normally scoops up LDL cholesterol particles that are traveling through the bloodstream and transports them to the liver for disposal. In people with the Apo E 4 genotype (found in 25 percent of the population), HDL is less effective at removing excessive LDL from the blood vessels. As a result, there's more LDL circulating in the bloodstream and a greater likelihood that bad cholesterol will penetrate the arterial walls and form plaque.

A low-fat diet (about 20 percent fat, from healthy oils) is the best cardiovascular defense for carriers of the Apo E 4 genotype. Switching to this eating plan was one of the lifestyle modifications that Berend used to dramatically turn his health around, despite having previously believed himself to be "doomed" to suffer a debilitating stroke or develop dementia, as his mother did. Like many other people with the Apo E 4 genotype, Berend had high triglycerides and other lipid abnormalities—problems that he has now conquered through a diet tailored to his DNA and other lifestyle modifications, including losing 30 pounds. In the next section of the chapter, we'll reveal the most-effective strategies to achieve—and maintain—a healthy weight.

How Apo E Genotype Affects Response to Diet and Exercise

	Apo E 2	Apo E 3	Apo E 4
Population prevalence estimates	10%	65%	25%
Carbohydrate-rich diet	may worsen lipids	neutral	may help lipids
High-fat diet (even good fats)	may help lipids	neutral	may worsen lipids

Daily moderate alcohol intake	may help lipids	neutral	may worsen lipids
Protein – low-fat protein	lower LDL	lower LDL	lower LDL
Exercise	extra benefit	neutral	moderate

Secrets of Long-Term Weight Loss

Americans have a huge problem: Currently, about 70 percent of adults (and nearly 32 percent of kids) in this country are overweight or obese. If you have a body mass index (BMI) of 25 to 29, you qualify as overweight, while a BMI of 30 or above is defined as obese. Your BMI is calculated by using this formula: Weight in pounds divided by height in inches squared, with the result of that calculation multiplied by a conversion factor of 703. Round off the result to the first decimal. For example, if you are 5'5" (65 inches) and weigh 160 pounds, you'd do the following calculation: $[160 \div (65)^2] \times 703 = 26.6$ (overweight).

If you're a woman who is 5'5", a healthy weight is 114 to 144 pounds, which corresponds to a BMI of 19 to 24. You're overweight at 150 pounds (a BMI of 25) and obese at 180 pounds (a BMI of 30). If you're a man who is 5'10", a healthy weight is 132 to 167 pounds, while you're overweight at 174 pounds and obese at 202. As we've emphasized in previous chapters, a large waistline, even if your weight is normal, is another indication that you need to slim down.

Obesity is rapidly overtaking smoking as the leading cause of preventable death in the United States. Here are some frightening ways carrying around too many pounds can steal your health:

- In the Framingham Heart Study, being overweight boosted risk for heart failure by 34 percent; being obese more than doubled it. For each one-point rise in BMI, the threat of heart failure rose by 5 to 7 percent. Obesity stresses the heart, because it has to work harder to supply blood to all the extra fatty tissue.

- Excess pounds in the abdomen double the threat of developing type 2 diabetes. Shedding as little as 10 to 15 pounds—and exercising more—can often prevent the disease, even if you're already prediabetic.

- If you're obese, your risk for high blood pressure—the leading risk factor for stroke—nearly triples. Obesity frequently sparks chronic inflammation—the fire in the arteries that ignites heart attacks and strokes—and also magnifies risk for metabolic syndrome, insulin resistance, high cholesterol, and sleep apnea. Slimming down, even a little bit, shrinks the danger.

New research suggests that banishing unwanted pounds for good could be less difficult than you think. The key is to outsmart your hunger hormones, by making easy changes in your daily habits that have proved highly effective in large, long-term studies. For example, the members of the National Weight Control Registry (NWCR), an ongoing study of more than 10,000 people, have lost an average of 66 pounds and kept it off for 5.5 years. Some members have dropped 200 or even 300 pounds.

How did they do it? Here's the skinny on seven science-backed weight-loss strategies that have proven remarkably successful in the NWCR and other studies:

1. Keep a food diary. One of our patients told us that she finally got her weight under control by going on what she calls "the BLT diet," recording every bite, lick, and taste of food she took during the day. A study by Kaiser Permanente's Center for Health Research reported that people who kept a daily food diary lost twice as much weight as those who didn't track what they consumed, probably because the act of recording holds you accountable for your food choices.

2. Avoid skipping meals. An 11-year study recently demonstrated that skipping meals *raises* risk for obesity, while an even newer study found that overweight or obese women who ate regular meals, while following a 12-month reduced-calorie diet and exercise program, dropped about eight more pounds than those who skipped meals. Breakfast is a particularly important meal: about 80 percent of the NWCR members report that they eat breakfast every day, reducing the temptation to overeat later in the day.

3. Eat more to weigh less. While that advice may sound counterintuitive, a review of 17 earlier studies reported that filling up on "low-density" foods (those with more water and fewer calories per serving, such as vegetables) is crucial to weight control, while trying to limit yourself to small portions of higher-calorie foods is a recipe for dieting failure. Another recent study found that people who ate a three-cup, low-density salad before a meal consumed 8 percent fewer calories during the meal than those who ate a smaller salad with high-fat ingredients. Drinking water before meals can also help curb your appetite.

4. Love your body. Being unhappy with what you see in the mirror can sabotage your efforts to slim down. Conversely, improving your body image—and learning to love your looks despite the extra pounds—can more than triple your success with a weight-loss program based on dieting and exercise, according to a 2011 study. While you might think that people who were unhappy with their appearance would be *more* motivated to lose weight, the researchers found that dieters who dislike their bodies are more prone to unhealthy eating patterns, such as binge eating and emotional overeating.

5. Have self-compassion. Being able to forgive yourself for indulging in a high-calorie treat helps you avoid the vicious cycle of negative feelings that can trigger emotional overeating and weight gain. An intriguing study at Wake Forest University looked at the effects of self-compassion on candy consumption. College students, including current dieters, were told they would be participating in a taste test of various candies. Some students were required to eat a donut before the taste test. Those who were encouraged to forgive themselves for downing the donut ate far less candy during the taste test than those who felt guilty about breaking their diet with the donut.

6. Weigh yourself regularly. About 75 percent of NWCR members checked their weight at least once a week to make sure they were still on track with their weight goal. Recording your weight in your food diary is another way to hold yourself accountable for your food choices—as well as to celebrate your successes.

7. Move more. Nine out of 10 NWCR members average an hour of exercise a day, and 62 percent watch fewer than 10 hours of TV a week. Daily physical activity is beneficial for all Apo E genotypes. To make exercise a daily habit, look for a variety of activities—dancing, playing tennis, cycling, or a Wii fitness game—you can enjoy regardless of the weather. If your lifestyle is currently sedentary, talk to your healthcare provider about the best ways to get in shape. Workouts need not be strenuous to keep your weight down and enhance your heart health: the most commonly reported physical activity in the NWCR was walking, which has truly amazing cardiovascular benefits.

As you'll discover in the next chapter, any form of physical activity, including sex, torches calories, and helps keep every cell in your body younger and healthier. We'll also tell you easy actions you can take on your own to enhance cardiovascular wellness.

An Easy Exercise to Add Years to Your Life

Workouts don't have to be long and grueling to improve your cardiovascular health—and significantly lengthen your life. In fact, a recent study of more than 416,000 men and women reported that those who exercised at moderate intensity for as little as 15 minutes a day lived an average of three years longer than people who were inactive. An even newer study found that getting 22 minutes of moderate exercise daily (or working out vigorously for 11 minutes) trims the risk of developing heart disease by 14 percent. The new research was based on an analysis of 33 earlier studies and was the first ever to quantify the exact amount of physical activity necessary to get a cardiovascular benefit.

Other studies suggest that for every minute you spend walking, you increase your life expectancy by 1.5 to 2 minutes. Many studies show that people who walk regularly weigh less, have lower blood pressure, live longer, and enjoy better moods and overall health than nonwalkers. Simply clipping on a pedometer can provide powerful motivation to move more: This easy action prompted people to take up to 2,491 extra steps per day (about 1.25 miles), according to a recent analysis of 26 earlier studies involving 2,767 people, most of whom were overweight and sedentary at the start of the research.

Here are seven compelling reasons, backed by solid science, to lace up your shoes and start walking, right now:

- A healthier heart. Middle-aged or older women who walked briskly for three or more hours weekly decreased their risk for heart disease by up to 40 percent, according to an analysis of health data from more than 72,000 women enrolled in the Harvard Nurses' Health Study. Another recent study found that for elderly men, brisk walking cuts risk for coronary heart disease by 50 percent.

- Reduced diabetes risk. Just 30 minutes of daily walking helps ward off type 2 diabetes—even in people at high risk for developing the disease, according to a 13-year study in which participants' blood-sugar levels were tracked with oral-glucose tolerance tests. If you already have diabetes, walking one or more miles daily cuts 10-year risk for death from *all* causes by 50 percent!

- Protection against stroke. A study of more than 11,000 Harvard alumni (average age: 58) reported that those who walked 12.5 or more miles per week had a 50-percent lower risk for stroke.

- Lower blood pressure and achieve a slimmer waist. In a twelve-week study, previously sedentary people who walked briskly for 30 minutes a day, five days a week, whittled their waist circumference by about an inch and enjoyed a six-point drop in systolic blood pressure (the top number). In addition, they also reduced their hip measurement by about an inch.

- Torching calories. Walking for 30 minutes a day burns about 150 calories. Over a year, that adds up to a weight loss of nearly 16 pounds.

- Sounder slumber. When overweight or obese women ages 50 to 74 began taking a brisk, 45-minute walk every morning, they reported a 70 percent improvement in sleep quality. The researchers theorized that morning walks help set the body's clocks for better rest at night.

- Dispelling tension and depression. Walking and other forms of exercise are also excellent stress-busters, reducing the toxic toll that chronic tension could otherwise take on your cardiovascular health. Research published in *British Journal of Sports Medicine* also reported that walking regularly boosted mood more quickly than did antidepressants (with fewer side effects).

Action Step: Lift Your Lifestyle to the Next Level

Did you know that sex, chocolate, listening to music, and watching comedies can all be prescriptions for a healthier heart? As you'll learn in the next chapter, a variety of simple lifestyle changes offer remarkably powerful protection against a heart attack, cutting risk by up to 800 percent. Some of the easy—often enjoyable—actions we suggest may surprise or even delight you. We'll also alert you to best—and worst—supplements for heart health and which medications may be prescribed if you have coronary artery disease or major risk factors that can't be adequately controlled with lifestyle alone.

If you smoke, you'll learn the most effective ways to kick the habit for good, including two highly successful tactics that you probably haven't tried before. You'll also discover which strategies work best to defuse stress, improve your mood, and help you get a better night's sleep. Go to the next page to learn how to relax and enjoy greater cardiovascular wellness.

Chapter 13

Lift Your Lifestyle to the Next Level

"Moderation in all things, including moderation."

—Attributed to Petronius, Roman writer, ca. A.D. 27–66

Alysia Buob's father suffered a heart attack when he was in his mid-40s, but until recently she didn't consider herself at risk. "My dad was husky, with a big, round belly, and used to smoke, so I've always assumed that was why he had a heart attack at such a young age." says the 44-year-old registered nurse, a non-smoker who stays lean and fit with daily jogging. "The heart attack happened while he was in his cardiologist's office, during a treadmill test. It was a miracle that he survived, because the blockage was in an area called the 'widow-maker.'"

After she turned 40, Alysia began noticing health glitches. During one annual checkup, her blood sugar measured in the prediabetic range. "That was very scary, knowing what my dad went through when he developed type 2 diabetes after the heart attack," recalls the RN. "I've always felt that diabetes seems like a slow-motion train wreck, because it can destroy people's health in so many terrible ways."

When her family doctor repeated the blood-sugar test a few months later, Alysia was extremely relieved when the results came back normal. But she remained concerned about her cholesterol levels, which were getting higher every year. "I felt I needed to be more proactive about my health," says the mom of two. She decided to follow the prevention plan we'd advised for her husband, Patrick, profiled in Chapter Twelve, who is unable to take cholesterol-lowering medication because of adverse reactions. Over the next six months, Alysia's total cholesterol dropped by 20 points.

In this chapter, you'll learn which supplements are best for the heart—including those that helped Alysia lower her cholesterol levels without medication—and which vitamins and minerals may actually be hazardous. Some of the options we suggest may surprise or even delight you, such as the daily "dose" of dark chocolate that we often "prescribe" to enhance cardiovascular wellness, based on recent studies documenting the sweet treat's many health benefits.

Why a Personalized Treatment Plan Is Important

Although Alysia was delighted to see her cholesterol numbers improve, she wondered if following a prevention plan we'd specifically designed for her husband was the best way to manage *her* cardiovascular risks. As it turned out, when she finally came to our clinic for a comprehensive evaluation, she had three disorders that *don't* affect Patrick:

- Insulin resistance (IR), the root cause of type 2 diabetes and 70 percent of heart attacks. In this chapter and the next one, we'll look at treatments for this extremely common condition, including the best workouts, a delicious spice that's probably already in your kitchen, and if necessary, medication. We also advise all of our patients with IR to "eat like a diabetic so you never become one," by watching carbs and limiting or avoiding sugary foods.

- An inherited cholesterol disorder. An advanced lipid profile test revealed that Alysia had high levels of lipoprotein (a), the "mass murderer" that triples heart attack risk. As discussed in earlier chapters, elevated levels of this cholesterol have been shown to cause heart attacks and strokes, often at an unusually young age. That meant Alysia's self-treatment was only addressing part of her cholesterol problem. Later in this chapter, you'll discover which inexpensive vitamin can be helpful for a lipoprotein (a) problem and other cholesterol issues.

- An autoimmune disease that can affect heart health. Alysia was under the care of a specialist for Hashimoto's disease, an autoimmune disorder triggered by inflammation of the thyroid, resulting in an underactive thyroid. As discussed in Chapter Twelve, having low levels of thyroid hormones more than doubled the threat of a cardiovascular event in one study, while another, much larger study found that over a 35-year-period, hypothyroidism boosted risk for a fatal heart attack by 50 percent. Adding to Alysia's danger, she had elevated levels of inflammatory markers, indicating "fire" in her arteries.

In some ways, however, Alysia and her husband were remarkably alike. They shared the same Apo E 3/3 genotype, explaining why Alysia had benefited from following the diet we'd advised for Patrick: by chance, she was eating the ideal diet for her DNA. The couple was also shocked to discover that, amazingly, they were both carriers of the 9P21 heart attack gene. Understandably, they were immediately concerned about their daughters: Maggie, 15, and Olivia, 12. "It was scary to think that we might have passed this terrible gene on to our girls, then we realized that by catching this potential risk so early, we could instill the healthiest possible habits as our girls were growing up," says Alysia.

When we checked Maggie's arterial health with a cIMT scan, the teen was already showing very early signs of being on the fast track to blood-vessel disease, despite being slim and athletic. At age 15, Maggie had an arterial age of 30—but no plaque in her arteries. The Buobs plan to bring both of their daughters to our clinic for a comprehensive cardiovascular evaluation that may include genetic testing when the girls reach age 18. Meanwhile, Maggie and Olivia's health, which is currently excellent, is being monitored by their pediatrician, who has been alerted to Maggie's cIMT results.

The entire family is now following an intensive personalized prevention plan that includes a diet based on their DNA and heart-healthy lifestyle changes discussed in this chapter. "Sometimes our girls gripe about not being able to eat fried foods, but the other day, Maggie told a friend that he should eat more vegetables—and less junk food—so while it's tough to change a kid's diet, the choices we're making as a family are having an impact on reducing our daughters' risk—and our own," says the mom. "We're very thankful to be empowered by this knowledge."

The Top 10 Ways to Boost Your Heart Health

Did you know that all five of your senses can play a role in enhancing your cardiovascular wellness? A variety of activities—from listening to your favorite music to watching a hilarious video on YouTube, or getting a relaxing massage with aromatherapy oils—can do your heart good. You'll also want to discover the surprising cardiovascular benefits of consuming moderate amounts dark chocolate.

If you smoke, please read our tips at the end of this section on the most effective ways to snuff out this deadly addiction that's responsible for 443,000 preventable deaths a year in the U.S. We've included some proven strategies to kick the tobacco habit that you probably *haven't* tried before and advice on how to avoid gaining weight when you quit.

Here's a look at 10 easy actions and lifestyle changes—many of which are relaxing and enjoyable—that do your heart good.

1. Sleep six to eight hours a night.

     Snoozing fewer than six hours a night doubles heart attack and stroke risk, and boosts the threat of congestive heart failure by 70 percent, compared to catching six to eight hours of ZZZ's per night, according to a 2012 study of more than 3,000 people. Other recent research links skimping on slumber to higher risk for obesity and diabetes. Among the best ways to improve sleep naturally are having a consistent bedtime and wake-up time, even on weekends; avoiding watching TV in the bedroom; dimming the lights and avoiding computer use during the hour before bed; taking a warm, relaxing bath in the evening and scenting your pillow with lavender, a soothing aroma with a well-deserved reputation for improving sleep quality. Sleep doctors call these relaxing rituals and habits "good sleep hygiene."

2. Nibble on dark chocolate.

   Amazing, but true: Eating dark chocolate could actually help save your life. A recent study published in *European Heart Journal* reports that people who ate an average of 7.5 grams of chocolate a day were 27 percent less likely to have heart attacks and 48 percent less likely to have strokes than those who ate less than one gram per day, even after risk factors were taken into account. The researchers tracked more than 19,000 people for an average of eight years. An even larger study reported that eating chocolate trimmed the risk for diabetes by 31 percent, while other studies found beneficial effects on cholesterol levels, blood pressure, and insulin resistance.

   We recommend eating one or two squares (7 to 10 grams) of dark chocolate that is at least 72 percent cocoa daily, a "prescription" for better heart health that the Buobs—and our other patients—are delighted to follow. Dark chocolate contains powerful disease-fighting antioxidants called flavonols, which are also found in tea, wine, and certain fruits and vegetables. Since the small amount of chocolate we recommend only contains 30 to 50 calories—and very little sugar—it's as healthy for people with insulin resistance, like Alysia. When we talk to patients about this "prescription," we often say, "Not all pills are hard to swallow." Don't bother with white or milk chocolate for health benefits, since they don't contain the flavonols you need.

3. Keep your cells young with at least 22 minutes of daily physical activity.

   Two groundbreaking new studies reveal *why* exercise offers powerful protection against chronic diseases like diabetes, cardiovascular disease, and cancer—and also helps people live longer and feel more youthful. Physical activity enhances "autophagy," the process cells use to clear out debris (such as broken-down cellular components) and recycle it as fuel. Without this housekeeping process, which literally means "self-eating," cells would become choked with trash and die. Slowing down of autophagy is linked to a wide range of diseases and also is believed to play a major role in aging.

   Exercise also helps our cells stay young in another way: by preventing premature cellular senescence, a form of accelerated aging. Senescence, a medical term meaning that cells have lost their ability to divide, is a normal aging process. As we get older, telomeres (caps at the end of chromosomes that protect DNA, much like the plastic caps on at the ends of shoelaces) become shorter and shorter, until the cells are no longer able to divide, leading to their death. Senescence can occur prematurely as a result of oxidative stress, the "rusting" process that produces health-damaging free radicals. This can happen to arterial cells, such as those in the endothelium and smooth muscle cells. That's dangerous, because senescence makes cells become highly inflammatory, which can drive the atherosclerotic disease process, leading to heart attacks and strokes at an unusually young age.

   These biochemical discoveries add to an important insight from the Women's Health Study. After observing that women who exercise regularly had a significantly lower risk of developing CVD, the researchers analyzed the reasons for this benefit. While physical activity improved both cholesterol levels and blood pressure, by far the biggest benefit of keeping fit was a dramatic reduction in inflammatory markers. This finding, taken together with the new research, suggests that regular physical activity enhances natural firefighting processes at the cellular level *and* keeps your body young.

4. Battle belly fat and insulin resistance with interval training.

If you have insulin resistance or metabolic syndrome (which often includes too much belly fat), research shows that the best way to combat these problems is interval training, in which you alternate bouts of more intense exercise with intervals of lighter activity. For example, you might include short bursts of jogging or sprinting in a brisk walk. In one recent study of obese and overweight people, this type of exercise resulted in overall weight loss, a slimmer waist, an improved triglyceride-to-HDL ratio, and a 32.5 percent reduction in rates of metabolic syndrome.

Concerned about risk for type 2 diabetes? You can reduce the threat by up to 70 percent by improving your fitness level, a recent study of nearly 5,000 men suggests. You should also realize that every extra 500 calories you burn up in a week reduces the risk of progressing to diabetes by 6 percent. Other research demonstrates that within a few months of starting a program of regular interval training, insulin sensitivity typically improves significantly. If you haven't been working out regularly, talk to your healthcare provider about what level of exercise intensity is appropriate for you.

5. Sexual activity is safe—and healthy—for most heart patients.

It's very common for people with cardiovascular disease (CVD), particularly those who have already suffered a heart attack or have undergone heart procedures, such as bypass surgery, to worry that engaging in sexual activity might be dangerous. Because of such fears, heart patients often assume, mistakenly in most cases, that they must resign themselves to a celibate life. A major reason for this common misconception, the American Heart Association reported in its first-ever scientific statement addressing this issue, is that healthcare providers rarely discuss sexual matters. In fact, during the year following a heart attack, one study reported that less than 40 percent of men and less than 20 percent of women talked to their provider about sexual activity.

"We would not want to see patients refraining from sex out of undue concern about precipitating a heart attack or sudden death," stated Dr. Glenn Levine, the lead author of the 2012 AHA statement, which addresses several topics that patients with CVD may be embarrassed to ask their healthcare provider. Among the highlights:

- It's usually safe for patients with stable CVD to have sex. The AHA encourages healthcare providers to evaluate patients after a CVD diagnosis and let them know if they're healthy enough to resume sexual activity.

- People with severe heart disease that triggers symptoms (such as chest pain) during minimal physical activity, such as walking short distances, or while they're at rest should refrain from sex until their symptoms have been treated and stabilized. In the next chapter, you'll find a guide to medications that are commonly used to treat heart disease and its major risk factors.

- Contrary to urban legend, the rate of cardiovascular events, such as chest pain or a heart attack, during sex is "miniscule," even among people with known CVD, the AHA emphasizes.

- Drugs to treat erectile dysfunction (such as Viagra, Levitra, and Cialis) are usually safe for men with stable CVD. Men who are receiving nitrate therapy for angina (chest pain due to coronary artery disease), however, should not use these medications because of potentially harmful drug interactions.

- It's usually safe for postmenopausal women with CVD to use topical estrogen cream to treat vaginal symptoms, such as dryness or pain during intercourse. Relatively little estrogen from topical vaginal cream is absorbed into the bloodstream, compared to taking estrogen orally in pill form.

6. Avoid sugary drinks.

A long-term study of more than 42,000 men, ages 40 to 75, found that those who swilled sugar-sweetened beverages the most often were 20 percent more likely to suffer heart attacks. The researchers also calculated that having just one 12-ounce sweet drink a daily boosted the relative risk of developing CVD by 19 percent—and was also linked to adverse changes in levels of HDL, triglycerides, and the inflammatory marker C-reactive protein. Another large study reported similar harm in women who consumed sugary beverages.

Nor are diet soft drinks a healthy alternative. Drinking these beverages daily was linked to a 43 percent rise in heart attack, stroke, and death from vascular disease during the 10-year study of 2,500 adults older than age 40. The diet-soda drinkers were also more likely to have high blood sugar, high blood pressure, and rather ironically, larger waistlines than those who abstained from diet drinks. Other studies link daily diet soda consumption to a 67 percent jump in diabetes risk and a 53 percent rise in risk for metabolic syndrome.

Which beverages are heart-healthy? We recommend drinking eight glasses of water daily for healthy hydration with zero calories. Coffee also has a remarkable array of health perks, including reduced risk for heart disease, stroke, atrial fibrillation, diabetes, gallstones, several forms of cancer, and even superbug infections like MRSA (methicillin-resistant *Staphylococcus aureus*). Caffeine is a powerful natural antioxidant that has proven beneficial in several cardiovascular studies. A recent review suggests that drinking up to four 8-ounce cups of coffee per day appears to be safe.

Another delicious and invigorating beverage is green tea, which not only improves the health of your blood vessel lining and fights inflammation, but also lowers risk for gum disease and at least nine forms of cancer. Green and black tea both come from the same plant, but green tea has three times more catechins, a type of disease-fighting antioxidant. Hibiscus tea is another thirst-quencher with cardiovascular benefits, since it's been shown to lower blood pressure significantly.

7. Feast on fiber.

Increasing the amount of fiber in your diet could add years to your life, suggests a recent nine-year study of nearly 400,000 adults ages 50 and older. Researchers from the National Institutes of Health reported that men who ate the most fiber were up to 56 percent less likely to die from CVD, infectious diseases, or respiratory disorders, compared to men who ate the least fiber. In women, a high-fiber diet cut risk for mortality from those causes by 58 percent.

Among the most beneficial sources of fiber are whole grains, fruits, and vegetables. In fact, for each additional serving of fruits and vegetables people eat daily, their risk of fatal cardiovascular disease drops by 4 percent, another large study found. Those who consumed at least eight servings of about three ounces apiece had a 25 percent drop in cardiovascular mortality, compared to people who ate fewer than three portions. Intriguingly, eating an apple a day really does keep the doctor away, since consuming white fruits and vegetables—including apples, pears, and cauliflower—was linked to a 52 percent drop in 10-year stroke risk in a recent European study.

8. Take vacations and relaxation breaks.

Research shows remarkably powerful cardiovascular benefits from taking time off from work to kick back and recharge. An analysis of Framingham Heart Study data found that women who take vacations once every six years—or less often—were nearly eight times more likely to suffer a heart attack or die from cardiac causes than those who vacationed at least twice a year, even when such factors as smoking and diabetes were taken into account. A nine-year study that tracked 12,000 middle-aged men at high risk for heart disease reported that those who regularly took annual getaways had a 29 percent lower rate of cardiovascular mortality. The researchers theorized that stress reduction may explain the benefits of annual vacations.

Since chronic stress takes a toll on cardiovascular health, it's also important to have coping strategies that you're able to use every day. Here are some stress-busters that do wonders for both your heart and your mood:

- Laughter. It's no joke: a good laugh expands blood vessels and increases blood flow to the heart, a recent study found. Laughter yoga, which combines deep yogic breathing and self-triggered mirth is also a great ways to relax after a stressful day. A recent study also found that after just three weeks of laughter yoga, study participants had significant drops in blood pressure.

- Have a cup of tea. British researchers found that people who drank black tea were able to relax after a stressful task more quickly than those who drank a fake tea substitute. In addition, the tea drinkers had lower levels of the stress hormone cortisol and less blood platelet activation (linked to blood clots and heart risk) after a tension-inducing event.

- Play your favorite song. Listening to enjoyable music (this will vary from one individual to another) can dilate (widen) arteries, increasing blood flow as much as statin medication or aerobic exercise, according to a study presented at the American Heart Association 2008 Scientific Sessions. Music also has beneficial effects on blood pressure and heart rate— but only if you listen to classical or meditation music. The study suggested that heavy metal or techno music is ineffective.

9. Get a flu shot.

   Adults who are vaccinated against influenza have a 50 percent reduction in cardiovascular mortality, a large study found. The researchers also report that up to 91,000 Americans die each year from cardiovascular events triggered by the flu. Another recent study reported that people who are vaccinated early in the flu season have a greater reduction in heart-attack risk than those who wait until mid-November to get the shot.

   And here's even more motivation to get immunized against flu: Doing so also lowers the risk of getting a blood clot in your lungs (pulmonary embolism) or in your legs (deep vein thrombosis). The Centers for Disease Control currently recommends an annual flu shot for everyone except infants under six months of age, but cautions that certain people should check with a healthcare provider before being immunized. These patients include those with a severe allergy to chicken eggs, people who have had a severe reaction to a flu shot, and patients who are ill with a fever (they should wait until they've recovered to get vaccinated).

   Based on the latest science, we also recommend two other vaccinations if you are 50 or older and have arterial disease. That's because any viral or bacterial infection sparks cause inflammation, the fire in the arteries that can cause the cat in the gutter to leap out and trigger a heart attack or stroke. Therefore, it's crucial to protect yourself against vaccine-preventable diseases that drive inflammation. If you *don't* have atherosclerosis, you should still get these shots, but at an older age, as discussed below.

   Everyone who is 60 or older—and those who are 50 or older with arterial disease—should get the herpes zoster vaccination against shingles. This shot protects against reactivation of the chickenpox virus that almost everyone was exposed to during childhood. The virus, which lies dormant in your nerve cells, can flare up, typically in older people, and cause a blistering skin rash that can lead to chronic nerve pain.

   Not only does vaccination reduce risk for shingles and its painful complications by about 70 percent, but it also helps protect against stroke. Two large studies report that people who develop shingles are at up to four times higher risk for stroke, highlighting the value of vaccination against the virus that causes this disease. While shingles usually targets people who are 60 or older, about 20 percent of cases occur in those who 50 to 59, which is why we advise being vaccinated at 50 if you have CVD.

If you're 65 or older, or younger with risk factors for pneumonia—such as heart failure, chronic pulmonary disease, or diabetes—the CDC advises being immunized against pneumococcal pneumonia. A study of more than 84,000 people found that those who had been vaccinated against this disease were at lower risk for both heart attack and stroke. Given these benefits, we recommend being vaccinated at age 50 if you have CVD.

10. Avoid secondhand smoke.

Secondhand smoke kills more than 42,000 nonsmokers a year, according to a scary 2012 University of California, San Francisco, study. Most of these fatalities (34,000) are due to heart disease, the researchers reported. More frightening facts: tobacco fumes contain hundreds of toxins, at least 70 of which are known to cause cancer. Exposure to secondhand smoke boosts risk for heart disease by up to 30 percent, while smoking quadruples the danger.

Surprising Ways to Quit Smoking

More than three million Americans kick the tobacco habit every year—and you can, too. Need some motivation? Within 20 minutes of quitting, your heart rate and blood pressure drop, and within 24 hours, carbon monoxide levels in your blood fall to normal. After one to nine months, shortness of breath decreases and you'll cough less. One year after you quit, your risk for heart disease is half that of a continuing smoker—and after five years, your risk for several types of cancer drops by 50 percent.

More reasons to stop playing with fire *right now*: smoking as little as one cigarette a day raises risk for heart disease by 63 percent and puffing 20 or more cigarettes daily more than quadruples it. Smoking also doubles stroke danger and accelerates aging and contributes to chronic inflammation. This deadly addiction also boosts the threat of developing peripheral artery disease (narrowed arteries that reduce blood flow to the extremities, such as the legs), abdominal aortic aneurysm (a weak, ballooning area in the heart's main artery that could rupture), diabetes, chronic obstructive lung disease (COPD), and cancer.

What's the best way to snuff out your last cigarette? It typically takes eight attempts to achieve success, so never give up trying. Also, 70 percent of smokers want to kick the habit, but don't know the most effective methods. While some people are able to quit cold turkey, the success rate is only 5 percent per attempt. Therefore, if this approach hasn't worked for you, we suggest that you talk to your healthcare provider about trying these following strategies, which have proven significantly more effective in large studies:

- Smoking cessation counseling. To find a program to help you quit smoking, try local hospitals, your health plan, the American Cancer Society, and other medical organizations; or ask your healthcare provider for recommendations. Generally, it's best to select a program that is at least four to eight weeks in length. The benefits of weekly counseling include support and actionable tips on how to combat cravings, cope with stress, and replace tobacco use with healthy habits.

- A smoking cessation program plus nicotine replacement. Combining nicotine replacement and a counseling program has a success rate of 20 to 40 percent, compared to a 10 percent success rate with nicotine replacement alone. Nicotine replacement can consist of a patch, gum, or spray used during the initial phase of quitting.

- Acupuncture. A 2012 review of 14 randomized clinical studies reported that smokers treated with acupuncture were 3.5 times more likely to be smoke-free 6 to 12 months later than those who received a fake treatment. These results compare favorably to medications for smoking cessation, which typically lift success rates by a factor of 2 to 2.5 (compared to taking a placebo). Acupuncture for smoking cessation typically involves treating specific acupoints on the ear, either with traditional thin needles or a laser that directs a low-energy beam at the area, creating a sensation of heat.

- Hypnosis. In the same review of studies, smokers treated with a few sessions of hypnotherapy were 4.5 times more likely to be abstinent from tobacco 6 to 12 months later than a control group who didn't receive treatment.

- Lifestyle modification. Regardless of which approach you use to quit, it's crucial to have strategies for curbing nicotine cravings. Among those most likely to be helpful are: replacing cigarette breaks with exercise breaks (such as a short, brisk walk) several times a day to cope with stress; munching on crunchy foods, such as carrot or celery sticks, sugar-free chewing gum or jellybeans; and drinking more water. Replace the "oral gratification" of smoking by taking excellent care of your teeth (with the dental care tips in the next chapter). Along with its many other health benefits, quitting smoking—or other forms of tobacco use, such as smokeless (chewing) tobacco—reduces risk for periodontal disease and brightens your smile.

The Best and Worst Supplements for Your Heart

Of the $20 billion Americans spend annually on dietary supplements, those promoted as good for the heart top the list. While some vitamins and minerals are extremely beneficial for cardiovascular health, others can be downright hazardous: In fact, one supplement that millions of Americans routinely pop can actually double the risk of dying from a heart attack, a 2012 study reported.

But it's not all bad news: as you'll discover in this section, one of the most beneficial supplements is an inexpensive vitamin that can dramatically improve cholesterol levels, combat chronic inflammation, and reduce risk for cardiovascular events by 90 percent, as we reported in a paper we published in *Journal of Cardiovascular Nursing*. Here are several supplements—including a delicious spice—with benefits supported by solid science, and three to avoid. *Before taking any dietary supplement, including vitamin pills, it's crucial to check with your healthcare provider, to make sure it's safe and appropriate for you. Some vitamins and supplements can have harmful interactions with certain medications.*

- Vitamins A and E

  Both of these antioxidant vitamins are essential for good health. However, when taken as supplements, they are not only ineffective for preventing cardiovascular disease but actually raise risk for early death, according to a review of 68 randomized trials involving 232,606 participants, published in *Journal of the American Medical Association (JAMA)*. Another alarming finding: In a placebo-controlled study of nearly 15,000 men, not only was there no cardiovascular benefit to taking 400 i.u. of vitamin E every other day, but supplement users had a significantly *higher* risk for hemorrhagic stroke during eight years of follow-up. And it gets worse: A 2005 study published in *Journal of the American Medical Association* linked vitamin E supplements to higher rates of heart failure during seven years of follow-up. Based on this research, we advise getting these vitamins through a healthy diet, rather than by popping supplements.

- Calcium

  Millions of postmenopausal women take calcium supplements to protect against osteoporosis (the brittle-bone disease that can lead to fracture in older people) and boost their bone health, but two large studies link these supplements to increased heart attack danger. A 2011 analysis of earlier studies, including data from about 30,000 women participating in the Women's Health Initiative, found that for every 1,000 women who popped calcium pills, there were six additional heart attacks or strokes, while only three fractures were prevented.

  After that study was published, we advised all of our patients to stop taking calcium supplements. Since then, evidence has continued to mount that taking calcium, with or without with vitamin D, can be hazardous. A large 2012 study reported that people taking supplements that included calcium were 86 percent more likely to have a heart attack, compared to people who didn't take any supplements, while participants who *only* took calcium had double the heart attack risk. Yet people who consumed a moderate amount of calcium in their diet had a 31 percent *lower* risk of heart attack.

  Confused? What this study is telling patients, in our opinion, is that getting too little or too much calcium is bad for your heart. Since calcium is a major building block of bone, with 99 percent of the body's calcium found in the skeleton, we recommend that you get this crucial mineral through your diet—not a pill. The best dietary sources include dairy products, canned fish with edible bones, green vegetables like broccoli, kale, and bok choy, nuts (especially almonds and Brazil nuts), and certain fruits, such as apricots, dried figs, and oranges. You can further protect your heart *and* bone health by avoiding smoking, which is a major risk factor for osteoporosis and osteopenia (bone thinning).

It's also imperative that both men and women get daily bone-building exercise, which can include a brisk walk, jogging, dancing, step aerobics, jumping rope, racquet sports, weight lifting, and other activities in which you work your muscles against gravity. We also recommend that women get a baseline DEXA (dual energy X-ray absorptiometry) scan prior to menopause to use as a baseline measurement, followed by periodic scans after menopause to check for bone loss. This test uses low-dose X-rays to measure bone density, typically in the hip and spine. Although osteoporosis is often thought of as a woman's disease, it can also affect men, particularly those with metabolic syndrome, insulin resistance, or type 2 diabetes. While there's no specific guideline for men, it's reasonable for men to have their bone density checked at age 60, or at a younger age if advised by their healthcare provider.

- Vitamin D

    For some people, preventing heart disease can be as simple as reversing vitamin D deficiency, which affects about 75 percent of U.S. adults and teens. A 2010 study reported that in 9,491 participants who were initially deficient in the sunshine vitamin, normalizing their D levels reduced one-year risk of heart failure, heart disease, and premature death by 30 percent. Another new study found that statin users with low levels of D are four times more likely to experience muscle pain (a common side effect of statin therapy). Treating the deficiency reduced symptoms in one-third of patients within eight weeks.

    Although the sunshine vitamin offers numerous heart-health benefits—including reducing arterial inflammation—it's also possible to get too much of a good thing, a recent study by researchers at Johns Hopkins found. A simple blood test is the best way to tell if a vitamin D supplement is likely to be helpful or harmful, since research shows that people with blood levels below 30 nanograms per milliliter (vitamin D deficiency) have increased cardiovascular risk, as do those with levels above 100 nmol.

    This inexpensive test, which is usually covered by insurance plans, revealed that the entire Buob family—particularly their kids—were vitamin D deficient, a problem they're now treating by taking supplements. Vitamin D is found in relatively few foods, such as cod liver oil, fatty fish, vitamin D–fortified milk, orange juice, or cereal, egg yolk, and cheese. Our bodies also produce D when we're out in the sun: In fact, 10 minutes in the sun provides as much vitamin D as 150 egg yolks! The vitamin D–boosting benefits of sun exposure, however, need to be balanced against the risk of skin cancer.

- Omega-3 Fatty Acids (Fish Oil)

  Supplementing with omega-3 fatty acids in the form of fish oil lowered the risk of heart disease and death from cardiovascular causes, especially in high-risk patients according to a review of 11 studies involving nearly 40,000 patients. The FDA has approved fish oil as a treatment for very high triglycerides, and we also recommend it for overall vascular wellness, based on large studies showing that it's beneficial for both primary prevention of heart disease and for reducing risk for cardiovascular events in people who already have arterial disease.

  We encourage our patients to get omega-3 fatty acid from eating fresh, fatty fish, such as salmon or herring, at least three times a week. Eating fish frequently has been shown to cut heart attack risk by one-third or more. For people who are unable to eat fish three or more times a week, we recommend daily omega-3 supplements containing up to two grams of combined EPA (eicosapentaenoic acid) and DHA (docosahexaenoic acid), the long-chain omega-3 fatty acids found in fish.

- Coenzyme Q-10 (CoQ-10)

  CoQ-10 is a vitamin-like compound with antioxidant properties that's found naturally in the body. It's an important element for cellular health. Supplements are sometimes necessary because some people have lower than normal levels, a problem that is particularly likely to occur in statin users. Several small clinical trials suggest that CoQ-10 supplements may help lower blood pressure, but it typically takes 4 to 12 weeks to notice any change. In studies of patients who have had a heart attack, those who took CoQ-10 daily, starting within three days of the event and continuing for one year, had significantly lower rates of chest pain, subsequent heart attacks, and deaths from heart disease. Two studies have found that daily CoQ-10 supplements improved blood-sugar levels in diabetics, while another study didn't find any effect. Along with being available as capsules, tablets, and a spray, CoQ-10 is also found in certain foods, including oily fish such as tuna and salmon, organ meats (like liver), and whole grains. There are two kinds of CoQ-10, ubiquinone and ubiquinol. We recommend that people on statins take a daily dose of ubiquinol of one mg per pound of the person's body weight. For example, if a patient weighed 200 pounds, we would recommend 200 mg of ubiquinol daily.

- Cinnamon

  Daily consumption of this tasty spice significantly reduced triglycerides, blood sugar, and LDL, while increasing good (HDL) cholesterol, in a very recent analysis that pooled results of 10 randomized studies involving 543 diabetic patients. Two studies published in 2009 found that cinnamon also improves insulin sensitivity in people without diabetes. Scientists at the Beltsville (Maryland) Human Nutrition Center have recently identified the compound in cinnamon responsible for this benefit, methylhydroxy chalcone polymer (MHCP), and report that it boosted glucose metabolism by about 20-fold in a test tube assay of fat cells. Glucose metabolism is the process in which cells convert blood sugar to energy. The scientists also demonstrated that MHCP has antioxidant properties. Based on this research, we recommend that patients with insulin resistance or diabetes take two grams of cinnamon daily, which is available in capsule form.

- Chromium

   This mineral helps control blood-sugar levels, so it can be helpful for people with insulin resistance or type 2 diabetes. Chromium plays a role in metabolism of proteins and fats, and transport of blood sugar to cells, where it's used for energy. Chromium is found in many foods, including brewer's yeast, liver, potatoes (especially the skin), cheese, molasses, whole grains, and some brands of cinnamon supplements or multivitamins.

- L-Carnitine

   Carnitine is naturally produced by the liver and kidneys. The body uses it to convert fat into energy. Several clinical trials show that L-carnitine supplements help reduce angina symptoms and increase the ability of patients with heart-related pain to exercise. A 2009 study reported that when patients took two grams of L-carnitine daily, along with the statin drug Zocor (simvastatin), for four months, levels of lipoprotein (a) were reduced by 30 percent. Lipoprotein (a), discussed in Chapter Eight, is the dangerous cholesterol we call "the mass murderer" because elevated levels triple risk for heart attacks. Since this inherited cholesterol disorder has also been shown, unequivocally, to actually cause heart attacks, you may be wondering if everybody with elevated Lp(a) should take L-carnitine. The answer is no. We only prescribe L-carnitine in the amount of two grams daily if a patient has elevated levels of lipoprotein (a) and also follows a strict vegan diet. Here's why we don't advise this supplement if you eat meat or dairy: Recent studies have shown that the oxidant trimethylamine N-oxide (TMAO) increases cardiovascular risk. People who are carnivores or eat dairy products produce bacteria in their gut that converts L-carnitine into TMAO. Therefore, they should avoid taking it.. Because L-carnitine can interact with certain medications, it's crucial to consult your healthcare provider before using this supplement, even if you are a vegan. Carnitine is found in red meat (particularly lamb), dairy products, fish, poultry, asparagus, wheat, avocados, and peanut butter.

- Niacin (vitamin B3)

   Unlike statin medications, which mainly reduce inflammation and levels of LDL "bad" cholesterol, niacin (vitamin B3) dramatically improves *all* lipid levels—including raising HDL "good" cholesterol and lowering levels of lipoprotein (a)—and also helps quell inflammation. Cholesterol-lowering treatment regimens that included niacin lowered risk of cardiovascular events by up to 90 percent in clinical trials (compared to the rate in people who took a placebo) and can also help slow progression of cardiovascular disease. Niacin is also a valuable treatment for most people with insulin resistance, since this inexpensive vitamin combats the vascular inflammation and complex lipid issues that often accompany insulin resistance.

Niacin, however, can have an uncomfortable (and usually temporary) side effect known as the "niacin flush." Medically termed "vasodilation," the niacin flush occurs when capillaries near the surface of the skin expand, creating a sensation of warmth that's often accompanied by blushing and reddening of skin all over the body. When used at therapeutic doses (500 to 2,000 mg), niacin should be taken under the supervision of a healthcare provider, who should monitor your response with lab tests and evaluation. Niacin can elevate blood sugar during the first three to six months of treatment, so it's important to track the effects on blood sugar, particularly if you are insulin resistant or diabetic. In most cases, blood sugar will subsequently return to the baseline level.

In the next chapter, we offer an in-depth patient guide to medications that are commonly prescribed for CVD or conditions that magnify the threat of developing it, such as high cholesterol, high blood pressure, insulin resistance/diabetes, and chronic inflammation. We'll also alert you to questions to ask before you swallow a pill, the pros and cons of various therapies, and which medications are likely to be most effective in common medical scenarios. You may also be startled to discover that many healthcare providers prescribe a newer heart medication even though an older one has been shown in multiple studies to offer superior heart-attack protection. And if you're taking medication because you're insulin resistant or prediabetic, you'll want to find out if you're taking the drug that has been shown to successfully halt progression to type 2 diabetes in 72 percent of cases, or one that only works 37 percent of the time.

Action Step: Find Out If You Need to Combine Lifestyle Changes with Medication

For many people, lifestyle modification is *not* enough, even for those as physically fit as our patient Wesley Robinson (also known as Superman, because of his muscular physique). As you read in an earlier chapter, his inflammatory markers soared when he quit taking his niacin (vitamin B3), putting him at high risk for a heart attack or stroke. That was a frightening wake-up call for Superman, who hadn't previously appreciated how even therapies as simple as a vitamin pill can dramatically decrease risk for cardiovascular events.

If you have arterial disease, the next chapter will alert you to four crucial treatments—including lifestyle changes—that can save your life. We'll also share one of our most remarkable success stories: how changes in medication helped one of our sickest patients avoid heart transplant surgery. A clinical trial involving nearly 500,000 patients showed that the strategy we advise—known as optimal medical care—was just as effective for preventing cardiovascular events and early death from cardiovascular disease as costly and potentially risky surgical procedures to reopen clogged arteries.

Whether you already have arterial disease or want to ensure that you never develop it, protecting your heart health requires individual management, using therapies specifically designed to help *you* achieve an optimal outcome. Keep reading to find out if you're getting the right treatments to conquer your cardiovascular risks.

14 Prescriptions for Better Cardiovascular Health

"A merry heart doeth good like medicine."

—King Solomon

Joe Inderman used to lead a very limited—and rather lonely—life. "People are meant to share their lives with others, but I didn't allow myself to even attempt a romantic relationship, because I wasn't healthy enough for *any* sustained physical activity, including sex or even going out on a date," says the divorced Texan, whom you met in Chapter Four. "I had such severe chest pain that I couldn't walk even one block without taking nitroglycerin—and I needed it so often that I actually had to ration the 100 nitroglycerin pills that my health plan let me have each month so I didn't run out."

Joe's symptoms were so severe that specialists advised heart transplant surgery. But the retired real estate broker balked. "I wasn't sold on the idea that I needed a new heart when I'd never had a heart attack," says Joe. However, he worried that he'd run out of other treatment options. After all, he'd already undergone quadruple bypass surgery, had dramatically improved his lifestyle, and was taking several medications, including drugs to lower his cholesterol and blood pressure—yet he kept getting sicker.

"My father had died from a heart attack five years after *his* quadruple bypass surgery—and I knew that if I didn't find the right treatment, I was rapidly reaching a point where my life would also be cut short," the dad of two adult sons recalls. Was there anything left to try, short of getting a new heart?

A Lifesaving Treatment Strategy

As you'll learn in this chapter, there's an excellent, but underused treatment for arterial disease. Known as "optimal medical therapy" (OMT) or optimal medial management, this approach combines an optimal lifestyle with drug therapy to treat both arterial disease *and* conditions that drive it, such as chronic inflammation and insulin resistance. Excellent studies have demonstrated that this treatment approach can save lives by preventing heart attacks and strokes. In fact, the scientific evidence is so overwhelming that we've been prescribing OMT for *all* patients with arterial disease since 2001.

OMT is sometimes confused with "aggressive treatment." For example, some researchers have theorized that the best way to manage such issues as high blood pressure, high cholesterol, or high blood sugar—all of which are discussed in this chapter—was to drive levels down as low as possible in all patients who have these disorders. When aggressive treatment, which typically involves taking high doses of medication or several powerful drugs at once, was tested in clinical trials, however, it was frequently found to be ineffective, dangerous, or, in some cases, even fatal for certain patients.

We define optimal medical therapy as "individualized medical therapy," in which medications are used cautiously in situations in which the benefits clearly outweigh the harms, such as treating cardiovascular disease (CVD), the leading killer of Americans. Treatment goals should always be personalized according to the patient's overall health and other medical conditions. It's also essential to identify and treat the root cause of the disease, along with any conditions that contribute to heart attack and stroke risk, such as high blood pressure or periodontal disease.

As discussed in an earlier chapter, it can often take a decade or more for medical guidelines to catch up with new science. In November, 2012, the four therapies described in the next section of this chapter, which we call the "cornerstones" of treating arterial disease, were formally endorsed in the new clinical practice guidelines issued jointly by the American College of Physicians, the American Heart Association, the American College of Cardiology Foundation, the Preventative Cardiovascular Nurses Association, and other leading medical societies, based on a "scientifically valid, high-quality review of the evidence."

All of these therapies have been rigorously evaluated in many excellent, peer-reviewed studies. The landmark 2007 COURAGE (Clinical Outcomes Utilizing Revascularization and Aggressive Drug Evaluation) trial demonstrated that OMT is just as effective at preventing attacks, strokes, and early death as subjecting patients to the risks and expense of balloon angioplasty and stent insertion, an invasive procedure that costs about $10,000.

These findings were confirmed with the 2009 BARI 2D study, the first clinical trial to compare treatment strategies for people with type 2 diabetes *and* heart disease. Half of the patients were treated with coronary bypass surgery (which costs about $60,000) or stents plus OMT, while the rest only received OMT, unless their symptoms got worse, in which case they were also treated surgically. After five years of follow-up, there were no significant differences in survival or rates of cardiovascular events in the two groups.

A 2011 analysis published in *Journal of the American Medical Association (JAMA)* reported that the main benefit of surgery is relieving symptoms like angina, the debilitating chest pain that left Joe Inderman unable to walk across our exam room without taking nitroglycerin during his first visit to our clinic. Symptomatic relief can also be achieved with OMT, however, at far lower cost, the researchers report, adding that optimal medical therapy, despite its thoroughly documented benefits, remains underused. In an interview on CardioExchange, two of the *JAMA* study authors theorize that the reasons include "economic incentives to preferentially treat with revascularization."

In other words, it's a lot more profitable to send a patient like Joe to the operating room for a $60,000 bypass surgery—or even an $800,000 heart transplant operation—than it would be for a healthcare provider to manage his complex medical issues with medications, given the need for frequent follow-up appointments and lab tests to make sure that the treatments were working. Even the most extensive surgery, however, doesn't cure cardiovascular disease or halt its progression. Since Joe's quadruple-bypass surgery didn't treat the root causes of his disease (insulin resistance and genetic susceptibility to chronic inflammation), the operation only brought him 18 months of symptomatic relief.

Had Joe gotten a heart transplant, his excruciating chest pain would have inevitably returned, because his coronary arteries would still have had blockages that obstructed blood flow to his new heart, leaving it deprived of oxygen and vital nutrients. The progression of the disease would have also put him at risk for such events as a heart attack, stroke, peripheral artery disease, and even vascular dementia. Instead of another costly—and potentially risky—trip to the operating room, he needed OMT to treat the disease in his arteries *and* its underlying causes.

Together, these four cornerstones discussed in the next section of this chapter serve as the foundation of our heart attack–and–stroke prevention plan for patients with diseased arteries. In some cases, as we'll explain in detail, these therapies can also be beneficial for people who *don't* have arterial disease, but are at high risk for developing it.

Questions to Ask Before You Take a Pill

If your healthcare provider advises taking medication, ask the following questions to make sure you understand why the therapy is being prescribed and how it will help manage your coronary artery disease or reduce your risk for a heart attack or stroke. Don't be shy about asking the provider to explain anything that is not clear. It's helpful to take notes to help you remember any important information about your treatment.

- Why do you recommend this medication and what does it treat?
- Could this medication interact with any of my other medications or supplements?
- How likely is this treatment to help me and how will I know if it's working?
- Should this medication be taken with food or on an empty stomach?
- Is there a certain time of day that I should take this medication?
- What are the potential side effects and which are serious?
- What should I do if I have a side effect?
- How do I reach you in an emergency?

- What are my other treatment options?

- What should I do if I miss a dose of my medication?

- Are there any foods, medications, supplements, or activities to avoid while I am taking this medication?

- When should I return for a follow-up appointment?

- Which lab tests will you do to see if this medication is helping or harming me?

- When should I expect to feel better? If this medication doesn't help me, what are the next steps?

The Four Cornerstones of Treating Arterial Disease

Picture plaque as a predatory cat hidden inside the walls of your arteries. How do you prevent it from attacking? Since it's not always possible to get rid of the cat, one option would be to trim its claws, so you won't get hurt if it pounces. That's the concept behind using antiplatelet medications, such as low-dose aspirin. By making platelets in your blood less likely to clump into clots, these drugs provide protection in the event of a plaque rupture, by reducing the risk of artery-blocking clots that could lead to a heart attack or stroke.

A second line of defense is medications that combat inflammation—the fire in the arteries that causes the cat to jump out. Keeping the arteries as "cool" as possible stabilizes plaque. It's like building a very strong cage so the wily predator can't escape. By combining both tactics—declawing and caging—you'll be well-protected against cardiovascular events. As we've emphasized throughout this book, however, treatment needs to be personalized. While the therapies discussed below have helped millions of people gain control of arterial disease—or even reverse it—these treatments may not be appropriate for certain patients.

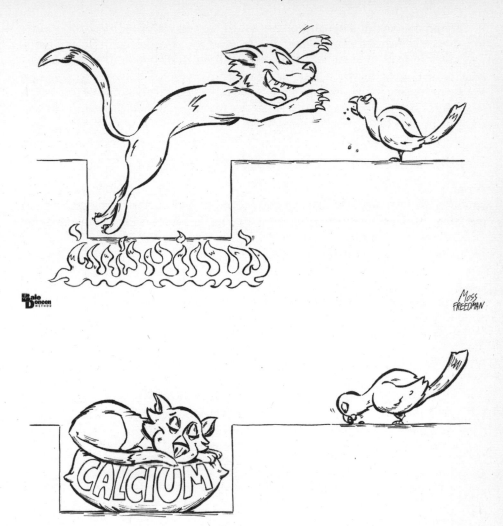

Discuss the risks and benefits of these medications with your medical provider and alert him or her if you are pregnant, planning to conceive, or have any medication allergies or intolerances. Depending on which disorders you have, it may also be necessary to layer additional treatments on top of the four cornerstones. We suggest using the information in this section as a springboard for a discussion with your doctor or nurse practitioner about the optimal medical therapy to protect you against heart attacks and strokes.

Cornerstone #1: Optimal Lifestyle

An optimal lifestyle is the strongest cornerstone of your prevention plan. Large studies show that taking excellent care of your heart through such simple steps as avoiding smoking, exercising regularly, getting adequate sleep, and managing stress can reduce risk for cardiovascular events by up to 80 percent. Along with a diet based on your DNA and the lifestyle recommendations described in the previous two chapters, we also advise optimal dental care to ward off periodontal disease, which can double or even triple the threat of a heart attack or stroke. In addition, studies have linked good oral health to a longer life and lower risk for a wide range of disorders from colds and flu to diabetes and even dementia.

To keep your teeth and gums healthy, follow these steps:

- Brush and floss twice a day. It takes at least 24 hours for oral bacteria to organize into dental plaque and then tartar, a hard mineral deposit that can cause gums to become swollen and inflamed, leading to the earliest stage of gum disease: gingivitis. Brushing and flossing twice a day dislodges debris and bacteria before they form plaque. We advise brushing for at least two minutes, preferable with a sonic toothbrush.

- Use the correct flossing technique: forming a C-shape with the floss and wrapping it around each tooth to clean the surface, rather than just snapping the floss up and down between the teeth, which doesn't clean the tooth structure properly.

- Go to bed with a clean mouth. Since you produce less saliva during sleep to wash the teeth and gums, it's particularly crucial to brush and floss thoroughly at bedtime. Dentists also suggest using a tongue scraper, so your mouth is as clean as possible before you go to sleep.

- Sugarless gum containing xylitol has an antimicrobial effect, so you may want to chew it between meals to reduce risk for gum disease. And here's another benefit: many studies show that xylitol products, such as chewing gum, lozenges, or toothpaste, help prevent cavities.

- Have a dental cleaning every three months, or as advised by your dental provider. If you have gum disease, treatment typically involves scaling and root planning (deep cleaning of root surfaces to remove plaque and tartar) or in severe cases, surgery. Your dentist may also advise medication, such as prescription antimicrobial mouthwash, dental trays with antimicrobial gel, or oral antibiotics.

Cornerstone #2: Low-Dose Aspirin

Aspirin is such a widely used over-the-counter drug that it's easy to underestimate both its amazing benefits and its potential for harm. Also known as acetylsalicylic acid, the familiar white pills found in almost everyone's medicine cabinet have been used since 1897 to combat fever, pain, and inflammation. Earlier versions derived from willow bark (which is rich in salicylic acid) have been prescribed since 400 B.C., when Hippocrates recommended it to treat aches and pains and as an analgesic for women in labor.

We often tell patients that if aspirin were invented today, it probably wouldn't receive FDA approval because of its powerful effects on bleeding. Aspirin, even in small doses, makes platelets less likely to form clots. This antiplatelet action is why low-dose aspirin therapy (taking one 81 mg tablet daily) is a cornerstone of treating arterial disease: it provides potentially lifesaving protection if plaque in the arterial wall ruptures, by reducing the risk that an artery-blocking clot will form and trigger a heart attack or stroke.

Many studies show that when patients with arterial disease take a low-dose aspirin a day, risk for both first-time and recurrent cardiovascular events drops dramatically. Other antiplatelet medications include Plavix, which is frequently prescribed for patients with stents in their arteries or those with peripheral artery disease (PAD, obstructed arteries in the legs); and Aggrenox, a combination of aspirin and extended release dipyridamole used for stroke prevention.

Serious side effects of aspirin include internal bleeding, stomach ulcers, and ringing in the ears. These problems are more likely to occur in people who frequently take full-strength aspirin, which is *not* recommended for treating arterial disease. That's because full-strength aspirin (325 mg) acts on two enzymes, COX-1 and COX-2, while tiny dose in baby aspirin only affects COX-1, the enzyme that spurs production of a chemical "glue" that makes platelets stick together and form clots. Inhibiting COX-1 is how low-dose aspirin helps prevent heart attacks and clot-related strokes.

While COX-2 stimulates production of chemicals that contribute to pain and fever, it also has *beneficial* effects on blood vessels, including widening arteries and fighting clots. Therefore medications that inhibit COX-2 may actually increase risk for heart attacks and strokes, which is why the selective COX-2 inhibitors Bextra and Vioxx were taken off the market. A recent review of more than 30 clinical trials involving 116,429 patients also reported that taking ibuprofen frequently can nearly triple stroke risk, for similar reasons. Aspirin, however, is 170 times more active against COX-1 than COX-2, explaining why low doses protect the heart by combating clots, but also boost risk for bleeding.

Given these risks and benefits, which patients should take baby aspirin for heart attack and stroke prevention? Since anyone with plaque is at risk for a clot-induced cardiovascular event, we consider aspirin to be a crucial foundational therapy for *all* patients with arterial disease, unless the patient is allergic, in which case we prescribe another antiplatelet medication, such as Plavix.

Standard care, however, bases the treatment decision on risk factor analysis, rather than the presence of disease in the arteries. The American Heart Association and American Stroke Association recommend aspirin to prevent cardiovascular events, including stroke, if patients have a 10-year risk of 6 to 10 percent or greater, based on their Framingham Risk Score. Both groups caution that for patients whose risk score is below this threshold, the harms of daily aspirin outweigh the benefits.

Risk factor analysis, however, can be dangerously misleading. For example, Camille's heart attack occurred a few months after she was told that her chances of having one in the next decade were less than 1 percent, according to her Framingham Risk Score. Juli Townsend's risk score was equally low, but the 37-year-old mom had *two* heart attacks. Based on risk factors alone, neither woman would have been considered a candidate for low-dose aspirin—a drug that costs about two cents a day—even though it might have prevented their heart attacks. Conversely, some people with lots of risk factors never suffer heart attacks or strokes, because they don't have disease in their arteries. Taking aspirin daily would put these patients at needless risk for bleeding or other side effects with no cardiovascular benefit.

Even when aspirin is appropriately prescribed, it helps some patients more than others. About 30 percent of the U.S. population has some degree of aspirin resistance, meaning that they don't get enough of an antiplatelet effect to prevent a clot—or a heart attack. Several studies have demonstrated that aspirin-resistant patients with arterial disease are up to 4 times more likely to suffer cardiovascular events than those who are not resistant, while one study reported that ischemic strokes are 14 times more likely to occur in people with aspirin resistance.

Despite the well-documented dangers of aspirin resistance, many doctors don't tell patients about a simple blood test to check for this problem. Although this test, which only needs to be done once in a lifetime, isn't routinely performed as part of standard cardiovascular care, it's widely available and only costs about $20. If you're taking daily aspirin for heart attack and stroke prevention, demand to be tested, to make sure your treatment is working. If you turn out to be aspirin resistant, your healthcare provider may increase your dose to two baby aspirin a day or switch you to a different antiplatelet medication, such as Plavix.

Cornerstone #3: Statin Therapy

Remember how Juli Townsend quit taking the statin medication her doctors had prescribed after her second heart attack? Because her healthcare providers didn't explain *why* this drug was advised, the 37-year-old mom—who had been told that her cholesterol levels were "beautiful, like a teenager's"—mistakenly assumed she was being treated for a problem she didn't have. Actually, Juli made an extremely dangerous mistake when she halted statin therapy without seeking medical advice.

Like most patients and some healthcare providers, Juli didn't know that statin drugs—sold under such brand names as Lipitor, Crestor, and Zocor, among others—can be potentially lifesaving after a heart attack, even for people with optimal cholesterol levels. There's also an excellent reason, backed by compelling science, why the Bale/Doneen Method advises that *all* patients with arterial disease, regardless of their lipid numbers, should be placed on statin therapy to prevent heart attacks and strokes, surprising as that recommendation may sound.

Statins, which block a liver enzyme that helps produce cholesterol, have been promoted for their ability to reduce "bad" LDL. On average, patients who take statins will see their LDL cholesterol drop by 40 to 60 percent, according to an analysis of 164 randomized, placebo-controlled clinical trials, published in *British Medical Journal*. The researchers, who only examined short-term studies, also reported that statin users had a 60 percent drop in heart attacks and 17 percent lower risk for stroke, compared to study participants who took a placebo.

And it's not just heart patients with an LDL problem who get extra insurance against cardiovascular events if they take a statin. Here's why: bad cholesterol doesn't cause the cat (plaque) to jump out of the gutter—inflammation sparks the leap. Therefore, the key to preventing heart attacks and strokes is to keep the arteries as "cool" as possible.

Statins are arguably the most-powerful firefighting medications we have, as a number of compelling studies show. A few highlights of recent research:

- Statins are extremely effective at reducing biomarkers that signal inflammation of the inside lining of the artery (high sensitivity C-reactive protein, also called hs CRP) and of the arterial wall (Lp-PLA2). A recent analysis of an excellent statin trial demonstrated the majority of the risk reduction from the statin was because of its lowering of Lp-PLA2 as opposed to its lowering of LDL.

- A 2012 study published in the journal *Circulation* also showed that statins reduced the oxidative stress that drives inflammation.

- Another exciting discovery was that these medications reduce the stickiness of platelets, lowering risk for artery-blocking clots that could lead to a heart attack or stroke.

These benefits help explain the startling results of earlier studies. In 2000, researchers demonstrated that if a statin was used, patients had an *equal* reduction in cardiovascular events and fatalities if their starting LDL level was 70 (ideal) or 170 (very high). That was a landmark realization because it challenged the very foundation on which statins had been marketed and prescribed. If the reason statins reduced heart attack and stroke risk was because they lower LDL, then people who already had optimal levels at the start of the trial should get no benefit—yet they actually got just as much protection as patients with sky-high LDL. Since then, many studies have confirmed these findings. One trial even found a wonderful cardiovascular risk reduction in people who entered the study with LDL levels below 60, a truly superb value.

Further evidence came from an excellent 2008 study called JUPITER, in which more than 17,000 participants with high levels of the inflammatory marker hs CRP but normal LDL were randomly assigned to either get a statin or a placebo.

Statin users had such a huge drop in heart attack and stroke risk that the study had to be stopped several years early since it would have been inhumane to leave the placebo group untreated. The results were so conclusive that the FDA approved the statin used in the study (Crestor) as a therapy for elevated hs CRP, regardless of the person's LDL level. This compelling science is why statin therapy is a cornerstone of therapy for arterial disease.

Does it matter which statin you take? Combined results of the large statin trials indicate that all of these medications are effective at reducing cardiovascular risk and vascular inflammation, but when you look at some of the better trials individually, it appears that one statin, Lipitor (atorvastin) may not be the best choice for women or people who are insulin resistant, including those with type 2 diabetes or metabolic syndrome. We advise women and insulin-resistant patients to discuss other statin options with their healthcare provider.

We also prescribe statins to patients who *don't* have a cat in the gutter, if there's evidence of arterial inflammation, their LDL levels are very high, or the person has a strong genetic predisposition to developing heart disease. Darren Liens, whom you met in Chapter Eleven, is a case in point, since he had high levels of inflammatory markers, was a carrier of the 9P21 "heart attack" gene, *and* had accelerated arterial aging (as measured by an cIMT scan of his neck arteries during his initial visit to our clinic)—indicating that at age 33, this muscular, athletic young man was already on the fast track to heart disease.

Dosing depends on the degree of inflammation in the artery. For example, if someone is recovering from a heart attack, research supports short-term high-dose statin therapy to quell the fire, while effective long-term disease management can usually be achieved with moderate to low doses, combined with a heart-healthy lifestyle. It's crucial to monitor arterial inflammation periodically, using the "fire panel" of blood and urine tests discussed in Chapter Seven. Dosage may need to be temporarily increased during an inflammatory crisis, such as a dental infection, injury, or surgery.

Side effects of statins can include muscle pain and weakness or, in rare cases, muscle breakdown. Oftentimes, statin-related myopathy (muscle pain) is driven by vitamin D deficiency, low level of Co-Q10, or even obstructive sleep apnea (OSA). In these cases, myopathy can be mitigated through using a statin at a very low dose, along with supplements to boost vitamin D or Co-Q10, or treating the OSA. Liver toxicity is also a risk, but can be prevented by monitoring liver function with blood tests and using the lowest-effective dose.

If high LDL remains an issue once the artery has been cooled with statin therapy, we may add niacin (vitamin B3) to the patient's therapy, or modestly increase the statin dose. Later in the chapter, we'll look at other treatments for high cholesterol, including therapies for people who don't have plaque in their arteries.

Cornerstone #4: Renin-Angiotensin Aldosterone System Inhibitors

The renin-angiotensin aldosterone system (RAAS) regulates blood pressure and the body's fluid balance. RAAS inhibitors reduce the effects of angiotensin, a hormone that constricts arteries and boosts blood pressure. By causing blood vessels to relax and widen, these drugs lower blood pressure. Since angiotensin also promotes blood clotting and can contribute to arterial wall inflammation, it's not surprising that medications that decrease the effects of this hormone have been shown in many studies to lower heart attack and stroke risk.

In fact, the scientific evidence is so overwhelming that in 2004, the American College of Physicians recommended this type of medication for all patients with known coronary artery disease. We certainly agree with this. We go a step further, however, and prescribe RAAS inhibitors for patients with plaque in *any* of their arteries (not just those that supply the heart). To us, it doesn't make sense to focus solely on heart attack prevention (by treating people with coronary artery disease) and ignore patients with plaque in their neck arteries that could lead to a devastating ischemic stroke.

RAAS inhibitors relax the wall of the artery, resulting in lower blood pressure. That's an important benefit, since high blood pressure is a leading cause of stroke (and a major risk factor for heart attack). A study of nearly 500,000 people demonstrated that each 10 mm hG drop in diastolic blood pressure (the lower number) yields an approximately 50 percent drop in stroke risk. However, just as statins are beneficial for patients with arterial disease—even if they have normal or optimal cholesterol levels—RAAS inhibitors have been shown to shrink cardiovascular risk in patients with blood pressure as low as 110/70. RAAS inhibitors also help promote nitric oxide to the artery wall, making it stronger and more resistant to plaque rupture.

There are three main types of RAAS inhibitors, all of which target the same process that constricts blood vessels. But each type inhibits or blocks a different step of the process.

Angiotensin-converting enzyme inhibitors

Also known as (ACE) inhibitors, these medications prevent an enzyme from converting the substance renin into angiotensin. We love the medical slang for these drugs, which are known as the ACEs, because we like having this ace up our sleeve! The ACEs are the oldest medications in this category and have a wealth of data showing significant reductions in heart attacks, strokes, heart failure and kidney failure. Another wonderful bonus of the ACEs is that they increase a substance called bradykinin, which in turn boosts nitric oxide—the best possible "food" for the inside lining of the artery.

Among the RAAS inhibitors, the ACEs have the best outcome data for preventing both cardiovascular events and fatalities. There are many different ACEs, but we feel that the one called ramipril has superior data, with the very large HOPE trial reporting a 32 percent drop in risk for stroke, 20 percent for heart attack, 26 percent for cardiovascular fatalities *and* a 34 percent decrease in new cases of diabetes. No other ACE has been shown to be nearly as effective for preventing diabetes. That's a very important benefit for our patients with arterial disease and/or high blood pressure, since many of them are also on the road to type 2 diabetes.

The ACEs do have some drawbacks, however. The most common side effect, occurring in about 10 percent of those who take this type of medication, is a dry, hacking cough. While nitric oxide is fabulous for the blood vessel lining, it can irritate the airway lining, leading to coughing. If this occurs, we switch patients to a different type of RAAS inhibitor, such as angiotensin receptor blockers (ARBs). The most serious side effect of the ACEs—affecting about one in 1,000 users—is sudden swelling of the mouth and back of the throat that demands immediate treatment in an emergency room. Like many drugs, ACEs are not safe during pregnancy.

We warn patients who are being treated with RAAS inhibitors not to take an antibiotic called "Septra" or "Bactrim." Combining these drugs can cause your potassium level to become dangerously high. This antibiotic is frequently ordered for bladder or kidney infections. Make sure any healthcare provider who treats you checks for potential drug interactions with your current therapies whenever any new medication is prescribed. Also keep a list of your medications (including dosages) in your wallet or stored on your mobile device, so it's handy for medical appointments or an emergency.

Angiotensin receptor blockers (ARBs)

Many healthcare providers prefer to prescribe angiotensin receptor blockers (ARBs) instead of ACES, because the ARBs don't cause coughing. Commonly prescribed ARBs include Benecar (olmesartan) and Diovan (valsartan). As the name suggests, ARBs block the action of angiotensin by preventing it from binding to receptors in blood vessels and other tissues, much as filling the lock on your front door with cement would render your house key useless. In effect, an ARB tells the body, "Make all the angiotensin you want. It doesn't matter, because I am going to stop its actions."

ARBs have been proven to significantly reduce stroke risk, but do not lower heart attack danger. They are effective at preventing and treating heart and kidney failure, with very few side effects. They also help prevent type 2 diabetes, but not as effectively as the ACEs. Taking an ARB trims the threat of new-onset diabetes by about 20 percent or less, compared to the 34 percent risk reduction associated with ACE use.

Renin Inhibitors

The latest type of medication to reduce the effects of angiotensin works by inhibiting renin. Currently, there is one medication in this category: Tekturna (aliskiren). While this type of drug may ultimately turn out to be an excellent way to reduce CV risk, it's so new that there are no studies yet demonstrating a definite reduction in heart attacks and stroke.

A very recent two-year study in people with heart disease, however, found that adding aliskiren to other standard treatments cut the risk of major cardiovascular events in half. Most of that benefit was driven by reductions in nonfatal heart attack. The study was too small to be definitive. Seventy-six percent of the patients taking aliskiren were already on an ACE or ARB. Another study in type 2 diabetics with significant kidney disease was halted early because of potential harm from combining aliskiren with an ACE or ARB. The jury is still out on the wisdom of adding this renin inhibitor to another RAAS medication.

We have some patients whose blood pressure is already so low that they cannot tolerate any type of RAAS inhibitor. In general, these medications need to be prescribed with caution and patients should be warned of the symptoms of excessively low blood pressure (hypotension), such as dizziness, fainting, blurred vision, and cold, clammy, pale skin. To reduce this risk, we start with the lowest dose and slowly increase it if necessary. We also caution patients that this medication can have a rare, but serious side effect: angioedema (swelling of tongue and throat that can affect breathing). In studies, this side effect was seen in 0.2 percent of African American patients and 0.09 percent of people of other ethnicities.

If you take blood pressure medication, talk to your healthcare provider about the best time to take your daily dose. Studies show that people with hypertension get significantly more protection from suffering a cardiovascular event if they take tat least one of their blood pressure medications in the evening as opposed to the morning.

Therapies for Insulin Resistance and Type 2 Diabetes

Since insulin resistance (IR)—the culprit in 70 percent of heart attacks—is the leading cause of both atherosclerosis and high blood pressure, it's essential to treat this condition. The reason Joe Inderman kept getting sicker, despite taking blood pressure and cholesterol medications, was that his IR had gone untreated for so long that he'd become prediabetic. Research shows that people with prediabetes can reduce the risk of progressing to type 2 diabetes by nearly 60 percent, by losing 7 percent of their body weight and exercising moderately 30 minutes a day, at least five days a week.

In some cases, diet and exercise aren't enough to halt further loss of insulin-producing beta cells in the pancreas and further damage to blood vessels. In this situation, we sometimes prescribe Actos (pioglitazone). It's important to realize, however, that this is an "off-label" use of this oral medication, meaning that the FDA has *not* approved Actos for this purpose. Actos *is* FDA-approved for treating high blood sugar associated with type 2 diabetes. Once a drug is FDA-approved for any purpose, healthcare providers can legally prescribe it for other medical uses. Because there are no drugs that are specifically FDA-approved for IR/prediabetes, the risks and benefits of using Actos off-label should be carefully weighed if your medical provider advises this option.

How likely is Actos to prevent diabetes if you're insulin resistant? A recent 2.4-year study of 602 prediabetic patients with impaired fasting glucose and/or impaired glucose tolerance reported that those treated with 30 to 45 mg of Actos daily were 72 percent less likely to progress to diabetes than those given a placebo. Those results are particularly impressive compared to those for metformin (Glucophage), a diabetes drug that stopped conversion to full-blown diabetes in only 37 percent of prediabetic patients in a different placebo-controlled study. Research shows that Actos has a variety of cardiovascular benefits, including these:

- Enhancing HDL's ability to remove cholesterol from the bloodstream during a six-week study.

- Reducing blood pressure by 3 mm hG in prediabetic patients. Remember that even a small drop in blood pressure has been linked to a surprisingly large reduction in stroke risk.

- Decreasing inflammatory markers in an amazingly rapid fashion. For example, in a study of high-risk diabetic patients with known coronary artery disease, levels of hs C-reactive protein dropped by 18 percent—after just three days of treatment.

- Improving insulin sensitivity and reducing triglycerides in nondiabetic patients.

- Reducing deaths and nonfatal heart attacks and strokes by 18 to 20 percent, in a study of high-risk diabetic patients. The researchers also found that treatment with Actos significantly reduced diabetic participants' need to migrate to insulin injections. Some diabetics treated with Actos, however, may need additional medications to optimize blood sugar control. Actos is also known to have many serious side effects, so, in our opinion, it should only be prescribed by a medical provider who is very familiar with the potential risk, fully informs patients, and follows them closely to make sure the medication is helping.

Medications to Combat Cardiovascular Risks

Along with following an optimal lifestyle, certain patients who *don't* have plaque in their arteries can benefit from two of the medications we recommend as cornerstones for treating cardiovascular disease: statins and RAAS inhibitors. Darren Liens, whom you met in Chapter Eleven, is a case in point since he had several disorders that made him an excellent candidate for both statin therapy and a RAAS inhibitor:

- Severe arterial inflammation. Darren had accelerated arterial aging (as measured by the cIMT ultrasound of the neck discussed in Chapter Six), signaling that he was on the fast track to heart disease. Statin therapy is arguably the best firefighting drug we have and can significantly reduce the threat of developing arterial disease.

- Elevated levels of lipoprotein (a), the "mass murderer" cholesterol that triples heart attack risk. As you learned in an earlier chapter, people with this inherited disorder benefit from keeping their LDL levels as low as possible. For both people with an Lp(a) problem and those with high LDL, statin therapy and niacin are both excellent ways to lower bad cholesterol if lifestyle changes alone aren't enough to solve the problem.

- High blood pressure, the leading risk factor for stroke. At 136/88, Darren's blood pressure was in the prehypertensive range—a level that doubles the danger of dying from cardiovascular causes. To combat this perilous pressure, we prescribed ramapril, an ACE inhibitor with excellent cardiovascular benefits.

- Because of a strong genetic risk for cardiovascular disease, Darren felt he was leading a "doomed existence" after watching his extremely physically fit father die from a heart attack at age 46. In addition, his uncle underwent quadruple-bypass surgery to treat severely clogged arteries at age 49. The combination of a statin and an ACE inhibitor have put out the blaze in Darren's arteries and cut his LDL and blood pressure to optimal levels. Getting his risks under control has also extinguished the insurance adjuster's terror of dying young now that he's found a path to enjoying a long and healthy future.

Treating high blood pressure can be tricky. For example, Joe Inderman had to try three blood pressure medications before he found the one that worked best for him. Along with the ACEs and ARBs discussed earlier in this chapter, commonly prescribed blood pressure medications include diuretics (water pills); beta blockers, such as metoprolol (Lopressor, Toprol XL), carvedilol (Coreg) and Bystolic (nebivolol); and calcium channel blockers, which include amlodipine (Norvasc), diltiazem (Cardizem, Dilacor XR), and nifedipine (Adalat, Procardia). Ultimately, ramipril successfully lowered Joe's blood pressure from a dangerously high reading of 150/90 to the normal range. That's a blood pressure he really can live with!

Nor did Joe need someone else's heart beating in his chest to overcome his debilitating symptoms. Thanks to optimal medical therapy, Joe no longer has to ration his nitroglycerin pills, because he almost never needs them. "I went from living a very restricted lifestyle—and not being able to walk for five minutes—to going on hikes and riding horses all day, without any chest pain," says the divorced Texan, who adds that his heart has healed in other ways. Now that he's healthy again, he has rediscovered the pleasures of romance—and sex. "I have a special friend and feel very happy and fulfilled to be sharing my life with someone I care deeply about."

Action Step:
Find Out If Your Treatment Is Working

Whether you are being treated with many of the therapies discussed in this chapter as Joe is, are taking a couple of medications, like Darren, or are striving to overcome your cardiovascular risks through an optimal lifestyle, it's crucial to schedule follow-up appointments with your healthcare provider to monitor your response to treatment, particularly the impact it's having on vascular inflammation. In the next chapter, we'll provide detailed guidance on how to tell if your treatment is working. We'll also share intriguing insights from our patients' diverse experiences to help you continue your journey to peak health without fear of a heart attack or stroke.

Chapter 15

Achieving and Maintaining Peak Health

"When you reach the top, keep climbing."

—Zen Proverb

Several months ago, our tallest patient, Kevin Fitzwilson, told us that he had an equally outsized ambition: The 6'8" tall investment manager wanted to climb Washington's highest mountain, Mt. Rainier. But he also had concerns. Would the arduous ascent to the 14,410-foot peak be safe for someone with vascular disease? "I don't want to risk having a heart attack or blowing out my neck arteries with a stroke," he told us. "Is this climb something an 83-year-old guy with heart problems should even consider?"

Actually, Kevin isn't an octogenarian. According to his birth certificate, he's only 41. But the financier from Bellevue, Washington, was shocked—and frightened—last year when a cIMT scan revealed that his neck arteries are more than twice as "old" as his chronological age. He was even more terrified when his family doctor diagnosed him with atherosclerosis: the disease that had killed his father, Jim, at age 53.

"My doctor kept saying that thankfully, we'd caught this in time, but I felt that if I didn't find the right treatment, I'd be dead in 10 years, like my father," Kevin recalled in a recent interview. The financier still gets furious remembering what happened to his dad. "He'd gone to doctors several times with chest pain, but first he was told it was gas, then he was treated for pleurisy (inflammation of the lungs). It never occurred to anyone that such a tall, fit man could have heart disease—until he was wheeled into the OR for triple-bypass surgery after a heart attack."

Initially, Jim seemed to recover fully from the open-heart operation. "A few weeks later, at Thanksgiving, he got very emotional, talking about how the experience had made him appreciate all the little things in life," recalls the financier, then 26. "The following February, my mom came home from shopping and found him dead on the basement floor. He'd gone through the hell of being sawed open for bypass surgery, only to die from another heart attack five months later," adds Kevin, who is convinced that his dad would be alive today if the older man's initial symptoms had been correctly diagnosed and treated.

After the funeral, "I had to step up and take care of my younger brother. I told him that we needed to be super-proactive about our health," adds Kevin, an outstanding athlete who had played division 1 basketball in college. "I started exercising like a madman, with a routine heavily based on weight training." He eliminated all fat and animal products from his diet, and got frequent checkups. "Doctors always told me that I was in great physical shape and my cholesterol was fine, so there was nothing to worry about."

But Kevin couldn't shake his fear that deadly danger lurked in his DNA—and insisted that his family doctor order a cIMT scan to check for arterial disease. After the scan detected plaque deposits, the investment manager was referred to a specialist for a stress test. "I maxed out on the treadmill test, running at the top speed without any chest pain," recalls Kevin. "I was told that I should consider starting on statins, but I felt there must be more I could do to save my life." When a friend told him about our comprehensive heart-attack-and-stroke-prevention method, he adds, "It sounded like exactly what I was searching for."

Are You Getting Effective Treatment?

Kevin's desire to climb Mt. Rainier turned out to be an excellent metaphor for the goal of his treatment, which included the "four cornerstones" discussed in the previous chapter: optimal lifestyle, statin therapy, daily low-dose aspirin, and RAAS inhibitors. Mt. Rainier is one of most dangerous volcanoes in the world, while our tests showed that Kevin had fire in his arteries: high levels of inflammatory markers that could trigger a plaque eruption, putting him at extreme risk for a heart attack or a stroke.

Yet Mt. Rainier is also the most glaciated (and highest) peak in the 48 contiguous states, spawning six major rivers fed by melting snow. To maintain a healthy flow of blood to Kevin's heart and brain, we needed to keep his arteries as "cold" as possible, much like the icy volcano he longed to climb, which hasn't erupted in more than a century. In other words, we wanted to "freeze" (stabilize) the soft, vulnerable plaque in his arteries, so it couldn't leap out and cause a heart attack or stroke.

Understandably, Kevin wanted to know how to tell if the treatment was working. After all, he had no symptoms and looked and felt fine. So what was the best way to determine if his 83-year-old arteries were getting younger and healthier? While the lab tests we use to monitor treatment response can vary according to which issues we're treating, the most important way to track progress is checking the patient's inflammatory markers periodically, with the "fire panel" of blood and urine tests described in Chapter Seven.

Of these tests, there are two that are especially valuable for monitoring treatment response, both for patients with arterial disease and those at risk for it because of inflamed arteries. As you learned earlier in this book, most healthcare providers don't use microalbumin/creatinine urine Ratio (MACR)—a urine test that costs just pennies and is covered by almost all health plans—to monitor the health of the arterial wall. There are compelling reasons, however, for patients to demand this simple test: MACR has been shown to be an independent biomarker that predicts risk for cardiovascular events. What's more, recent evidence from the large Framingham Offspring study shows that women whose MACR was above 7.5 and men with a ratio higher than 4 had *nearly triple* the risk for heart attacks, strokes, and other cardiovascular events. Therefore, it's crucial for patients to find out if their MACR is signaling danger—and if so, for their healthcare providers to reevaluate their treatment plan.

The other test we particularly recommend for monitoring inflammation is the Lp-PLA2 blood test, which checks an enzyme that has recently been identified as both a biomarker of arterial wall inflammation *and* a direct player in arterial disease. A recent study suggests that Lp-PLA2 contributes to plaque formation and the risk that plaque will rupture explosively—and spark a heart attack or stroke. Think of it Lp-PLA2 as a volcano warning. In some cases, it's also valuable to track levels of the inflammatory marker C-reactive protein (CRP).

Also discuss the other "fire panel" tests that we've detailed in Chapter Seven with your healthcare provider to find out which are most appropriate for you—and how often these tests should be repeated. We typically repeat the tests at least once a year—and retest high-risk patients (those with inflamed plaque) every three months to monitor their treatment response. The wonderful news is that with the right treatment, elevated levels of inflammatory markers typically drop quickly, indicating that the patient is no longer on the fast track to a heart attack or stroke. For example, in just a few months, Kevin showed a dramatic decrease, signaling that the plaque "volcanoes" in his arteries were no longer on the verge of erupting.

Along with monitoring inflammation with blood or urine tests, we also advise patients with vascular disease or accelerated arterial aging to have their arteries directly examined with an imaging test, such as a cIMT ultrasound scan of the neck arteries, once a year. If the treatment is effective, then there should be no *new* plaque "volcanoes" (soft plaque deposits), while existing ones should be stabilizing, as evidenced by calcification (flecks of calcium forming a protective crust over the plaque, like molten lava cooling into solid rock).

During the first annual imaging checkup, it's important to be cautious in drawing any conclusion about changes in the size of existing plaque or the thickness of the lining of your neck arteries. Even if the plaque looks a little bigger or your arterial lining has gotten a little thicker, your treatment could still be effectively stabilizing the plaque. The main problems to watch for are existing plaque that shows no sign of calcifying or new areas of soft plaque, which are indications that your healthcare provider may need to make changes in your treatments or order additional tests to find out why you're not responding to the therapies you're using.

If your arterial age is significantly higher than your chronological age, over time, with the right treatment, your arteries should gradually become "younger." Even if you're getting optimal medical care and following an outstanding lifestyle, however, it may take several years to achieve an arterial age that's similar to the one on your driver's license. Remember that arterial disease develops over many years and stabilizing—or better still, reversing it—requires patience and a long-term commitment.

Finally, if your treatment is working, there should also be improvements in any targeted cardiovascular issues, such as your cholesterol levels, blood pressure, blood sugar, or oral health. In Kevin's case, a combination of medications and lifestyle changes, including a diet based on his DNA, revamping his workout to focus on aerobic exercises like hiking and running, and learning healthy ways to cope with stress, proved amazingly effective. In just 12 months, his arterial age fell from 83 to 53 and his blood pressure—which tended to spike as high as 140/90 when his heart was stressed by tense days at work or intense bouts of weight training—consistently measured in the normal range.

Over the summer, Kevin and two of his friends literally had a peak experience. He e-mailed us a spectacular video he'd taken, showing the sun rising over the majestic peak of Mt. Rainier. "Here we are, on top of the world," he announced, in a voice that sounded amazingly young for someone who once called himself "an 83-year-old guy with heart problems." He later told us that climbing Mt. Rainier was the adventure of a lifetime. "At times, I was screaming with excitement as I celebrated this awesome milestone of getting my health back. It was dangerous as hell being up there on the glacier, but incredibly exhilarating. I've never felt so happy—or so alive."

Six Lessons to Take to Heart

In many ways, healing the heart is like Kevin's alpine adventure: It can take a long, challenging climb to achieve younger, healthier arteries and free yourself from the fear of a heart attack or stroke. And just as Kevin didn't try to ascend Mt. Rainier on his own, improving your heart health is a team effort: You need healthcare providers who are committed to giving you optimal care to monitor your progress, alert you to potential pitfalls along the way, and keep you focused on reaching your goal.

We love the Zen proverb that tells people, "After you reach the top, keep climbing." For patients, it's an inspiring reminder that ultimately, achieving peak health means being determined to always take that next step forward. For healthcare providers, it means going the extra mile to embrace the latest science and improve clinical practice. We firmly believe that every patient deserves optimal care. With perseverance, and right personalized therapies, the reward could be like Kevin's mountaintop epiphany: Achieving peak health and watching the dawn of a brighter tomorrow.

Here are six key insights to help you reach your health goals, as you continue your journey to the top.

1. Even supermen—and superwomen—can have kryptonite in their arteries.
   Throughout this book, you've heard the stories of patients whose true cardiovascular danger was missed, simply because they looked too young and healthy to have heart disease, lacked the classic Framingham risk factors that healthcare providers typically check for, or didn't have signs of arterial disease that show up on indirect tests of heart health. For example,

at 52, David Bobbett was so fit that he could run on a treadmill until the motor burned out and always passed his annual stress test with "flying colors."

Only by chance did David hear about an imaging test—coronary artery calcium score—that revealed that his arteries were so severely clogged that he was at extreme risk for a fatal heart attack. In fact, the nonsmoking CEO turned out to have a calcium score that identified him as being in 10 times more danger than a smoker without calcified plaque in the arteries. "Keeping patients in the dark about a lifesaving test is murder," contends David, who was told his risk for a heart attack was so high that he needed emergency bypass surgery. Instead, he had the wisdom to "look for [healthcare providers] whose patients don't have heart attacks." He now credits optimal medical care with saving his life.

Similarly, Camille Zaleski was assured that based on her Framingham risk factors, there was less than a 1 percent probability that she'd suffer a heart attack in the next 10 years—a few months before she keeled over at work with a massive heart attack. Like another mom you met in these pages, Juli Townsend, Camille's symptoms were initially brushed off, because all too often, doctors still think that young women don't have heart attacks. In fact, when Camille literally collapsed on her doctor's doorstep three years before her heart attack, with symptoms that would have almost certainly prompted an immediate cardiac workup in a man, she was given a prescription for an antianxiety drug for her "panic attack."

Juli was sent home from the emergency room with antibiotics when her first heart attack was misdiagnosed as pneumonia, only to suffer a second heart attack less than a week later. Even though both women knew something was terribly wrong during their heart attacks, neither of them picked up the phone and called 911, because they didn't trust their gut instincts after healthcare professionals had discounted their symptoms. Women and their healthcare providers need to know that cardiovascular disease kills more women than men, in part because CVD *still* goes unrecognized in women. We urge you to remember the list of women's heart disease symptoms in Chapter Five—and get immediate emergency care if you experience any of them. If that occurs, women should tell ER physicians, "I think I'm having a heart attack" and insist on getting a thorough evaluation.

Younger men, such as Kevin and Darren Liens, both of whom lost their seemingly healthy, physically fit fathers to previously undiagnosed heart disease, may also struggle to find a doctor who takes their concerns seriously if they look too young and healthy to be considered candidates for a heart attack or stroke. It was only when Kevin demanded that his family physician order a cIMT test that he received the right diagnosis. Without it, he says, "I would have probably had a heart attack by now." All patients deserve optimal care, and we hope the information in this book will empower you to be your own healthcare advocate.

The message we emphasize to all patients—regardless of age, gender or risk factors—and to the healthcare providers who attend our continuing medical education courses is that it's time to stop basing cardiovascular care on dangerously unreliable guesswork. Instead of analyzing risk factors or how long and fast patients can jog on a treadmill during a stress test, we now have marvelous imaging technology to "look" through the skin and see if the arteries are diseased. Risk factors don't stop the flow of blood to your heart—or your brain—but an eruption of inflamed plaque can. Therefore, even if you've dodged such "bullets" as obesity, smoking, high blood pressure, and high cholesterol, please follow Kevin and David's example and *demand* to have your arteries directly checked for disease, with a cIMT scan or one of the other imaging tests discussed in Chapter Six. Finding if your arteries harbor silent, deadly plaque—and if so, getting the right treatment—could save your life.

2. Insulin icebergs can sink your cardiovascular health.

Tens of millions of Americans are walking around with perilously high blood sugar that has gone undiagnosed and untreated. David, Camille, Juli, and Berend Friehe were shocked to find out that they had prediabetes. Often times, as discussed in Chapter Nine, prediabetes or even full-blown diabetes goes undetected until the patient suffers a cardiovascular event. And even then, insulin resistance (IR)—the root cause of 70 percent of heart attacks and many ischemic strokes—may be overlooked. The discovery that a patient has IR, however, opens the door to additional therapies that can dramatically turn around the person's heart health.

In Joe Inderman's case, the solution to an apparent medical mystery—why his CVD kept getting worse despite quadruple bypass surgery, lifestyle improvement, and medication—was in his medical records. Results of a blood-sugar test performed several years earlier showed that he was prediabetic. Yet none of his healthcare providers had picked up on the root cause of the disease that left him so debilitated that he couldn't even walk across a room without popping a nitroglycerin tablet. Instead of prescribing medication and an optimal lifestyle to get Joe's prediabetes under control, specialists told him that he needed an $800,000 heart transplant, because he'd supposedly exhausted all other treatment options. Actually, as you read in the last chapter, Joe is now living very happily with his own heart, which is a lot healthier now that his blood sugar is in the normal range.

Have *you* had your blood sugar checked with the highly accurate two-hour oral glucose tolerance test (OGTT)? If not, don't let your healthcare provider tell you that other blood-sugar tests, such as A1C blood test or the fasting plasma glucose test are just as good. Review the medical evidence we present in Chapter Nine and decide if you want to be checked with tests that have been shown, in multiple studies, to be unreliable predictors of problematic blood sugar—and can miss up to 63 percent of those with prediabetes. We're confident that you'll conclude that investing two hours of your time—the length of an average movie—to get an OGTT, endorsed by the American Diabetes Association as "the gold standard" of blood-sugar testing, is the way to go.

While IR is marked by elevated blood sugar, the real menace of this disorder is the underlying arterial inflammation it sparks—damaging blood vessels for years, even before type 2 diabetes sets in. Picture high blood sugar as gasoline that feeds the fire of inflammation. The sooner this dangerous disorder is detected and treated, the safer you'll be from a heart attack or stroke. If you think you don't need a blood-sugar test because you feel fine, here's what you need to know: In our presentations to medical providers, we show them drawings depicting two "insulin icebergs" to illustrate the point that subtle warning signs of this dangerous disorder can easily be missed.

If you have any of conditions listed below, you could have IR and should get an OGTT:

- High triglycerides or low HDL (good) cholesterol.

- A large waist or big belly.

- A sleep disorder.

- A family history of diabetes.

- Dark, velvety patches on your skin (ancanthosis nigrans).

- Numbness or tingling in your feet.

- High blood pressure.

- An inactive lifestyle or obesity.

- Arterial disease.

- Erectile dysfunction.

- Polycystic ovary syndrome.

- You feel "fine." Many people with IR have no warning signs, which is why everyone older than 40, or younger people with any of the red flags listed above, should get an OGTT, even if they've been checked with other blood-sugar tests.

3. Firefighting is the secret of cardiovascular wellness.

Our patients are often surprised that we back our results with a written, money-back guarantee, stating that should they suffer a heart attack or stroke while under our care, we will refund 100 percent of the fees paid that year. To date, we've had to give only one refund. The secret of our guarantee is monitoring the health of our patient's arterial wall with the "fire panel" of blood and urine tests discussed earlier in this chapter.

If you have arterial disease or are at high risk for developing it, any rise in inflammation or persistently elevated markers is a fire alarm, warning of a hidden blaze smoldering in the arteries. For example, as you read earlier in this book, these tests alerted us that Wesley Robinson (also known as Superman) remained at high risk for a heart attack or stroke despite a year of treatment. That's when we discovered that without consulting us, he'd quit taking the niacin we had prescribed, after experiencing a minor side effect: flushing. We had to enlist the help of Superman's worried wife to persuade him that flushing wouldn't kill him, but inflamed plaque might.

Similarly, Juli put her health—and even her life—at risk by discontinuing her statin therapy after her second heart attack, because she was unaware that this medication is the best firefighting drug available. We cannot emphasize enough how crucial it is to get chronic inflammation under control. A growing body of scientific evidence suggests that this fiery process may at the root of all chronic diseases, so arguably the single most important thing you can do to attain a long and healthy life is to keep your arteries as "cool" as possible.

The wonderful news is that there is much you can do on your own to combat and quell inflammation, including daily exercise, maintaining a healthy weight, and getting optimal dental care. After Superman resumed taking his niacin, his inflammatory markers remained high when he was retested, alerting us that the fire in his arteries had a second point of origin. Further investigation, using the OralDNA tests discussed in Chapter Ten, identified the arsonist: periodontal disease. Once this issue had been addressed—again with help from Superman's wife, a dentist—the Man of Steel finally began to win the battle against the kryptonite in his arteries.

4. Genetic knowledge is power.

If you haven't had the genetic tests we recommend yet, perhaps because you're afraid of what you might find out or think there's nothing you can do to counteract threats that may lurk in your DNA, consider the stories of Darren and Berend. When they were in the dark about their genetics, both men believed that they were leading "doomed" existences. After suffering a ministroke, Berend was in such a state of panic, thinking that he might be destined to develop dementia, a memory-robbing disorder that runs in his family, that he couldn't sleep at night. Darren used to dread his birthday, feeling that each year he was getting closer to his "expiration date" of 46, the age at which his father had died from a heart attack.

In their zeal to ward off calamity, the two men started following highly restrictive eating plans that they thought would improve their heart health. But genetic tests showed that both were actually eating the worst possible diet for their ApoE genotype. Now that they know what their genotypes, they've switched to diets based on their DNA and are protecting their cardiovascular health with other personalized therapies. Darren has a roadmap to guide the way to optimal health and no longer fears the future. In fact, he told us that these days, he feels empowered and at peace. And Berend also rests easy at night, knowing that he's armed with the best weapons to fight the threats in his DNA.

In Berend's case, the discovery that he had genetic threats prompted his wife, Carla, and their daughter, Katharina, to be tested as well. As you read in Chapter Ten, the fun-loving blonde was shocked to discover that she was a carrier of a high-risk ApoE genotype. At 25, Katharina was already well on the fast track to heart disease. In fact, her arterial age of 55 was "older" than her mom's chronological age!

Katharina is thankful to have this knowledge—and has totally transformed her lifestyle to avoid developing plaque in her arteries. For the Friehe family, the lesson learned is that it's never to soon—or too late—to turn your cardiovascular health around. They're using genetic knowledge to achieve a truly optimal lifestyle: the most powerful defense against heart attacks and strokes.

5. The heart has an amazing ability to heal—at any age.

Jack Grayson recalls waking up after an angiogram to find four cardiologists "so eager to start cutting that they were practically sharpening their knives" at his hospital bedside? The Texas businessman, then 83, was advised that he urgently needed surgery to insert stents because one of his major coronary arteries was 100 percent blocked and three others, including his "widow-maker" artery (the left anterior ascending artery) were 70 to 90 obstructed.

Instead, Jack opted to be treated with the Bale/Doneen Method. After nearly six years of managing his disease with medications and an optimal lifestyle, we sent him to the heart catheterization lab for a repeat angiogram to evaluate the impact of eight years of these therapies on Jack's cardiovascular system. The results were among the most miraculous we've ever seen: X-rays of his heart and coronary arteries demonstrated an astonishing amount of angiogenesis, meaning that new vessels had formed to route blood around the blocked areas.

The Texas cardiologist who performed the angiogram, Dr. Amit Manhas, told us that Jack's arteries looked so healthy that "stenting can be reserved for a time when he has more symptoms and limitations, if that ever occurs." In effect, Jack's nearly 90-year-old arteries had grown their own natural bypasses, much like a river carving a new channel if the original one becomes dammed.

While we can't promise that everyone will get such marvelous results, Jack is *not* the only patient whose diseased heart is healing itself through angiogenesis. David Bobbett was also deemed a candidate for emergency surgery after an angiogram revealed 100 percent blockage of one coronary artery and areas of 70 percent obstruction in another. In both men's cases, angiogenesis appears to have begun even before they started treatment, probably because of their excellent lifestyle, and their blood flow has continued to improve since then.

To us, witnessing the miracle of angiogenesis in an 89-year-old heart is living proof that medical therapy, plus an optimal lifestyle, can help a diseased heart recover at any age. When patients who truly need medication are reluctant to take it, because drug therapy is not "natural," we explain that the true value of medication is enhancing the body's natural ability to heal itself. Jack, an avid adventurist who recently celebrated his 90th birthday by skydiving, takes his test results as further evidence that he's well on his way to achieving an ambition that's long been dear to his heart: living to 113—or beyond.

6. Go forward with vigilance, not fear.

Very few people would consider having a heart attack to be "almost a blessing," but Camille does. Why? "I survived it—and I'm stronger now," says the 50-year-old mom from Peoria, Arizona, who has lost 60 pounds and is so fit that she now competes in half-marathons. But hers is *not* a happily-ever-after story. Like many heart patients, she has experienced a variety of challenges and setbacks.

Eight years ago, Camille was under intense stress, because she'd just bought a new house, three days before her husband was laid off from his job. Shortly before her heart attack, she was consumed with worry about how she'd pay the mortgage. This year, in a span of just six months, Camille lost her home to foreclosure and her husband left her. She's now faced with ongoing legal, financial, and custody battles over the couple's son—and has recently learned that she might be laid off from her job.

Wisely recognizing the parallels between her current situation and the extreme anxiety she was experiencing before her heart attack, she alerted us to the upheaval in her life and asked to be evaluated. The results of her fire panel of tests were quite alarming, since a spike in her inflammatory markers signaled that the plaque in her arteries was blazing hot. To prevent a heart attack, we made immediate changes in her treatment that have successfully extinguished the fire.

As we continue to track her health closely, Camille has found coping strategies. "An airline pilot told me that in an emergency, always put on your own oxygen mask on first, before you try to help anyone else. I've applied that concept to my life, by focusing on what I *can* control: my health." To soothe her body and spirit, adds Camille, "I try to find inspiration and be thankful. Exercise helps me keep my sanity and I make sure I'm eating well. I prioritize and tackle one problem at a time."

And while her financial future remains uncertain, she's even found a reason to be optimistic. "When kids play a video game, sometimes, if they're lucky, they get a bonus round. Even with all my problems, life is a wonderful thing. I just have to keep going forward, making the most of *my* bonus round." Camille's strength and courage during adversity inspires us, as do the stories of all of the patients you've met in these pages. Their journey to peak health—to reaching that mountaintop and watching a brighter day dawn—is ongoing. The opportunity to make a real difference to their health, by helping them live well without constant fear of a heart attack or stroke, is what fuels our passion.

As you strive to improve your heart health, using the program in this book, we urge you to follow the sage advice of Abraham Lincoln, "Beware of rashness, but with energy and sleepless vigilance, go forward and give us victories."

Afterword:
Letter to the Reader

We hope you've enjoyed our book and that it has helped you to become an empowered patient as you strive to improve the health of your most important muscle, your heart, and your most important organ, your brain. If you have any questions or comments, or would like to share your experiences with the Bale/Doneen Method, you can contact us via our website, www.baledoneen.com.

While we cannot offer specific medical advice about your individual case, we encourage you to be proactive about your health. We suggest that you use the recommendations in this book in addition to your regular medical care and that you partner with your healthcare provider to receive the optimal personalized care that every patient deserves.

You may also want to remind your provider that we offer an American Academy of Family Physicians–accredited two-day course for clinicians several times a year in cities around the U.S. The course, which covers the essentials of the Bale/Doneen Method and the latest science on cardiovascular care, is approved for a significant amount of Continuing Medical Education (CME) credit. We would love the opportunity to influence your medical care through interactions with your provider.

As new research offers further insights into the best ways to maintain cardiovascular wellness, our evidence-based prevention plan will continue to evolve. We suggest visiting our website and blog regularly for the latest news about how to protect your cardiovascular system. Our goal is to help you lead a long and healthy life by maintaining optimal arterial health.

—Bradley Bale, MD, Nashville, Tennessee, and
Amy Doneen, ARNP, Spokane, Washington

Acknowledgments

Raising awareness and helping patients receive optimal care for cardiovascular disease is a team effort. We would like to acknowledge the wonderful support, encouragement, and inspiration we've received from our families, friends, colleagues, and patients for this book.

We would like to thank our marvelous agent, Jessica Papin, for her belief in our message that all heart attacks and strokes are preventable and for securing John Wiley & Sons as our publisher. We also thank Thomas Miller, former Executive Editor for John Wiley & Sons, for his excitement and commitment to our project. We greatly appreciate our editors, Constance Santisteban and Christina Roth, for their immediate enthusiasm and for guiding our book to publication. We give special thanks to our illustrator, Moss Freedman, for his amazing ability to grasp complex scientific concepts and illustrate them into desirable and tangible images. His intelligence and artistic ability continue to amaze us. Thank you, Moss!

Special recognition must be given to David Levesque from Sonosite), who had the wisdom to connect us with Lisa Collier Cool. Her background in healthcare writing coupled with her superb intelligence and writing skills have enabled us to bring the Bale/Doneen Method to the public. We will be forever indebted to her. We are honored and proud to have her as our co-author. If possible, we would bestow on her an honorary medical degree.

Thanks to our patients Alysia and Patrick Buob; David Bobbett; Suzanne Dills; Carla, Berend, and Katharina Friehe; Kevin Fitzwilson; Jack Grayson; Joe Inderman; Darren Liens; Lauralee Nygaard, DDS; Juli Townsend; Wesley Robinson (aka Superman); and Camille Zaleski, for so generously sharing their stories in our book. We were deeply saddened that our patient Henry Nugent, whose cardiovascular story appears on these pages, died from cancer at age 75 as we were writing this book. We offer our heartfelt condolences to his beautiful widow, Mickey.

Thanks also to the many healthcare providers who have attended our continuing medical education programs and are now forging ahead with incorporating the Bale/Doneen Method into their clinical practices. We are elated by your successes and warmly appreciate the lovely testimonials you have provided.

We mourn the loss of our patient and cardiovascular pioneer, Dr. Lloyd Rudy, whose remarkable surgical skills allowed the removal of a thrombus from a patient having a heart attack. This retrieval confirmed Dr. Marcus DeWood's theory, published in *New England Journal of Medicine* in 1980, that a blood clot, not cholesterol, blocks the flow of blood during a heart attack. By revolutionizing scientific understanding of how these catastrophic events actually occur, Dr. DeWood—a strong supporter of our method as well as one of the most famous cardiologists in the world—and Dr. Rudy, one of Washington's leading cardiovascular surgeons, helped launch our paradigm of stabilizing vascular disease to prevent an artery-blocking clot.

A huge thanks to our families, including those who are now part of our "office family": Zoann Atwood, chief operating officer of Bale/Doneen, LLC, and Brittany

Bale Woodcock, RN, BSN, who is helping carry our passion for heart attack and stroke prevention forward to the next generation of patients. Our lead nurse, Pamela Edstrom, RN, BSN, has been the heart of our team for nearly a decade. Together, the three of you keep the spirit of the Bale/Doneen Method vibrant and thriving every day.

A special acknowledgement and thank you from Bradley Bale, MD: Words cannot express my gratitude to my partner, Amy Doneen, ARNP. Her knowledge, energy, and dedication have been critical: She has truly put her heart and soul into the book. Anyone reading it will realize and respect her vast wisdom and caring nature via the patient stories. Her heart beats strong and lovingly throughout these pages. Many lives will be enhanced from her stellar contributions to both this book and the field of medicine.

A special acknowledgment and thank you from Amy Doneen, ARNP: I am forever grateful for my partner, Dr. Bradley Bale, for his unwavering commitment to our work. His partnership has both inspired me and shaped my personal clinical focus and career. It is his persistent optimism and focus that keep us inspired as we strive to create a change in the standard of care, making the Bale/Doneen Method available to patients everywhere. His contributions to this book enhance the depth and clarity of the science.

Medical Testimonials for the Bale/Doneen Method

Since cofounding the Bale/Doneen Method in 2001, we've given more than 1,200 speeches and presentations about our prevention strategies and research to some 60,000 medical providers around the world. In 2006, we launched a preceptorship program, accredited for continuing medical education (CME) by the American Academy of Family Physicians, to train healthcare providers on how to use our method to provide optimal cardiovascular care. The course is offered several times a year in cities around the United States.

Here are some of the testimonials we've received from the hundreds of medical providers who have attended our training program—many of whom have subsequently opened their own heart attack–and–stroke prevention clinics. Please visit our websites, www.baledoneen.com and beattheheartattackgene. com, to learn more about the course and our heart attack–and–stroke prevention method.

"Throw out what you learned in medical school and start over with the Bale/Doneen Method. A must for every primary care physician."

—Bryan Glick, DO [doctor of osteopathy], Arizona

"This course is the most important event I have ever attended in my 22 years of practice! It elegantly and practically presented a powerful model of how to diagnose early and very effectively treat the most important and prevalent human disease, atherosclerosis! Every primary care doctor in the United States should attend this course!"

—Gary Blume, MD, PhD, Washington

"It was the education of a lifetime . . . I quickly recognized that it is the only totally comprehensive program in the world for the prevention of this disease."

—Joe Turnbow, MD, Cardiovascular Disease Prevention [formerly Emergency Medicine], Colorado

"An incredible resource on advanced, but very personalized treatment of vascular risk."

—Richard Mattis, MD, Idaho

"This was a moving, motivating session. I believe it will help me save lives and deliver medical care second to none. The course empowered me with the knowledge to educate my patients, which will help to keep them motivated for real lifestyle changes."

—Randy Baggesen, MD, Virginia

"This high-energy, intensive, evidence-based two-day course makes a compelling case that heart attacks and strokes can be prevented by individualized assessment of the high-risk factors and indicators. My patients will appreciate the application of this approach in my office practice. Thank you Dr. Bale and Ms. Doneen."

—Ed Friedler, MD, Virginia

"This course is designed to comprehensively improve one's identification of those at risk for CAD/CVD risk and absolutely control the outcomes of their patients in such a life-altering way. This is the best course I've ever attended with regard to the protection of my patients from the devastating effects of CAD/CVD. I would recommend this course only to those who are serious about improving the longevity of their patients."

—David Izenberg, DO, Arizona

"I am pleased to have found people who are as interested in atherosclerosis and have figured it out. They have stayed on top of the scientific developments and are able to integrate it together in a way that I can bring it directly to my practice."

—Stanley Sharp, MD, Kansas

"After meeting Bale and Doneen, I no longer feel that we have to practice preventative medicine at the edge of a cliff."

—Ryan Dirks, PA-C [physician assistant–certified], Washington

"I found the course invaluable and feel it should be mandatory for all physicians and primary care practitioners to attend to help decrease CHD/CVD."

—Rakesh C. Patel, MD, Arizona

"This week has been exhilarating and exhausting. It seems as though the majority of my patients (and I see 35–40 per day) need to be 'recalibrated' per the Bale/Doneen Method . . . My patients' eyes are wide open and jaws are dropping as I blow them away with triple the passion, enthusiasm, and evidence that I normally show . . . I've been running more than an hour later than usual every day, but the payoff this week was when a longstanding, overweight, midlife, female patient with multiple unaddressed risk factors calmly looked at her watch after I concluded my comments and said, '*Wow, doctor, you've never spent that much time with me. . . .*'" In the hallway of my office I have a huge picture of some beautiful sand dunes with a caption that says, '*A mind once stretched by a new idea never regains its original dimension.*' . . . As I walked past it for the millionth time on Monday, I glanced at it and smiled to myself, knowing that, after this weekend, it now carries a very different meaning . . . I am very grateful for the vast amount of time, thought, effort, and passion you both have put into this."

—David Garza, DO, Arizona

"[This] is a well-organized, nonbiased course to assist physicians in providing a rational, evidence-based, comprehensive approach to correcting the underlying causes which drive heart disease and stroke. I would recommend this course to any physician interested in providing better care for their patients."

—Marina Johnson, MD, Texas, author of *Outliving Your Ovaries: An Endocrinologist Weighs the Risks and Rewards of Treating Menopause with Hormone Replacement Therapy*

"This my third [time taking the Bale/Doneen] course . . . what brought me originally is that I have done several thousand open hearts including all of these coronary artery bypasses and [began] to think, 'What can I do to keep these people from coming back?'...I had lots of patients I did every 10 years... All you cardiologists ought to be referring patients right and left to this clinic, high time, because I know you are not doing the things that Brad and Amy do to prevent people from either accelerating . . . their disease or developing the disease."

—Lloyd Rudy, MD, Washington

"This course shows a clear pathway to coronary disease prevention and stabilization that I will apply to every patient I see. I'm worried about my colleagues who don't take the course!"

—Bruce R. McCurdy, MD, Maryland

"The ideal would be if every CEO in America would actually say to their medical staff, 'I am going to bring the Bale/Doneen course to this facility' . . . when we hand these tools to the family physician, the internist, the cardiologist, the lipidologist, we will start to see our population be healthier and happier and in this economic environment it will be less expensive . . . I do believe [Bradley and Amy] harbor the secret of success for treating patients with cardiovascular illness."

—Melissa Walton-Shirley, MD, Kentucky

Resources

Chapter One

Borden, W. B., Redberg, R. F., Mushlin, A. I., Dai, D., Kaltenbach, L. A., & Spertus, J. A. (2011). Patterns and intensity of medical therapy in patients undergoing percutaneous coronary intervention. *JAMA*, 305(18), 1882–1889. doi: 10.1001/jama.2011.601

Cook, N. R., Paynter, N. P., Eaton, C. B., Manson, J. E., Martin, L. W., Robinson, J. G., . . . Ridker, P. M. (2012). Comparison of the Framingham and Reynolds Risk Scores for Global Cardiovascular Risk Prediction in the Multiethnic Women's Health Initiative. *Circulation*, 125(14), 1748–1756. doi: 10.1161/circulationaha.111.075929

DECODE study group. (2001). Glucose tolerance and mortality: comparison of WHO and American Diabetic Association diagnostic criteria. *The Lancet*, 354(9179), 617-621. doi: http://dx.doi.org/10.1016/S0140-6736(98)12131-1

DeFronzo, R. A. (2009). From the Triumvirate to the Ominous Octet: A New Paradigm for the Treatment of Type 2 Diabetes Mellitus. *Diabetes*, 58(4), 773–795. doi: 10.2337/db09-9028

Expert Panel on, Detection, Evaluation, & and Treatment of High Blood Cholesterol in Adults. (2001). Executive summary of the third report of the national cholesterol education program (ncep) expert panel on detection, evaluation, and treatment of high blood cholesterol in adults (adult treatment panel iii). *JAMA*, 285(19), 2486–2497. doi: 10.1001/jama.285.19.2486

Haffner, S. M., Lehto, S., Rönnemaa, T., Pyörälä, K., & Laakso, M. (1998). Mortality from Coronary Heart Disease in Subjects with Type 2 Diabetes and in Nondiabetic Subjects with and without Prior Myocardial Infarction. *N Engl J Med*, 339(4), 229–234. doi: 10.1056/NEJM199807233390404

Iakoubova, O. A., Sabatine, M. S., Rowland, C. M., Tong, C. H., Catanese, J. J., Ranade, K., . . . Braunwald, E. (2008). Polymorphism in KIF6 gene and benefit from statins after acute coronary syndromes: results from the PROVE IT-TIMI 22 study. *J Am Coll Cardiol*, 51(4), 449-455. doi: 10.1016/j.jacc.2007.10.017

Iakoubova, O. A., Tong, C. H., Rowland, C. M., Kirchgessner, T. G., Young, B. A., Arellano, A. R., . . . Sacks, F. M. (2008). Association of the Trp719Arg Polymorphism in Kinesin-Like Protein 6 With Myocardial Infarction and Coronary Heart Disease in 2 Prospective Trials: The CARE and WOSCOPS Trials. *J Am Coll Cardiol*, 51(4), 435–443. doi: http://dx.doi.org/10.1016/j.jacc.2007.05.057

Lloyd-Jones, D. M., Nam, B., D'Agostino, Sr, R. B., et al. (2004). Parental cardiovascular disease as a risk factor for cardiovascular disease in middle-aged adults: A prospective study of parents and offspring. *JAMA*, 291(18), 2204–2211. doi: 10.1001/jama.291.18.2204

Mozaffarian, D., Marfisi, R., Levantesi, G., Silletta, M. G., Tavazzi, L., Tognoni, G., . . . Marchioli, R. (1992). Incidence of new-onset diabetes and impaired fasting glucose in patients with recent myocardial infarction and the effect of clinical and lifestyle risk factors. *The Lancet*, 370(9588), 667–675. doi: http://dx.doi.org/10.1016/S0140-6736(07)61343-9

Okosieme, O. E., Peter, R., Usman, M., Bolusani, H., Suruliram, P., George, L., & Evans, L. M. (2008). Can Admission and Fasting Glucose Reliably Identify Undiagnosed Diabetes in Patients With Acute Coronary Syndrome? *Diabetes Care*, 31(10), 1955–1959. doi: 10.2337/dc08-0197

Palomaki, G. E., Melillo, S., & Bradley, L. A. (2010). Association between 9p21 genomic markers and heart disease: A meta-analysis. *JAMA*, 303(7), 648–656. doi: 10.1001/jama.2010.118

Reis, J. P., Loria, C. M., Lewis, C. E., et al. (2013). Association between duration of overall and abdominal obesity beginning in young adulthood and coronary artery calcification in middle age. *JAMA*, 310(3), 280–288. doi: 10.1001/jama.2013.7833

Sidney, S., Rosamond, W. D., Howard, V. J., & Luepker, R. V. (2013). The "Heart Disease and Stroke Statistics—2013 Update" and the Need for a National Cardiovascular Surveillance System. *Circulation*, 127(1), 21–23. doi: 10.1161/circulationaha.112.155911

Valderrama, A. L., Loustalot, F., Gillespie, C., George, M. G., Schooley, M., Briss, P., . . . Yoon, P. W. (2011). Million Hearts: Strategies to Reduce the Prevalence of Leading Cardiovascular Disease Risk Factors—United States, 2011. *MMWR*, 60(36), 1248–1251.

Chapter Two

Arbab-Zadeh, A., Nakano, M., Virmani, R., & Fuster, V. (2012). Acute coronary events. *Circulation*, 125(9), 1147–1156. doi: 10.1161/CIRCULATIONAHA.111.047431

Austin, M. A., Breslow, J. L., Hennekens, C. H., Buring, J. E., Willett, W. C., & Krauss, R. M. (1988). Low-density lipoprotein subclass patterns and risk of myocardial infarction. *JAMA*, 260(13), 1917–1921. doi: 10.1001/jama.1988.03410130125037

Bale, B. F., D. A. L. (2013). Autophagy, Senescence, and Arterial Inflammation: Relationship to Arterial Health and Longevity. *Altern Ther Health Med*, 19(4), 8–10.

Boden, W. E., O'Rourke, R. A., Teo, K. K., Hartigan, P. M., Maron, D. J., Kostuk, W. J., . . . Weintraub, W. S. (2007). Optimal Medical Therapy with or without PCI for Stable Coronary Disease. *N Engl J Med*, 356(15), 1503–1516. doi: 10.1056/NEJMoa070829

Burke, A. P., Kolodgie, F. D., Farb, A., Weber, D. K., Malcom, G. T., Smialek, J., & Virmani, R. (2001). Healed Plaque Ruptures and Sudden Coronary Death : Evidence That Subclinical Rupture Has a Role in Plaque Progression. *Circulation*, 103(7), 934–940. doi: 10.1161/01.cir.103.7.934

Cabin, H. S. (1992). The heart and circulation. *Yale University School of Medicine heart book*. New York: Hearst Books, 5.

Canoy, D., Boekholdt, S. M., Wareham, N., Luben, R., Welch, A., Bingham, S., . . . Khaw, K. T. (2007). Body fat distribution and risk of coronary heart disease in men and women in the European Prospective Investigation Into Cancer and Nutrition in Norfolk cohort: a population-based prospective study. *Circulation*, 116(25), 2933–2943. doi: 10.1161/CIRCULATIONAHA.106.673756

Davies, M. J. (1996). The contribution of thrombosis to the clinical expression of coronary atherosclerosis. *Thromb Res*, 82(1), 1–32. doi: http://dx.doi.org/10.1016/0049-3848(96)00035-7

de Koning, L., Malik, V. S., Kellogg, M. D., Rimm, E. B., Willett, W. C., & Hu, F. B. (2012). Sweetened Beverage Consumption, Incident Coronary Heart Disease, and Biomarkers of Risk in Men. *Circulation*, 125(14), 1735–1741. doi: 10.1161/circulationaha.111.067017

DeWood, M. A., Spores, J., Notske, R., Mouser, L. T., Burroughs, R., Golden, M. S., & Lang, H. T. (1980). Prevalence of Total Coronary Occlusion during the Early Hours of

Transmural Myocardial Infarction. *N Engl J Med,* 303(16), 897–902. doi: 10.1056/NEJM198010163031601

Dhingra, R., Sullivan, L., Jacques, P. F., Wang, T. J., Fox, C. S., Meigs, J. B., . . . Vasan, R. S. (2007). Soft Drink Consumption and Risk of Developing Cardiometabolic Risk Factors and the Metabolic Syndrome in Middle-Aged Adults in the Community. *Circulation,* 116(5), 480–488. doi: 10.1161/circulationaha.107.689935

Doneen, A. L., & Bale, B. F. (2013). Carotid intima-media thickness testing as an asymptomatic cardiovascular disease identifier and method for making therapeutic decisions. *Postgrad Med,* 125(2), 108–123. doi: 10.3810/pgm.2013.03.2645

Falk, E., Shah, P. K., & Fuster, V. (1995). Coronary Plaque Disruption. *Circulation,* 92(3), 657–671. doi: 10.1161/01.cir.92.3.657

Fischer, L. M., Schlienger, R. G., Matter, C., Jick, H., & Meier, C. R. (2004). Effect of rheumatoid arthritis or systemic lupus erythematosus on the risk of First-Time acute myocardial infarction. *Am J Cardiol,* 93(2), 198–200. doi: http://dx.doi.org/10.1016/j.amjcard.2003.09.037

Helgadottir, A., Thorleifsson, G., Magnusson, K. P., Gretarsdottir, S., Steinthorsdottir, V., Manolescu, A., . . . Stefansson, K. (2008). The same sequence variant on 9p21 associates with myocardial infarction, abdominal aortic aneurysm and intracranial aneurysm. *Nat Genet,* 40(2), 217–224. doi: 10.1038/ng.72

IL6R Genetics Consortium Emerging Risk Factors Collaboration. (2012). Interleukin-6 receptor pathways in coronary heart disease: a collaborative meta-analysis of 82 studies. *The Lancet,* 379(9822), 1205–1213. doi: 10.1016/s0140-6736(11)61931-4

The Interleukin-6 Receptor Mendelian Randomisation Analysis (IL6R MR) Consortium. (2012). The interleukin-6 receptor as a target for prevention of coronary heart disease: a mendelian randomisation analysis. *The Lancet,* 379(9822), 1214–1224. doi: http://dx.doi.org/10.1016/S0140-6736(12)60110-X

Investigators, H. H.-T. S. (2005). Long-Term Effects of Ramipril on Cardiovascular Events and on Diabetes: Results of the HOPE Study Extension. *Circulation,* 112(9), 1339–1346. doi: 10.1161/circulationaha.105.548461

Kaffashian, S., Dugravot, A., Elbaz, A., Shipley, M. J., Sabia, S., Kivimaki, M., & Singh-Manoux, A. (2013). Predicting cognitive decline: a dementia risk score vs. the Framingham vascular risk scores. *Neurology,* 80(14), 1300–1306.

Khot, U. N., Khot, M. B., Bajzer, C. T., et al. (2003). Prevalence of conventional risk factors in patients with coronary heart disease. *JAMA,* 290(7), 898–904. doi: 10.1001/jama.290.7.898

Kolata, Gina. New Heart Studies Question the Value of Opening Arteries. *New York Times,* March 21, 2004, http://www.nytimes.com/2004/03/21/us/new-heart-studies-question-the-value-of-opening-arteries.html?pagewanted=all&src=pm

Lee, Y. L., Hu, H. Y., Huang, N., Hwang, D. K., Chou, P., & Chu, D. (2013). Dental prophylaxis and periodontal treatment are protective factors to ischemic stroke. *Stroke,* 44(4), 1026–1030. doi: 10.1161/STROKEAHA.111.000076

Lockhart, P. B., Bolger, A. F., Papapanou, P. N., Osinbowale, O., Trevisan, M., Levison, M. E., . . . Council on Clinical, C. (2012). Periodontal disease and atherosclerotic vascular disease: does the evidence support an independent association?: a scientific statement from the American Heart Association. *Circulation,* 125(20), 2520–2544. doi: 10.1161/CIR.0b013e31825719f3

McEvoy, J. W., Blaha, M. J., Rivera, J. J., Budoff, M. J., Khan, A. N., Shaw, L. J., . . . Nasir, K. (2012). Mortality Rates in Smokers and Nonsmokers in the Presence or Absence of

Coronary Artery Calcification. *JACC: Cardiovascular Imaging,* 5(10), 1037–1045. doi: http://dx.doi.org/10.1016/j.jcmg.2012.02.017

Nelson, R. G. (2008). Periodontal disease and diabetes. *Oral Diseases,* 14(3), 204–205. doi: 10.1111/j.1601-0825.2008.01443.x

Orth, M., Weng, W., Funke, H., Steinmetz, A., Assmann, G., Nauck, M., . . . Luley, C. (1999). Effects of a Frequent Apolipoprotein E Isoform, ApoE4Freiburg (Leu28 Pro), on Lipoproteins and the Prevalence of Coronary Artery Disease in Whites. *Arterioscler Thromb Vasc Bio,* 19(5), 1306–1315. doi: 10.1161/01.atv.19.5.1306

Ridker, P. M. (2009). The JUPITER Trial: Results, Controversies, and Implications for Prevention. *Circ Cardiovasc Qual Outcomes,* 2(3), 279–285. doi: 10.1161/circoutcomes.109.868299

Rioufol, G., Finet, G., Ginon, I., André-Fouët, X., Rossi, R., Vialle, E., . . . Tabib, A. (2002). Multiple Atherosclerotic Plaque Rupture in Acute Coronary Syndrome: A Three-Vessel Intravascular Ultrasound Study. *Circulation,* 106(7), 804–808. doi: 10.1161/01.cir.0000025609.13806.31

Roger, V. L., Go, A. S., Lloyd-Jones, D. M., Benjamin, E. J., Berry, J. D., Borden, W. B., . . . Stroke Statistics, S. (2012). Heart disease and stroke statistics—2012 update: a report from the American Heart Association. *Circulation,* 125(1), e2–e220. doi: 10.1161/CIR.0b013e31823ac046

Ross, R. (1999). Atherosclerosis—An Inflammatory Disease. *N Engl J Med,* 340(2), 115–126. doi: 10.1056/NEJM199901143400207

Rothwell, P. M., Fowkes, F. G. R., Belch, J. F. F., Ogawa, H., Warlow, C. P., & Meade, T. W. Effect of daily aspirin on long-term risk of death due to cancer: analysis of individual patient data from randomised trials. *The Lancet,* 377(9759), 31–41. doi: http://dx.doi.org/10.1016/S0140-6736(10)62110-1

Russo, C., Jin, Z., Homma, S., Elkind, M. S. V., Rundek, T., Yoshita, M., . . . Di Tullio, M. R. (2013). Subclinical Left Ventricular Dysfunction and Silent Cerebrovascular Disease: The Cardiovascular Abnormalities and Brain Lesions (CABL) Study. *Circulation,* 128, 1105–1111. doi: 10.1161/circulationaha.113.001984

Schoenhagen, P., Ziada, K. M., Kapadia, S. R., Crowe, T. D., Nissen, S. E., & Tuzcu, E. M. (2000). Extent and Direction of Arterial Remodeling in Stable Versus Unstable Coronary Syndromes: An Intravascular Ultrasound Study. *Circulation,* 101(6), 598–603. doi: 10.1161/01.cir.101.6.598

Taylor, A. J., Cerqueira, M., Hodgson, J. M., Mark, D., Min, J., O'Gara, P., & Rubin, G. D. (2010). ACCF/SCCT/ACR/AHA/ASE/ASNC/NASCI/SCAI/SCMR 2010 Appropriate Use Criteria for Cardiac Computed Tomography: A Report of the American College of Cardiology Foundation Appropriate Use Criteria Task Force, the Society of Cardiovascular Computed Tomography, the American College of Radiology, the American Heart Association, the American Society of Echocardiography, the American Society of Nuclear Cardiology, the North American Society for Cardiovascular Imaging, the Society for Cardiovascular Angiography and Interventions, and the Society for Cardiovascular Magnetic Resonance. *J Am Coll Cardiol,* 56(22), 1864–1894. doi: 10.1016/j.jacc.2010.07.005

Teo, K. K., Ounpuu, S., Hawken, S., Pandey, M. R., Valentin, V., Hunt, D., . . . Yusuf, S. Tobacco use and risk of myocardial infarction in 52 countries in the INTERHEART study: a case-control study. *The Lancet,* 368(9536), 647–658. doi: http://dx.doi.org/10.1016/S0140-6736(06)69249-0

Tricoci, P., Allen, J. M., Kramer, J. M., Califf, R. M., & Smith, S. C. (2009). Scientific evidence underlying the acc/aha clinical practice guidelines. *JAMA, 301*(8), 831–841. doi: 10.1001/jama.2009.205

U.S. Preventive Services Task Force. (2004). Screening for Coronary Heart Disease: Recommendation Statement. *Ann Intern Med, 140*(7), 569–572.

_____. USPSTF Prevention&Screening Recommendations. (2012). < treadmill testing not recommended by USPSTF.pdf > .

Varbo, A., Benn, M., Tybjaerg-Hansen, A., & Nordestgaard, B. G. (2013). Elevated Remnant Cholesterol Causes Both Low-Grade Inflammation and Ischemic Heart Disease, While Elevated Low-Density Lipoprotein Cholesterol Causes Ischemic Heart Disease without Inflammation. *Circulation.* doi: 10.1161/circulationaha.113.003008

Wang, J.-S., Lee, I.-T., Lee, W.-J., Lin, S.-Y., Fu, C.-P., Ting, C.-T., . . . Sheu, W. H.-H. (2013). Performance of HbA1c and Fasting Plasma Glucose in Screening for Diabetes in Patients Undergoing Coronary Angiography. *Diabetes Care, 36*(5), 1138–1140. doi: 10.2337/dc12-1434

Wang, T. J., Gona, P., Larson, M. G., Tofler, G. H., Levy, D., Newton-Cheh, C., . . . Vasan, R. S. (2006). Multiple Biomarkers for the Prediction of First Major Cardiovascular Events and Death. *N Engl J Med, 355*(25), 2631–2639. doi: 10.1056/NEJMoa055373

Yeboah, J., McClelland, R. L., Polonsky, T. S., et al. (2012). Comparison of novel risk markers for improvement in cardiovascular risk assessment in intermediate-risk individuals. *JAMA, 308*(8), 788–795. doi: 10.1001/jama.2012.9624

Chapter Three

Cappuccio, F. P., D'Elia, L., Strazzullo, P., & Miller, M. A. (2010). Quantity and Quality of Sleep and Incidence of Type 2 Diabetes: A systematic review and meta-analysis. *Diabetes Care, 33*(2), 414–420. doi: 10.2337/dc09-1124

Celano, C. M., Suarez, L., Mastromauro, C., Januzzi, J. L., & Huffman, J. C. (2013). Feasibility and Utility of Screening for Depression and Anxiety Disorders in Patients With Cardiovascular Disease. *Circ Cardiovasc Qual Outcomes.* doi: 10.1161/circoutcomes.111.000049

Cereda, C. W., Tamisier, R., Manconi, M., Andreotti, J., Frangi, J., Pifferini, V., & Bassetti, C. L. (2013). Endothelial dysfunction and arterial stiffness in ischemic stroke: the role of sleep-disordered breathing. *Stroke, 44*(4), 1175–1178. doi: 10.1161/STROKEAHA.111.000112

Eke, P. I., Dye, B. A., Wei, L., Thornton-Evans, G. O., Genco, R. J., & Cdc Periodontal Disease Surveillance workgroup: James Beck, G. D. R. P. (2012). Prevalence of periodontitis in adults in the United States: 2009 and 2010. *J Dent Res, 91*(10), 914–920. doi: 10.1177/0022034512457373

Engdahl, J., Andersson, L., Mirskaya, M., & Rosenqvist, M. (2013). Stepwise screening of atrial fibrillation in a 75-year-old population: implications for stroke prevention. *Circulation, 127*(8), 930–937. doi: 10.1161/CIRCULATIONAHA.112.126656

Faraco, G., & Iadecola, C. (2013). Hypertension: A Harbinger of Stroke and Dementia. *Hypertension.* doi: 10.1161/HYPERTENSIONAHA.113.01063

Fifer, K. M., Qadir, S., Subramanian, S., Vijayakumar, J., Figueroa, A. L., Truong, Q. A., . . . Tawakol, A. (2011). Positron emission tomography measurement of periodontal (18) f-fluorodeoxyglucose uptake is associated with histologically determined carotid plaque inflammation. *J Am Coll Cardiol, 57*(8), 971–976. doi: 10.1016/j.jacc.2010.09.056

Friedewald, V. E., Kornman, K. S., Beck, J. D., Genco, R., Goldfine, A., Libby, P., . . . Journal of, P. (2009). The American Journal of Cardiology and Journal of Periodontology editors' consensus: periodontitis and atherosclerotic cardiovascular disease. *J Periodontol,* 80(7), 1021–1032. doi: 10.1902/jop.2009.097001

Gelfand, J. M., Neimann, A. L., Shin, D. B., Wang, X., Margolis, D. J., & Troxel, A. B. (2006). RIsk of myocardial infarction in patients with psoriasis. *JAMA,* 296(14), 1735–1741. doi: 10.1001/jama.296.14.1735

Grau, A. J., Becher, H., Ziegler, C. M., Lichy, C., Buggle, F., Kaiser, C., . . . Dorfer, C. E. (2004). Periodontal disease as a risk factor for ischemic stroke. *Stroke,* 35(2), 496–501. doi: 10.1161/01.STR.0000110789.20526.9D

Higgins, P., MacFarlane, P. W., Dawson, J., McInnes, G. T., Langhorne, P., & Lees, K. R. (2013). Noninvasive Cardiac Event Monitoring to Detect Atrial Fibrillation After Ischemic Stroke: A Randomized Controlled Trial. *Stroke.* doi: 10.1161/strokeaha.113.001927

Homma, S., & Di Tullio, M. R. (2010). Patent foramen ovale and stroke. *Journal of Cardiology,* 56(2), 134–141.

Hossein-nezhad, A., & Holick, M. F. (2013). Vitamin D for Health: A Global Perspective. *Mayo Clin Proc,* 88(7), 720–755.

Iwasaki, Y. K., Nishida, K., Kato, T., & Nattel, S. (2011). Atrial fibrillation pathophysiology: implications for management. *Circulation,* 124(20), 2264–2274. doi: 10.1161/CIRCULATIONAHA.111.019893

Jackson, C. A., & Mishra, G. D. (2013). Depression and Risk of Stroke in Midaged Women: A Prospective Longitudinal Study. *Stroke.* doi: 10.1161/STROKEAHA.113.001147

Jelic, S., Lederer, D. J., Adams, T., Padeletti, M., Colombo, P. C., Factor, P. H., & Le Jemtel, T. H. (2010). Vascular inflammation in obesity and sleep apnea. *Circulation,* 121(8), 1014–1021. doi: 10.1161/CIRCULATIONAHA.109.900357

Kennedy, J., Hill, M. D., Ryckborst, K. J., Eliasziw, M., Demchuk, A. M., & Buchan, A. M. (2007). Fast assessment of stroke and transient ischaemic attack to prevent early recurrence (FASTER): a randomised controlled pilot trial. *The Lancet Neurology,* 6(11), 961–969. doi: http://dx.doi.org/10.1016/S1474-4422(07)70250-8

Kurth, T., Gaziano, J., Cook, N. R., Logroscino, G., Diener, H., & Buring, J. E. (2006). Migraine and risk of cardiovascular disease in women. *JAMA,* 296(3), 283–291. doi: 10.1001/jama.296.3.283

Lavie, C. J., Lee, J. H., & Milani, R. V. (2011). Vitamin D and Cardiovascular Disease: Will It Live Up to its Hype? *J Am Coll Cardiol,* 58(15), 1547–1556. doi: http://dx.doi.org/10.1016/j.jacc.2011.07.008

Lloyd-Jones, D. M., Nam, B., D'Agostino, Sr, R. B., et al. (2004). Parental cardiovascular disease as a risk factor for cardiovascular disease in middle-aged adults: A prospective study of parents and offspring. *JAMA,* 291(18), 2204–2211. doi: 10.1001/jama.291.18.2204

Nasr, N., Ruidavets, J. B., Farghali, A., Guidolin, B., Perret, B., & Larrue, V. (2011). Lipoprotein (a) and carotid atherosclerosis in young patients with stroke. *Stroke,* 42(12), 3616–3618. doi: 10.1161/STROKEAHA.111.624684

Nordestgaard, B. G., Chapman, M. J., Ray, K., Borén, J., Andreotti, F., Watts, G. F., . . . Panel, f. t. E. A. S. C. (2010). Lipoprotein(a) as a cardiovascular risk factor: current status. *Eur Heart J.* doi: 10.1093/eurheartj/ehq386

Ornstein, D. L., & Cushman, M. (2003). Factor V Leiden. *Circulation,* 107(15), e94–e97. doi: 10.1161/01.cir.0000068167.08920.f1

Paganini-Hill, A., White, S. C., & Atchison, K. A. (2011). Dental health behaviors, dentition, and mortality in the elderly: the leisure world cohort study. *J Aging Res,* 156061. doi: 10.4061/2011/156061

Rundek, T., Gardener, H., Xu, Q., et al. (2010). Insulin resistance and risk of ischemic stroke among nondiabetic individuals from the northern manhattan study. *Archives of Neurology,* 67(10), 1195–1200. doi: 10.1001/archneurol.2010.235

Sidney, S., Rosamond, W. D., Howard, V. J., & Luepker, R. V. (2013). The "Heart Disease and Stroke Statistics—2013 Update" and the Need for a National Cardiovascular Surveillance System. *Circulation,* 127(1), 21–23. doi: 10.1161/circulationaha.112.155911

Vlachopoulos, C. V., Terentes-Printzios, D. G., Ioakeimidis, N. K., Aznaouridis, K. A., & Stefanadis, C. I. (2013). Prediction of Cardiovascular Events and All-Cause Mortality With Erectile Dysfunction: A Systematic Review and Meta-Analysis of Cohort Studies. *Circ Cardiovasc Qual Outcomes,* 6(1), 99–109. doi: 10.1161/circoutcomes.112.966903

Wheeler, J. G., Juzwishin, K. D., Eiriksdottir, G., Gudnason, V., & Danesh, J. (2005). Serum uric acid and coronary heart disease in 9,458 incident cases and 155,084 controls: prospective study and meta-analysis. *PLoS Med,* 2(3), e76. doi: 10.1371/journal.pmed.0020076

Chapter Four

Berman, D. S., Wong, N. D., Gransar, H., Miranda-Peats, R., Dahlbeck, J., Hayes, S. W., . . . Rozanski, A. (2004). Relationship between stress-induced myocardial ischemia and atherosclerosis measured by coronary calcium tomography. *J Am Coll Cardiol,* 44(4), 923–930. doi: 10.1016/j.jacc.2004.06.042

Canoy, D., Boekholdt, S. M., Wareham, N., Luben, R., Welch, A., Bingham, S., . . . Khaw, K. T. (2007). Body fat distribution and risk of coronary heart disease in men and women in the European Prospective Investigation Into Cancer and Nutrition in Norfolk cohort: a population-based prospective study. *Circulation,* 116(25), 2933–2943. doi: 10.1161/CIRCULATIONAHA.106.673756

Casalino, L. P., Dunham, D., Chin, M. H., et al. (2009). Frequency of failure to inform patients of clinically significant outpatient test results. *Arch Intern Med,* 169(12), 1123–1129. doi: 10.1001/archinternmed.2009.130

Coutinho, T., Goel, K., Correa de Sa, D., Carter, R. E., Hodge, D. O., Kragelund, C., . . . Lopez-Jimenez, F. (2013). Combining body mass index with measures of central obesity in the assessment of mortality in subjects with coronary disease: role of "normal weight central obesity." *J Am Coll Cardiol,* 61(5), 553–560. doi: 10.1016/j.jacc.2012.10.035

Ervin, R. B. (2009). Prevalence of metabolic syndrome among adults 20 years of age and over, by sex, age, race and ethnicity, and body mass index: United States, 2003–2006. *Natl Health Stat Report* (13), 1–7.

Gami, A. S., Witt, B. J., Howard, D. E., Erwin, P. J., Gami, L. A., Somers, V. K., & Montori, V. M. (2007). Metabolic syndrome and risk of incident cardiovascular events and death: a systematic review and meta-analysis of longitudinal studies. *J Am Coll Cardiol,* 49(4), 403–414. doi: 10.1016/j.jacc.2006.09.032

Grundy, S. M., Brewer, H. B., Cleeman, J. I., Smith, S. C., Lenfant, C., & Participants, f. t. C. (2004). Definition of Metabolic Syndrome: Report of the National Heart, Lung, and Blood Institute/American Heart Association Conference on Scientific Issues Related to Definition. *Circulation,* 109(3), 433–438. doi: 10.1161/01.cir.0000111245.75752.c6

Hsu, C., McCulloch, C. E., Darbinian, J., Go, A. S., & Iribarren, C. (2005). Elevated blood pressure and risk of end-stage renal disease in subjects without baseline kidney disease. *Arch Intern Med,* 165(8), 923–928. doi: 10.1001/archinte.165.8.923

Isomaa, B., Almgren, P., Tuomi, T., Forsen, B., Lahti, K., Nissen, M., . . . Groop, L. (2001). Cardiovascular morbidity and mortality associated with the metabolic syndrome. *Diabetes Care,* 24(4), 683–689.

Ivey, F. M., Ryan, A. S., Hafer-Macko, C. E., Garrity, B. M., Sorkin, J. D., Goldberg, A. P., & Macko, R. F. (2006). High prevalence of abnormal glucose metabolism and poor sensitivity of fasting plasma glucose in the chronic phase of stroke. *Cerebrovasc Dis,* 22(5-6), 368–371. doi: 10.1159/000094853

Jacobs, E. J., Newton, C. C., Wang, Y., et al. (2010). Waist circumference and all-cause mortality in a large us cohort. *Arch Intern Med,* 170(15), 1293-1301. doi: 10.1001/archinternmed.2010.201

Kim, T. N., Kim, S., Yang, S. J., Yoo, H. J., Seo, J. A., Kim, S. G., . . . Choi, K. M. (2010). Vascular Inflammation in Patients With Impaired Glucose Tolerance and Type 2 Diabetes: Analysis With 18F-Fluorodeoxyglucose Positron Emission Tomography. *Circulation: Cardiovascular Imaging,* 3(2), 142–148. doi: 10.1161/circimaging.109.888909

Lakka, H., Laaksonen, D. E., Lakka, T. A., et al. (2002). The metabolic syndrome and total and cardiovascular disease mortality in middle-aged men. *JAMA,* 288(21), 2709–2716. doi: 10.1001/jama.288.21.2709

Lawes, C. M. M., Hoorn, S. V., & Rodgers, A. Global burden of blood-pressure-related disease, 2001. *The Lancet,* 371(9623), 1513–1518. doi: http://dx.doi.org/10.1016/S0140-6736(08)60655-8

Lee, M., Saver, J. L., Chang, B., Chang, K. H., Hao, Q., & Ovbiagele, B. (2011). Presence of baseline prehypertension and risk of incident stroke: a meta-analysis. *Neurology,* 77(14), 1330–1337. doi: 10.1212/WNL.0b013e3182315234

Lewington, S., Clarke, R., Qizilbash, N., Peto, R., & Collins, R. (2002). Age-specific relevance of usual blood pressure to vascular mortality: a meta-analysis of individual data for one million adults in 61 prospective studies. *Lancet,* 360(9349), 1903–1913.

Liao, Y., Kwon, S., Shaughnessy, S., Wallace, P., Hutto, A., Jenkins, A. J., . . . Garvey, W. T. (2004). Critical evaluation of adult treatment panel III criteria in identifying insulin resistance with dyslipidemia. *Diabetes Care,* 27(4), 978–983.

Ma, W.-Y., Yang, C.-Y., Shih, S.-R., Hsieh, H.-J., Hung, C. S., Chiu, F.-C., . . . Li, H.-Y. (2013). Measurement of Waist Circumference: Midabdominal or iliac crest? *Diabetes Care,* 36(6), 1660–1666. doi: 10.2337/dc12-1452

Navar-Boggan, A. M., Boggan, J. C., Stafford, J. A., Muhlbaier, L. H., McCarver, C., & Peterson, E. D. (2012). Hypertension control among patients followed by cardiologists. *Circ Cardiovasc Qual Outcomes,* 5(3), 352–357. doi: 10.1161/CIRCOUTCOMES.111.963488

O'Donnell, M. J., Xavier, D., Liu, L., Zhang, H., Chin, S. L., Rao-Melacini, P., . . . Yusuf, S. Risk factors for ischaemic and intracerebral haemorrhagic stroke in 22 countries (the INTERSTROKE study): a case-control study. *The Lancet,* 376(9735), 112–123. doi: http://dx.doi.org/10.1016/S0140-6736(10)60834-3

Okosieme, O. E., Peter, R., Usman, M., Bolusani, H., Suruliram, P., George, L., & Evans, L. M. (2008). Can Admission and Fasting Glucose Reliably Identify Undiagnosed Diabetes in Patients With Acute Coronary Syndrome? *Diabetes Care,* 31(10), 1955–1959. doi: 10.2337/dc08-0197

Payne, A. H., & Hales, D. B. (2004). Overview of Steroidogenic Enzymes in the Pathway from Cholesterol to Active Steroid Hormones. *Endocrine Reviews,* 25(6), 947–970. doi: 10.1210/er.2003-0030

Pletcher, M. J., Bibbins-Domingo, K., Lewis, C. E., Wei, G. S., Sidney, S., Carr, J. J., . . . Hulley, S. B. (2008). Prehypertension during young adulthood and coronary calcium later in life. *Ann Intern Med,* 149(2), 91–99.

Prior, J. O., Quiñones, M. J., Hernandez-Pampaloni, M., Facta, A. D., Schindler, T. H., Sayre, J. W., . . . Schelbert, H. R. (2005). Coronary Circulatory Dysfunction in Insulin Resistance, Impaired Glucose Tolerance, and Type 2 Diabetes Mellitus. *Circulation,* 111(18), 2291–2298. doi: 10.1161/01.cir.0000164232.62768.51

Qureshi, A. I., Suri, M. F. K., Kirmani, J. F., Divani, A. A., & Mohammad, Y. (2005). Is Prehypertension a Risk Factor for Cardiovascular Diseases? *Stroke,* 36(9), 1859–1863. doi: 10.1161/01.STR.0000177495.45580.f1

Reduction in the Incidence of Type 2 Diabetes with Lifestyle Intervention or Metformin. (2002). *N Engl J Med,* 346(6), 393–403. doi: 10.1056/NEJMoa012512

Studies to Treat or Prevent Pediatric Type 2 Diabetes Prevention Study, G. (2008). Prevalence of the metabolic syndrome among a racially/ethnically diverse group of U.S. eighth-grade adolescents and associations with fasting insulin and homeostasis model assessment of insulin resistance levels. *Diabetes Care,* 31(10), 2020–2025. doi: 10.2337/dc08-0411

Tankó, L. B., Bagger, Y. Z., Alexandersen, P., Larsen, P. J., & Christiansen, C. (2003). Peripheral Adiposity Exhibits an Independent Dominant Antiatherogenic Effect in Elderly Women. *Circulation,* 107(12), 1626–1631. doi: 10.1161/01.cir.0000057974.74060.68

Chapter Five

AACE Menopause Guidelines Revision Task Force. (2006). American Association of Clinical Endocrinologists medical guidelines for clinical practice for the diagnosis and treatment of menopause. *Endocrine Practice,* 12, 315–337.

Abbas, A., Fadel, P., Wang, Z., et al. (2004). Contrasting effects of oral versus transdermal estrogen on serum amyloid A (SAA) and high-density lipoprotein-SAA in postmenopausal women. *Arterioscler Thromb Vasc Bio,* 24: e164–e167.

Banks, E., Beral V., Reeves G., et al. (2004). Fracture incidence in relation to the pattern of use of hormone therapy in postmenopausal women. *JAMA,* 291(18), 2212–2220.

Boostanfar, R. S., Saada T., Poysky J., et al. (June 2002). Serum endocrine markers and psychosocial mood in postmenopausal women: The difference between transdermal and oral HRT. Presented at 10th World Congress on Menopause; Berlin, Germany.

Brinton, L. A., Barrett, R. J., Berman, M. L., Mortel, R., Twiggs, L. B., Wilbanks, G. D. (1993). Cigarette smoking and the risk of endometrial cancer. *Am J Epidemiology,* 137, 281–291.

Chu, M., Cosper, P., Nakhuda, G. S., et al. (2006). A comparison of oral and transdermal short-term estrogen therapy in postmenopausal women with metabolic syndrome. *Fertility and Sterility* 86, 1669–1675.

Chu, M. C., Cosper, P., Lobo, R. A. (2005). Comparison of oral and transdermal estradiol therapy on insulin resistance parameters in postmenopausal women. *Fertility and Sterility,* 84(supp 1), S121.

Chu, M. C., Cosper, P., Nakhuda, G. S., et al. (2006). A comparison of oral and transdermal short-term estrogen therapy in postmenopausal women with metabolic syndrome. *Fertility and Sterility,* 86(6), 1669–1675.

Chu, M. C., Cushman, M., Solomon, R., et al. (2008). Metabolic syndrome in postmenopausal women: the influence of oral or transdermal estradiol on inflammation and coagulation markers. *Am J Obstet Gynecol,* 199, 526.e1–526.e7.

Cirillo, D. J., Wallace, R. B., and Rodabough, R. J. (2005). Effect of estrogen therapy on gallbladder disease. *JAMA,* 295, 330–339.

Clendenen, T. V., Koenig, K. L., Shore, R. E., et al. (2009). Postmenopausal levels of endogenous sex hormones and risk of colorectal cancer. *Cancer Epidemiology, Biomarkers & Prevention,* 18(1), 275–281.

Colao, A., Spiezia, S., et al. (2005). Circulating insulin-like growth factor-1 levels are correlated with the atherosclerotic profile in healthy subjects independently of age. *J Endocrinol Invest,* 28, 440–448.

Colbert, J., Martin, B. J., Hauer, T., Haykowsky, M., Austford, L., Arena, R., . . . Stone, J. (2013). Cardiac Rehabilitation Referral and Attendance in Women: A High-risk Population with Two Strikes Against It. *J Am Coll Cardiol,* 61(10_S). doi: 10.1016/S0735-1097(13)61414X

Darling, G. M., Johns, J. A., McCloud, P. I., et al. (1997). Estrogen and progestin compared with simvastatin for hypercholesterolemia in postmenopausal women. *N Engl J Med,* 337(9), 595–601.

DeCarlo, C., Tommaselli, G., et al. (2004). Serum leptin levels and body composition in postmenopausal women: effects of hormone therapy. *Menopause,* 11(4), 466–473.

Dennison, E, Mohamed, M. A., Cooper, C. (2006). Epidemiology of Osteoporosis. *Rheumatic Disease Clinics of North America,* 32(4), 617–780.

Elavsky, Steriani, Gonzales, Joaquin U., Proctor, David N., Williams, Nancy, Henderson, Victor W. (2012). Effects of physical activity on vasomotor symptoms: examination using objective and subjective measures. *Menopause.* doi: 10.1097/gme.0b013e31824f8fb8

Field, C. S., Ory, S. J., Wahner, H. W., et al. (1993). Preventive effects of transdermal 17B-estradiol on osteoporotic changes after surgical menopause: a two-year placebo-controlled trial. *Am J Obstet Gynecol,* 168, 114.

Gao, Y., Pacifici R. (2004). Key Mechanism in Estrogen's Role in Preventing Bone Loss. *Proceedings of the National Academy of Sciences of the United States of America.*

Gaudet, M. M., Gapstur, S. M., Sun, J., et al. (2013). Active Smoking and breast cancer risk: original cohort data and meta-analysis. *J Natl Cancer Inst,* 105(8), 15–25. doi: 10.1093/jknci/djt023. Epub (2013 Feb 28). http://www.ncbi.nlm.nih.gov/pubmed/23449445

Goodman, M. P. (2009). Is there any role for oral estrogen therapy?: The Case for Transdermal Therapy as of 2009. Abstract Presented at the 20th Annual Meeting of the North America Menopause Society, San Diego, California.

Hanington, E., Jones, R., Amess, J. (1982). Platelet aggregation in response to 5HT in migraine patients taking oral contraceptives. *The Lancet,* 1, 967–968.

Herrington, D. M., Parks, J. S. (2004). Estrogen and HDL: all that glitters is not gold. *Arterioscler Thromb Vasc Biol,* 24, 1741–1742.

Hollenbach, K. A., Barrett-Connor, E., Edelstein, S. L., Holbrook, T. Cigarette Smoking and Bone Mineral Density in Older Men and Women. *Am Journal of Public Health* 83(9),

1265–1270. http://www.ncbi.nlm.nih.gov/pmc/articles/PMC1694953/pdf/amjph00533-0075.pdf

Indiana University. (2013, 3 July). Older women who quit smoking can cut heart disease risk regardless of diabetes status. *ScienceDaily.* http://www.sciencedaily.com / releases/2013/07/130703101444.htm

Jessel, R. H., Nachtigall, M. J., Nachtigall, L. E. (October 2009). Obstetrics and Gynecology, NYU School of Medicine, New York, NY, two cases of endometrial adenocarcinoma in postmenopausal women on bioidentical hormone replacement therapy. Clinical Poster Presentation at the 20th Annual Meeting of the North American Menopause Society Annual Meeting.

Johnson, S. P., Hundborg, H. H, et al. (2005). Insulin-like growth factor (IGF-1) I-II and IGF binding protein-3 and risk of ischemic stroke. *J Clin Endocrinol Metab,* 90, 5937–5941.

Kleppinger, A., Kulidorff, M. (2003). Ultralow-dose micronized 17 B-estradiol and bone density and bone metabolism in older women. *JAMA,* 290(8), 1042–1048.

L'Hermite, M. L., Simoncini, T., Fuller, S., et al. (2002). Could transdermal estradiol + progesterone be a safer postmenopausal HRT?: A Review. *Maturitas,* 60, 185–201.

Liu, B., Beral, V., Balkwill, A., et al. (2008). Gallbladder disease and use of transdermal versus oral hormone replacement therapy in postmenopausal women: prospective cohort study. *BMJ,* 337, a386.

Lobo, R. A. (May 2013). Where Are We 10 years After the Women's Health Initiative? *J Clin Endocrinol Metab,* 98(5), 1771–1780. http://jcem.endojournals.org/content/98/5/1771.full.pdf + html

Lufkin, E. G., Wahner, H. W., Judd, H. L., et al. (1992). Treatment of postmenopausal osteoporosis with transdermal estrogen. *Ann Intern Med,* 117(1), 1–9.

Luo, Juhua, Rossouw, Jacques, Margolis, Karen L. (2013). Smoking Cessation, Weight Change, and Coronary Heart Disease Among Postmenopausal Women With and Without Diabetes: Coronary Heart Disease Among Postmenopausal Women. *JAMA,* 310(1), 94. doi: 10.1001/jama.2013.6871

Lwin, R., Darnell, B., Oster, R., et al. (2008). Effect of oral estrogen on substrate utilization in postmenopausal women. *Fertility and Sterility,* 90(4), 1275–1278.

Martin, V. T., Behbehani, M. (2006). Ovarian hormones and migraine headache: understanding mechanisms and pathogenesis. *Headache,* 46(3), 365–386.

Modena, M. G., Bursi, F., Fantini, G., et al. (2002). Effects of hormone replacement therapy on c-reactive protein levels in healthy postmenopausal women: comparison between oral and transdermal administration of estrogen. *Am J Med,* 113, 331–334.

Modena, M. G., Sismondi, P., et al. (2005). New evidence regarding hormone replacement therapies is urgently required transdermal postmenopausal hormone therapy differs from oral hormone therapy in risks and benefits. *Maturitas,* 52(1), 1–10.

Moyer, V. A. (2013). Menopausal Hormone Therapy for the Primary Prevention of Chronic Conditions: U.S. Preventive Services Task Force Recommendation Statement. *Ann Intern Med,* 158, 47–54. http://www.uspreventiveservicestaskforce.org/uspstf12/menohrt/menohrtfinalrs.pdf

Nachtigall, L. E., Raju, U., Banerjee, S., et al. (2000). Serum estradiol-binding profiles in postmenopausal women undergoing three common estrogen replacement therapies: associations with sex hormone binding globulin, estradiol, and estrone levels. *Menopause,* 7, 243–250.

Nappi, R. E., Polatti, F. (2009). The use of estrogen therapy in women's sexual functioning. *J Sex Med,* 6(3), 603–616.

O'Connell, M. B., (1995). Pharmacokinetic and pharmacologic variation between different estrogen products. *J Clin Pharmacol,* 35 (suppl), 18S–24S.

O'Sullivan, A. J., Crampton, L. J., Freund, et al. (1998). The route of estrogen replacement therapy confers divergent effects on substrate oxidation and body composition in post-menopausal women. *J Clin Invest,* 102, 1035–1040.

Parajuli, R., Bjerkaas, E., Gram, I. T., et al. (2013). The increased risk of colon cancer due to cigarette smoking may be greater in women than men. *Cancer Epidemiol Biomarkers Prev,* 5, 862–871. doi: 10.1158/1055-9965.EPI-12-1351. Epub (2013 Apr 30). http://www.ncbi.nlm.nih.gov/pubmed/23632818

Parente, R. C., Faerstein, E., Celeste, R. K., Werneck, G. L. (2008). The relationship between smoking and age at the menopause: a systematic review. *Maturitas,* 61, 287–298.

Parker, W. H., Feskanich, D., Manson, J. E., et al. (2013). Long-Term Mortality Associated With Oophorectomy Compared With Ovarian Conservation in the Nurses' Health Study. *Obstet Gynecol,* 21(4), 709–716. doi: 10.1097/AOG.0b013e3182864350

Penn State. (2012, June 27). Menopausal women could "work out" their hot flashes. *Science-Daily.* http://www.sciencedaily.com/releases/2012/06/120627122254.htm

Prentice, R. L., et al. (2009). Benefits and risks of postmenopausal hormone therapy when it is initiated soon after menopause. *Am J Epidemiol,* 170, 12.

Prince, R. L., Smith, M., Dick, I. M., et al. (1991). Prevention of postmenopausal osteoporosis: a comparative study of exercise, calcium supplementation, and hormone-replacement therapy. *N Engl J Med,* 325, 1189.

Ropponen, A., Aittomaki, K., Vihma, V., et al. (2005). Effects of oral and transdermal estradiol administration on levels of sex hormone-binding globulin in postmenopausal women with and without a history of intrahepatic cholestatis of pregnancy. *J Clin Endocrinol Metab,* 90(6)x, 3431–3434.

Rossouw, J. E., Prentice, R. L., Manson, J. E., et al. (2007). Postmenopausal hormone therapy and risk of cardiovascular disease by age and years since menopause. *JAMA,* 297(13), 1465–1477.

Sandhu, R., Jimenez, M. C., Chiuve, S. E., et al. (2012, December 11). Smoking, Smoking Cessation and Risk of Sudden Cardiac Death in Women. *Circ Arrhythm Electrophysiol.* http://circep.ahajournals.org/content/early/2012/11/16/CIRCEP.112.975219.abstract

Sare, G. M., Gray, L. J., Bath, P. M. W. (2008). Association between hormone replacement therapy and subsequent arterial and venous vascular events: a meta-analysis. *Eur Heart J,* 29, 2031–2041.

Sarrel, P. M., Njike, V. Y., Vinate, V., Katz, D. L. (September 2013). The Mortality Toll of Estrogen Avoidance: An Analysis of Excess Deaths Among Hysterectomized Women Aged 50-59. *Am J Public Health,* 103(9), 1583–1588. http://ajph.aphapublications.org/doi/pdf/10.2105/AJPH.2013.301295

Scarabin, P. Y., Oger, E., Plu-Bureau, G. (2003). Estrogen and thromboembolism risk study group: Differential association of oral and transdermal oestrogen-replacement therapy with venous thromboembolism risk. *The Lancet,* 362, 428–432.

Shifren, J., Desindes, S., et al. (2007). A randomized, open-label, crossover study comparing the effects of oral versus transdermal estrogen therapy on serum androgens, thyroid hormones, and adrenal hormones in naturally menopausal women. *Menopause,* 14(6), 985–994.

Shifren, J. L. (2008). A comparison of the short-term effects of oral conjugated equine estrogens versus transdermal estradiol on C-reactive protein, other serum markers of inflammation, and other hepatic proteins in naturally menopausal women. *J Clin Endocrinol Metab,* 9(5), 1702–1710.

Shrifrin, J. L., Desindes, S., McIlwain, M., Doros, G., Mazer, N. A. (2007). A randomized, open-label crossover study comparing the effects of oral versus transdermal estrogen therapy on serum androgens, thyroid hormones, and adrenal hormones in naturally menopausal women. *Menopause,* 14: 985–994.

Shriver, S. P., Bourdeau, H. A., Gubish, C. T., et al. (2000). Sex-Specific Expression of Gastri-Releasing Peptide Receptor: Relationship to Smoking history and Risk of Lung Cancer. *J Natl Cancer Inst,* 92(1), 24–33. doi: 10.1093/jnci/92.1.24 http://jnci.oxfordjournals.org/content/92/1/24.short

Simon, Stacy. (2013, February 28). Study Links Smoking to Breast Cancer Risk. *Cancer.org.* http://www.cancer.org/cancer/news/study-links-smoking-to-breast-cancer-risk

Slater, C. C., Hodis, H. N., Mack, W. J., et al. (2001). Markedly elevated levels of estrone sulfate after long-term oral, but not transdermal, administration of estradiol in postmenopausal women. *Menopause,* 8, 200–203.

Straczek, C., Oger, E., Yon de Jonage-Canonico, M. B., et al. (2005). Prothrombotic mutations, hormone therapy, and venous thromboembolism among postmenopausal women: impact of the route of estrogen administration. *Circulation,* 11, 3495–3500.

Sun, L., Tan, L., Yang, F., et al. Meta-analysis Suggests that Smoking is Associated with an Increased Risk of Early Natural Menopause. *Menopause,* 19(2), 126–132. http://www.medscape.com/viewarticle/757803_2

The Writing Group for the PEPI. (1996). Effects of hormone therapy on bone mineral density: results from the postmenopausal estrogen/progestin interventions (PEPI) trial. *JAMA,* 276, 1389.

Turgeon, J. L., McDonnell, D. P., Wise, K. A., Wise, P. M. (2004). Hormone therapy: physiological complexity belies therapeutic simplicity. *Science,* 304, 1269–1273.

Uhler, M. L., Marks, J. W., Voigt, B. J., Judd, H. L. (1998). Comparison of the impact of transdermal versus oral estrogen on biliary markers of gallstone formation in postmenopausal women. *J Clin Endocrinol Metab,* 83(2), 410–414.

Vehkavaara, S., Hakala-Ala-Pietila, T., Virkamaki, A., et al. (2000). Differential effects of oral and transdermal estrogen replacement therapy on endothelial function in postmenopausal women. *Circulation,* 102, 2687–2693.

Vehkavaara, S., Silveira, A., Hakala-ala-Pietila, T., et al. (2001). Effects of oral and transdermal estrogen replacement therapy on markers of coagulation, fibrinolysis, inflammation and serum lipids and lipoproteins in postmenopausal women. *Thromb Haemost,* 85, 619–625.

Villareal, D. T., Binder, E. F., Williams, D. B., et al. (2001). Bone mineral density response to estrogen replacement in frail elderly women: a randomized controlled trial. *JAMA,* 286(7), 815–820.

Vongpatanasin, W., Tuncel, M., Mansour, Y., Arbique, D., Victor, R. G. (2001). Transdermal estrogen replacement therapy decreases sympathetic activity in postmenopausal women. *Circulation,* 103, 2903–2908.

Walsh, B. W., Schiff, I., Rosner, B., et al. (1991). Effects of postmenopausal estrogen replacement on the concentrations and metabolism of plasma lipoproteins. *N Engl J Med,* 325(17), 1196–1204.

Wren, B. G., Champion, S. M., Willetts, K., Manga, R. Z., Eden, J. A. (2003). Transdermal progesterone and its effect on vasomotor symptoms, blood lipid levels, bone metabolic markers, moods, and quality of life for postmenopausal women. *Menopause,* 10, 13–18.

Wren, B. G., McFarland, K., Edwards, L. (1999). Micronised transdermal progesterone and endometrial response. *The Lancet,* 354, 1447–1448.

Writing Group for the Women's Health Initiative Investigators. (2004). Effects of conjugated equine estrogen in postmenopausal women with hysterectomy. *JAMA,* 291, 1701–1712.

____. (2002). Risks and benefits of estrogen plus progestin in healthy postmenopausal women: principal results from the Women's Health Initiative randomized controlled trial. *JAMA,* 88, 321–333.

Chapter Six

Adult participation in aerobic and muscle-strengthening physical activities - United States, 2011. (2013). *MMWR,* 62(17), 326–330.

Allison, M. A., Hiatt, W. R., Hirsch, A. T., Coll, J. R., & Criqui, M. H. (2008). A High Ankle-Brachial Index Is Associated With Increased Cardiovascular Disease Morbidity and Lower Quality of Life. *J Am Coll Cardiol,* 51(13), 1292–1298. doi: http://dx.doi.org/10.1016/j.jacc.2007.11.064

Baldassarre, D., Hamsten, A., Veglia, F., de Faire, U., Humphries, S. E., Smit, A. J., . . . Group, I. S. (2012). Measurements of carotid intima-media thickness and of interadventitia common carotid diameter improve prediction of cardiovascular events: results of the IMPROVE (Carotid Intima Media Thickness [IMT] and IMT-Progression as Predictors of Vascular Events in a High Risk European Population) study. *J Am Coll Cardiol,* 60(16), 1489–1499. doi: 10.1016/j.jacc.2012.06.034

Belcaro, G., Nicolaides, A. N., Ramaswami, G., Cesarone, M. R., De Sanctis, M., Incandela, L., . . . Martines, G. (2001). Carotid and femoral ultrasound morphology screening and cardiovascular events in low risk subjects: a 10-year follow-up study (the CAFES-CAVE study). *Atherosclerosis,* 156(2), 379–387. doi: http://dx.doi.org/10.1016/S0021-9150(00)00665-1

Bluemke, D. A., Achenbach, S., Budoff, M., Gerber, T. C., Gersh, B., Hillis, L. D., . . . Woodard, P. K. (2008). Noninvasive Coronary Artery Imaging: Magnetic Resonance Angiography and Multidetector Computed Tomography Angiography: A Scientific Statement From the American Heart Association Committee on Cardiovascular Imaging and Intervention of the Council on Cardiovascular Radiology and Intervention, and the Councils on Clinical Cardiology and Cardiovascular Disease in the Young. *Circulation,* 118(5), 586–606. doi: 10.1161/circulationaha.108.189695

Bourque, J. M., Patel, C. A., Ali, M. M., Perez, M., Watson, D. D., & Beller, G. A. (2013). Prevalence and Predictors of Ischemia and Outcomes in Outpatients With Diabetes Mellitus Referred for Single-Photon Emission Computed Tomography Myocardial Perfusion Imaging. *Circulation: Cardiovascular Imaging,* 6(3), 466–477. doi: 10.1161/circimaging.112.000259

Budoff, M. J., Achenbach, S., Blumenthal, R. S., Carr, J. J., Goldin, J. G., Greenland, P., . . . Wiegers, S. E. (2006). Assessment of Coronary Artery Disease by Cardiac Computed Tomography: A Scientific Statement From the American Heart Association Committee on Cardiovascular Imaging and Intervention, Council on Cardiovascular Radiology and

Intervention, and Committee on Cardiac Imaging, Council on Clinical Cardiology. *Circulation*. doi: 10.1161/circulationaha.106.178458

Candell-Riera, J., Ferreira-González, I., Marsal, J. R., Aguadé-Bruix, S., Cuberas-Borrós, G., Pujol, P., . . . García-Dorado, D. (2013). Usefulness of Exercise Test and Myocardial Perfusion–Gated Single Photon Emission Computed Tomography to Improve the Prediction of Major Events. *Circulation: Cardiovascular Imaging, 6*(4), 531–541. doi: 10.1161/circimaging.112.000158

Cobble, M., & Bale, B. (2010). Carotid intima-media thickness: knowledge and application to everyday practice. *Postgrad Med, 122*(1), 10–18. doi: 10.3810/pgm.2010.01.2091

Criqui, M. H., Alberts, M. J., Fowkes, F. G. R., Hirsch, A. T., O'Gara, P. T., Olin, J. W., & American Heart Association Writing Group 2. (2008). Atherosclerotic Peripheral Vascular Disease Symposium II: Screening for Atherosclerotic Vascular Diseases: Should Nationwide Programs Be Instituted? *Circulation, 118*(25), 2830–2836. doi: 10.1161/circulationaha.108.191172

De Michele, M., Zaccaro, D. J., & Bond, G. (2006). Assessment of carotid intima–media thickness in subjects with ischemic cerebrovascular events undergoing endarterectomy. *Nutrition, Metabolism and Cardiovascular Diseases, 16*(8), 536–542. doi: http://dx.doi.org/10.1016/j.numecd.2005.10.002

Einstein, A. J. (2013). Radiation from cardiac imaging tests: questions you should ask. *Circulation, 127*(11), e495–497. doi: 10.1161/CIRCULATIONAHA.112.146043

Einstein, A. J., Henzlova, M. J., & Rajagopalan, S. (2007). Estimating risk of cancer associated with radiation exposure from 64-slice computed tomography coronary angiography. *JAMA, 298*(3), 317–323. doi: 10.1001/jama.298.3.317

Eisenberg, M. J., Afilalo, J., Lawler, P. R., Abrahamowicz, M., Richard, H., & Pilote, L. (2011). Cancer risk related to low-dose ionizing radiation from cardiac imaging in patients after acute myocardial infarction. *CMAJ, 183*(4), 430–436. doi: 10.1503/cmaj.100463

Feinstein, M., Ning, H., Kang, J., Bertoni, A., Carnethon, M., & Lloyd-Jones, D. M. (2012). Racial differences in risks for first cardiovascular events and noncardiovascular death: the Atherosclerosis Risk in Communities study, the Cardiovascular Health Study, and the Multi-Ethnic Study of Atherosclerosis. *Circulation, 126*(1), 50–59. doi: 10.1161/CIRCULATIONAHA.111.057232

Galluzzi, L., & Kroemer, G. (2012). Autophagy mediates the metabolic benefits of endurance training. *Circ Res, 110*(10), 1276–1278. doi: 10.1161/RES.0b013e318259e70b

Gottlieb, I., Miller, J. M., Arbab-Zadeh, A., Dewey, M., Clouse, M. E., Sara, L., . . . Rochitte, C. E. (2010). The absence of coronary calcification does not exclude obstructive coronary artery disease or the need for revascularization in patients referred for conventional coronary angiography. *J Am Coll Cardiol, 55*(7), 627–634. doi: 10.1016/j.jacc.2009.07.072

Hankey, G. J., Norman, P. E., & Eikelboom, J. W. (2006). Medical treatment of peripheral arterial disease. *JAMA, 295*(5), 547–553. doi: 10.1001/jama.295.5.547

Harris, C. D., et al. (2013). Adult Participation in Aerobic and Muscle-Strengthening Physical Activities--United States, 2011. *Morb Mortal Wkly Rep, 62*, 326–330.

Hiatt, W. R. (2001). Medical Treatment of Peripheral Arterial Disease and Claudication. *N Engl J Med, 344*(21), 1608–1621. doi: 10.1056/NEJM200105243442108

Hiatt, W. R., Goldstone, J., Smith, S. C., Jr., McDermott, M., Moneta, G., Oka, R., . . . American Heart Association Writing, G. (2008). Atherosclerotic Peripheral Vascular Disease Symposium II: nomenclature for vascular diseases. *Circulation, 118*(25), 2826–2829. doi: 10.1161/CIRCULATIONAHA.108.191171

Hirsch, A. T., Criqui, M. H., Treat-Jacobson, D., et al. (2001). Peripheral arterial disease detection, awareness, and treatment in primary care. *JAMA, 286*(11), 1317–1324. doi: 10.1001/jama.286.11.1317

Interleukin-6 receptor pathways in coronary heart disease: a collaborative meta-analysis of 82 studies. *The Lancet, 379*(9822), 1205–1213. doi: http://dx.doi.org/10.1016/S0140-6736(11)61931-4

Kent, K. C., Zwolak, R. M., Jaff, M. R., Hollenbeck, S. T., Thompson, R. W., Schermerhorn, M. L., . . . Cronenwett, J. L. (2004). Screening for abdominal aortic aneurysm: A consensus statement. *J Vasc Surg, 39*(1), 267–269. doi: http://dx.doi.org/10.1016/j.jvs.2003.08.019

Lederle, F. A., Larson, J. C., Margolis, K. L., Allison, M. A., Freiberg, M. S., Cochrane, B. B., . . . Curb, J. D. (2008). Abdominal aortic aneurysm events in the women's health initiative: cohort study. *Bmj, 337*, a1724. doi: 10.1136/bmj.a1724

Martin, S. S., Blaha, M. J., Blankstein, R., Agatston, A. S., Rivera, J. J., Virani, S. S., . . . Nasir, K. (2013). Dyslipidemia, Coronary Artery Calcium, and Incident Atherosclerotic Cardiovascular Disease: Implications for Statin Therapy from the Multi-Ethnic Study of Atherosclerosis. *Circulation.* doi: 10.1161/circulationaha.113.003625

Members, C., Gibbons, R. J., Balady, G. J., Beasley, J. W., FAAFP, Bricker, J. T., . . . Members, T. F. (1997). ACC/AHA Guidelines for Exercise Testing: Executive Summary: A Report of the American College of Cardiology/ American Heart Association Task Force on Practice Guidelines (Committee on Exercise Testing). *Circulation, 96*(1), 345–354. doi: 10.1161/01.cir.96.1.345

Naghavi, M., Falk, E., Hecht, H. S., Jamieson, M. J., Kaul, S., Berman, D., . . . Shah, P. K. (2006). From Vulnerable Plaque to Vulnerable Patient—Part III: Executive Summary of the Screening for Heart Attack Prevention and Education (SHAPE) Task Force Report. *Am J Cardiol, 98*(2, Supplement 1), 2–15. doi: http://dx.doi.org/10.1016/j.amjcard.2006.03.002

Nambi, V., Chambless, L., Folsom, A. R., He, M., Hu, Y., Mosley, T., . . . Ballantyne, C. M. (2010). Carotid intima-media thickness and presence or absence of plaque improves prediction of coronary heart disease risk: the ARIC (Atherosclerosis Risk In Communities) study. *J Am Coll Cardiol, 55*(15), 1600–1607. doi: 10.1016/j.jacc.2009.11.075

Patel, M. R., Peterson, E. D., Dai, D., Brennan, J. M., Redberg, R. F., Anderson, H. V., . . . Douglas, P. S. (2010). Low Diagnostic Yield of Elective Coronary Angiography. *N Engl J Med, 362*(10), 886–895. doi: 10.1056/NEJMoa0907272

Polak, J. F., Pencina, M. J., O'Leary, D. H., & D'Agostino, R. B. (2011). Common Carotid Artery Intima-Media Thickness Progression as a Predictor of Stroke in Multi-Ethnic Study of Atherosclerosis. *Stroke, 42*(11), 3017–3021. doi: 10.1161/strokeaha.111.625186

Rotter, M. A., Schnatz, P. F., Currier, A. A., Jr., & O'Sullivan, D. M. (2008). Breast arterial calcifications (BACs) found on screening mammography and their association with cardiovascular disease. *Menopause, 15*(2), 276–281. doi: 10.1097/gme.0b013e3181405d0a

Smith, S. C., Greenland, P., & Grundy, S. M. (2000). Prevention Conference V: Beyond Secondary Prevention: Identifying the High-Risk Patient for Primary Prevention: Executive Summary. *Circulation, 101*(1), 111–116. doi: 10.1161/01.cir.101.1.111

Steg, P., Bhatt, D. L., Wilson, P. F., et al. (2007). One-year cardiovascular event rates in outpatients with atherothrombosis. *JAMA, 297*(11), 1197–1206. doi: 10.1001/jama.297.11.1197

The Society of Atherosclerosis, I., & Prevention. (2011). Appropriate use criteria for carotid intima media thickness testing. *Atherosclerosis, 214*(1), 43–46. doi: http://dx.doi.org/10.1016/j.atherosclerosis.2010.10.045

Vidal, J.-S., Sigurdsson, S., Jonsdottir, M. K., Eiriksdottir, G., Thorgeirsson, G., Kjartansson, O., . . . Launer, L. J. (2010). Coronary Artery Calcium, Brain Function and Structure: The AGES-Reykjavik Study. *Stroke, 41*(5), 891–897. doi: 10.1161/strokeaha.110.579581

Vliegenthart, R., Oudkerk, M., Hofman, A., Oei, H.-H. S., van Dijck, W., van Rooij, F. J. A., & Witteman, J. C. M. (2005). Coronary Calcification Improves Cardiovascular Risk Prediction in the Elderly. *Circulation, 112*(4), 572–577. doi: 10.1161/circulationaha.104.488916

Weintraub, W. S., Karlsberg, R. P., Tcheng, J. E., Boris, J. R., Buxton, A. E., Dove, J. T., . . . Shahian, D. M. (2011). ACCF/AHA 2011 key data elements and definitions of a base cardiovascular vocabulary for electronic health records: a report of the American College of Cardiology Foundation/American Heart Association Task Force on Clinical Data Standards. *J Am Coll Cardiol, 58*(2), 202-222. doi: 10.1016/j.jacc.2011.05.001

Wen, M., & Kowaleski-Jones, L. (2012). Sex and ethnic differences in validity of self-reported adult height, weight and body mass index. *Ethn Dis, 22*(1), 72–78.

Wolff, T., Guirguis-Blake, J., Miller, T., Gillespie, M., & Harris, R. (2007). Screening for Carotid Artery Stenosis: An Update of the Evidence for the U.S. Preventive Services Task Force. *Ann Intern Med, 147*(12), 860–870. doi: 10.7326/0003-4819-147-12-200712180-00006

Yeboah, J., McClelland, R. L., Polonsky, T. S., et al. (2012). Comparison of novel risk markers for improvement in cardiovascular risk assessment in intermediate-risk individuals. *JAMA, 308*(8), 788–795. doi: 10.1001/jama.2012.9624

Chapter Seven

Abdelbaky, A., Corsini, E., Figueroa, A. L., Fontanez, S., Subramanian, S., Ferencik, M., . . . Tawakol, A. (2013). Focal Arterial Inflammation Precedes Subsequent Calcification in the Same Location: A Longitudinal FDG-PET/CT Study. *Circulation: Cardiovascular Imaging, 6*(5), 747–754. doi: 10.1161/circimaging.113.000382

Allison, M., Jensky, N., Marshall, S., Bertoni, A., & Cushman, M. (2012). Sedentary behavior and adiposity-associated inflammation: the Multi-Ethnic Study of Atherosclerosis. *Am J Prev Med, 42*, 8–13.

Amar, S., Gokce, N., Morgan, S., Loukideli, M., Van Dyke, T., & Vita, J. (2003). Periodontal disease is associated with brachial artery endothelial dysfunction and systemic inflammation. *Arterioscler Thromb Vasc Biol, 23*, 1245–1249.

Ärnlöv, J., Evans, J. C., Meigs, J. B., Wang, T. J., Fox, C. S., Levy, D., . . . Vasan, R. S. (2005). Low-Grade Albuminuria and Incidence of Cardiovascular Disease Events in Nonhypertensive and Nondiabetic Individuals: The Framingham Heart Study. *Circulation, 112*(7), 969–975. doi: 10.1161/circulationaha.105.538132

Bale, B. F., D. A. L. (2013). Autophagy, Senescence, and Arterial Inflammation: Relationship to Arterial Health and Longevity. *Altern Ther Health Med, 19*(4), 8–10.

Berk, M., Williams, L., Jacka, F., O'Neil, A., Pasco, J., Moylan, S., . . . Maes, M. (2013). So depression is an inflammatory disease, but where does the inflammation come from? *BMC Medicine, 11*(1), 200.

Brilakis, E. S., McConnell, J. P., Lennon, R. J., Elesber, A. A., Meyer, J. G., & Berger, P. B. (2005). Association of lipoprotein-associated phospholipase A2 levels with coronary artery disease risk factors, angiographic coronary artery disease, and major adverse events at follow-up. *Eur Heart J,* 26(2), 137–144. doi: 10.1093/eurheartj/ehi010

Chae, C. U., Lee, R. T., Rifai, N., & Ridker, P. M. (2001). Blood Pressure and Inflammation in Apparently Healthy Men. *Hypertension,* 38(3), 399–403. doi: 10.1161/01.hyp.38.3.399

Chrysohoou, C., Panagiotakos, D., Pitsavos, C., Das, U., & Stefanadis, C. (2004). Adherence to the Mediterranean diet attenuates inflammation and coagulation process in healthy adults: The ATTICA Study. *J Am Coll Cardiol,* 44, 152–158.

Coussens, L. M., & Werb, Z. (2002). Inflammation and cancer. *Nature,* 420(6917), 860-867. doi: 10.1038/nature01322

Daskalopoulou, S. S., Delaney, J. A. C., Filion, K. B., Brophy, J. M., Mayo, N. E., & Suissa, S. (2008). Discontinuation of statin therapy following an acute myocardial infarction: a population-based study. *Eur Heart J.* doi: 10.1093/eurheartj/ehn346

de Heredia, F., Gomez-Martinez, S., & Marcos, A. (2012). Obesity, inflammation and the immune system. *Proc Nutr Soc,* 71, 332–338.

Emerging Risk Factors, C., Kaptoge, S., Di Angelantonio, E., Pennells, L., Wood, A. M., White, I. R., . . . Danesh, J. (2012). C-reactive protein, fibrinogen, and cardiovascular disease prediction. *N Engl J Med,* 367(14), 1310–1320. doi: 10.1056/NEJMoa1107477

Estacio, R. O., Dale, R. A., Schrier, R., & Krantz, M. J. (2012). Relation of reduction in urinary albumin excretion to ten-year cardiovascular mortality in patients with type 2 diabetes and systemic hypertension. *Am J Cardiol,* 109(12), 1743–1748. doi: 10.1016/j.amjcard.2012.02.020

Ferguson, J. F., Hinkle, C. C., Mehta, N. N., Bagheri, R., Derohannessian, S. L., Shah, R., . . . Reilly, M. P. (2012). Translational studies of lipoprotein-associated phospholipase A(2) in inflammation and atherosclerosis. *J Am Coll Cardiol,* 59(8), 764–772. doi: 10.1016/j.jacc.2011.11.019

Fibrinogen Studies Collaboration. (2005). Plasma fibrinogen level and the risk of major cardiovascular diseases and nonvascular mortality: An individual participant meta-analysis. *JAMA,* 294(14), 1799–1809.

Garate, I., Garcia-Bueno, B., Madrigal, J., Caso, J., Alou, L., Gomez-Lus, M., . . . Leza, J. (2013). Stress-induced neuroinflammation: role of the Toll-like receptor-4 pathway. *Biol Psychiatry,* 73, 32–43.

Gogebakan, O., Kohl, A., Osterhoff, M. A., van Baak, M. A., Jebb, S. A., Papadaki, A., . . . DiOgenes. (2011). Effects of weight loss and long-term weight maintenance with diets varying in protein and glycemic index on cardiovascular risk factors: the diet, obesity, and genes (DiOGenes) study: a randomized, controlled trial. *Circulation,* 124(25), 2829–2838. doi: 10.1161/CIRCULATIONAHA.111.033274

Goldstein, L. B., Bushnell, C. D., Adams, R. J., Appel, L. J., Braun, L. T., Chaturvedi, S., . . . Outcomes, R. (2011). Guidelines for the primary prevention of stroke: a guideline for healthcare professionals from the American Heart Association/American Stroke Association. *Stroke,* 42(2), 517–584. doi: 10.1161/STR.0b013e3181fcb238

Greenland, P., Alpert, J. S., Beller, G. A., Benjamin, E. J., Budoff, M. J., Fayad, Z. A., . . . American Heart, A. (2010). 2010 ACCF/AHA guideline for assessment of cardiovascular risk in asymptomatic adults: a report of the American College of Cardiology Foundation/American Heart Association Task Force on Practice Guidelines. *J Am Coll Cardiol,* 56(25), e50-103. doi: 10.1016/j.jacc.2010.09.001

Hamer, M., Sabia, S., Batty, G. D., Shipley, M. J., Tabak, A. G., Singh-Manoux, A., & Kivimaki, M. (2012). Physical activity and inflammatory markers over 10 years: follow-up in men and women from the Whitehall II cohort study. *Circulation,* 126(8), 928–933. doi: 10.1161/CIRCULATIONAHA.112.103879

The interleukin-6 receptor as a target for prevention of coronary heart disease: a mendelian randomisation analysis. *The Lancet,* 379(9822), 1214–1224. doi: http://dx.doi.org/10.1016/S0140-6736(12)60110-X

Interleukin-6 receptor pathways in coronary heart disease: a collaborative meta-analysis of 82 studies. *The Lancet,* 379(9822), 1205–1213. doi: http://dx.doi.org/10.1016/S0140-6736(11)61931-4

Jelic, S., Lederer, D. J., Adams, T., Padeletti, M., Colombo, P. C., Factor, P. H., & Le Jemtel, T. H. (2010). Vascular inflammation in obesity and sleep apnea. *Circulation,* 121(8), 1014–1021. doi: 10.1161/CIRCULATIONAHA.109.900357

Kamer, A. R., Craig, R. G., Dasanayake, A. P., Brys, M., Glodzik-Sobanska, L., & de Leon, M. J. (2008). Inflammation and Alzheimer's disease: Possible role of periodontal diseases. *Alzheimer's & Dementia,* 4(4), 242–250. doi: http://dx.doi.org/10.1016/j.jalz.2007.08.004

Kempf, K., Herder, C., Erlund, I., Kolb, H., Martin, S., Carstensen, M., . . . Tuomilehto, J. (2010). Effects of coffee consumption on subclinical inflammation and other risk factors for type 2 diabetes: a clinical trial. *Am J Clin Nutr,* 91(4), 950–957. doi: 10.3945/ajcn.2009.28548

Kim, T. N., Kim, S., Yang, S. J., Yoo, H. J., Seo, J. A., Kim, S. G., . . . Choi, K. M. (2010). Vascular Inflammation in Patients With Impaired Glucose Tolerance and Type 2 Diabetes: Analysis With 18F-Fluorodeoxyglucose Positron Emission Tomography. *Circulation: Cardiovascular Imaging,* 3(2), 142–148. doi: 10.1161/circimaging.109.888909

Koenig, W., Twardella, D., Brenner, H., & Rothenbacher, D. (2006). Lipoprotein-Associated Phospholipase A2 Predicts Future Cardiovascular Events in Patients With Coronary Heart Disease Independently of Traditional Risk Factors, Markers of Inflammation, Renal Function, and Hemodynamic Stress. *Arterioscler Thromb Vasc Bio,* 26(7), 1586–1593. doi: 10.1161/01.ATV.0000222983.73369.c8

Lavi, S., Prasad, A., Yang, E. H., Mathew, V., Simari, R. D., Rihal, C. S., . . . Lerman, A. (2007). Smoking Is Associated With Epicardial Coronary Endothelial Dysfunction and Elevated White Blood Cell Count in Patients With Chest Pain and Early Coronary Artery Disease. *Circulation,* 115(20), 2621–2627. doi: 10.1161/circulationaha.106.641654

Libby, P. (2012). Inflammation in atherosclerosis. *Arterioscler Thromb Vasc Biol,* 32(9), 2045-2051. doi: 10.1161/ATVBAHA.108.179705

____. (2013). Mechanisms of Acute Coronary Syndromes and Their Implications for Therapy. *N Engl J Med,* 368(21), 2004–2013. doi:10.1056/NEJMra1216063

Maki-Petaja, K. M., Elkhawad, M., Cheriyan, J., Joshi, F. R., Ostor, A. J., Hall, F. C., . . . Wilkinson, I. B. (2012). Anti-tumor necrosis factor-alpha therapy reduces aortic inflammation and stiffness in patients with rheumatoid arthritis. *Circulation,* 126(21), 2473–2480. doi: 10.1161/CIRCULATIONAHA.112.120410

Meuwese, M. C., Stroes, E. S., Hazen, S. L., van Miert, J. N., Kuivenhoven, J. A., Schaub, R. G., . . . Boekholdt, S. M. (2007). Serum myeloperoxidase levels are associated with the future risk of coronary artery disease in apparently healthy individuals: the EPIC-Norfolk Prospective Population Study. *J Am Coll Cardiol,* 50(2), 159–165. doi: 10.1016/j.jacc.2007.03.033

Montecucco, F., & Mach, F. (2009). Update on statin-mediated anti-inflammatory activities in atherosclerosis. *Semin Immunopathol,* 31(1), 127–142. doi: 10.1007/s00281-009-0150-y

Morrow, J. D. (2005). Quantification of Isoprostanes as Indices of Oxidant Stress and the Risk of Atherosclerosis in Humans. *Arterioscler Thromb Vasc Bio,* 25(2), 279–286. doi: 10.1161/01.ATV.0000152605.64964.c0

Nicholls, S. J., & Hazen, S. L. (2005). Myeloperoxidase and Cardiovascular Disease. *Arterioscler Thromb Vasc Bio,* 25(6), 1102–1111. doi: 10.1161/01.ATV.0000163262.83456.6d

Pejcic, A., Kesic, L. J., & Milasin, J. (2011). C-reactive protein as a systemic marker of inflammation in periodontitis. *Eur J Clin Microbiol Infect Dis,* 30(3), 407–414. doi: 10.1007/s10096-010-1101-1

Pignatelli, P., Carnevale, R., Pastori, D., Cangemi, R., Napoleone, L., Bartimoccia, S., . . . Violi, F. (2012). Immediate antioxidant and antiplatelet effect of atorvastatin via inhibition of Nox2. *Circulation,* 126(1), 92–103. doi: 10.1161/CIRCULATIONAHA.112.095554

Ridker, P. M. (2009). The JUPITER Trial: Results, Controversies, and Implications for Prevention. *Circ Cardiovasc Qual Outcomes,* 2(3), 279–285. doi: 10.1161/circoutcomes.109.868299

Ridker, P. M., Rifai, N., Rose, L., Buring, J. E., & Cook, N. R. (2002). Comparison of C-Reactive Protein and Low-Density Lipoprotein Cholesterol Levels in the Prediction of First Cardiovascular Events. *N Engl J Med,* 347(20), 1557–1565. doi: 10.1056/NEJMoa021993

Rosa Neto, J. C., Lira, F. S., Venancio, D. P., Cunha, C. A., Oyama, L. M., Pimentel, G. D., . . . de Mello, M. T. (2010). Sleep deprivation affects inflammatory marker expression in adipose tissue. *Lipids Health Dis,* 9, 125. doi: 10.1186/1476-511X-9-125

Rosenson, R. S., & Tangney, C. C. (1998). Antiatherothrombotic properties of statins: Implications for cardiovascular event reduction. *JAMA,* 279(20), 1643–1650. doi: 10.1001/jama.279.20.1643

Sabatine, M. S., Morrow, D. A., Jablonski, K. A., Rice, M. M., Warnica, J. W., Domanski, M. J., . . . Investigators, f. t. P. (2007). Prognostic Significance of the Centers for Disease Control/American Heart Association High-Sensitivity C-Reactive Protein Cut Points for Cardiovascular and Other Outcomes in Patients With Stable Coronary Artery Disease. *Circulation,* 115(12), 1528–1536. doi: 10.1161/circulationaha.106.649939

Serruys, P. W., García-García, H. M., Buszman, P., Erne, P., Verheye, S., Aschermann, M., . . . Investigators, I. S.-. (2008). Effects of the Direct Lipoprotein-Associated Phospholipase A2 Inhibitor Darapladib on Human Coronary Atherosclerotic Plaque. *Circulation,* 118(11), 1172–1182. doi: 10.1161/circulationaha.108.771899

Shishehbor, M. H., Zhang, R., Medina, H., Brennan, M. L., Brennan, D. M., Ellis, S. G., . . . Hazen, S. L. (2006). Systemic elevations of free radical oxidation products of arachidonic acid are associated with angiographic evidence of coronary artery disease. *Free Radic Biol Med,* 41(11), 1678–1683. doi: 10.1016/j.freeradbiomed.2006.09.001

Simpson, N., & Dinges, D. (2007). Sleep and inflammation. *Nutr Rev,* 65, S244–252.

Smith, J. D. (2010). Myeloperoxidase, inflammation, and dysfunctional high-density lipoprotein. *J Clin Lipidol,* 4(5), 382–388. doi: 10.1016/j.jacl.2010.08.007

Smith, S. C., Jr., Anderson, J. L., Cannon, R. O., 3rd, Fadl, Y. Y., Koenig, W., Libby, P., . . . AHA. (2004). CDC/AHA Workshop on Markers of Inflammation and Cardiovascular Disease: Application to Clinical and Public Health Practice: report from the clinical practice discussion group. *Circulation,* 110(25), e550–553. doi: 10.1161/01.CIR.0000148981.71644.C7

Tang, W. H., Katz, R., Brennan, M. L., Aviles, R. J., Tracy, R. P., Psaty, B. M., & Hazen, S. L. (2009). Usefulness of myeloperoxidase levels in healthy elderly subjects to predict risk of developing heart failure. *Am J Cardiol,* 103(9), 1269–1274. doi: 10.1016/j.amjcard.2009.01.026

Tang, W. H. W., Iqbal, N., Wu, Y., & Hazen, S. L. (2013). Usefulness of Cardiac Biomarker Score for Risk Stratification in Stable Patients Undergoing Elective Cardiac Evaluation Across Glycemic Status. *Am J Cardiol,* 111(4), 465–470. doi: http://dx.doi.org/10.1016/j.amjcard.2012.10.027

Varbo, A., Benn, M., Tybjærg-Hansen, A., & Nordestgaard, B. G. (2013). Elevated Remnant Cholesterol Causes Both Low-Grade Inflammation and Ischemic Heart Disease, Whereas Elevated Low-Density Lipoprotein Cholesterol Causes Ischemic Heart Disease Without Inflammation. *Circulation,* 128(12), 1298–1309. doi: 10.1161/circulationaha.113.003008

Wang, T. J., Gona, P., Larson, M. G., Tofler, G. H., Levy, D., Newton-Cheh, C., . . . Vasan, R. S. (2006). Multiple Biomarkers for the Prediction of First Major Cardiovascular Events and Death. *N Engl J Med,* 355(25), 2631–2639. doi: 10.1056/NEJMoa055373

Wu, B. J., Chen, K., Barter, P. J., & Rye, K.-A. (2012). Niacin Inhibits Vascular Inflammation via the Induction of Heme Oxygenase-1. *Circulation,* 125(1), 150–158. doi: 10.1161/circulationaha.111.053108

Yang, E. H., McConnell, J. P., Lennon, R. J., Barsness, G. W., Pumper, G., Hartman, S. J., . . . Lerman, A. (2006). Lipoprotein-Associated Phospholipase A2 Is an Independent Marker for Coronary Endothelial Dysfunction in Humans. *Arterioscler Thromb Vasc Bio,* 26(1), 106–111. doi: 10.1161/01.ATV.0000191655.87296.ab

Chapter Eight

Acharjee, S., Boden, W. E., Hartigan, P. M., Teo, K. K., Maron, D. J., Sedlis, S. P., . . . Weintraub, W. S. (2013). Low Levels of High Density Lipoprotein Cholesterol and Increased Risk of Cardiovascular Events in Stable Ischemic Heart Disease Patients: A Post Hoc Analysis from the COURAGE Trial. *J Am Coll Cardiol.* doi: 10.1016/j.jacc.2013.07.051

Ahn, J., Lim, U., Weinstein, S. J., Schatzkin, A., Hayes, R. B., Virtamo, J., & Albanes, D. (2009). Prediagnostic total and high-density lipoprotein cholesterol and risk of cancer. Cancer Epidemiol Biomarkers. *Prev,* 18(11), 2814–2821. doi: 10.1158/1055-9965.EPI-08-1248

Alsheikh-Ali, A. A., Maddukuri, P. V., Han, H., & Karas, R. H. (2007). Effect of the Magnitude of Lipid Lowering on Risk of Elevated Liver Enzymes, Rhabdomyolysis, and Cancer: Insights From Large Randomized Statin Trials. *J Am Coll Cardiol,* 50(5), 409–418. doi: http://dx.doi.org/10.1016/j.jacc.2007.02.073

Alsheikh-Ali, A. A., Trikalinos, T. A., Kent, D. M., & Karas, R. H. (2008). Statins, Low-Density Lipoprotein Cholesterol, and Risk of Cancer. *J Am Coll Cardiol,* 52(14), 1141–1147. doi: http://dx.doi.org/10.1016/j.jacc.2008.06.037

Aune, D., Chan, D. S., Lau, R., Vieira, R., Greenwood, D. C., Kampman, E., & Norat, T. (2011). Dietary fibre, whole grains, and risk of colorectal cancer: systematic review and dose-response meta-analysis of prospective studies. *Bmj,* 343, d6617. doi: 10.1136/bmj.d6617

Batic-Mujanovic, O., Zildzic, M., Beganlic, A., & Kusljugic, Z. (2006). The effect of cigarette smoking on HDL-cholesterol level. *Med Arh,* 60(6 Suppl 2), 90–92.

Boekholdt, S. M., Arsenault, B. J., Hovingh, G. K., Mora, S., Pedersen, T. R., Larosa, J. C., . . . Kastelein, J. J. (2013). Levels and Changes of HDL Cholesterol and Apolipoprotein A-I in Relation to Risk of Cardiovascular Events among Statin-Treated Patients: A Meta-Analysis. *Circulation.* doi: 10.1161/CIRCULATIONAHA.113.002670

Clarke, R., Emberson, J. R., Parish, S., et al. (2007). Cholesterol fractions and apolipoproteins as risk factors for heart disease mortality in older men. *Arch Intern Med,* 167(13), 1373–1378. doi: 10.1001/archinte.167.13.1373

Clarke, R., Peden, J. F., Hopewell, J. C., Kyriakou, T., Goel, A., Heath, S. C., . . . Farrall, M. (2009). Genetic Variants Associated with Lp(a) Lipoprotein Level and Coronary Disease. *N Engl J Med,* 361(26), 2518–2528. doi: 10.1056/NEJMoa0902604

Dey, A., Aggarwal, R., & Dwivedi, S. (2013). Cardiovascular Profile of Xanthelasma Palpebrarum. *BioMed Research International,* 2013, 3. doi: 10.1155/2013/932863

Djordjevic, V. B., Cosic, V., Stojanovic, I., Kundalic, S., Zvezdanovic, L., Deljanin-Ilic, M., . . . Popovic, L. (2011). Lipoprotein(a) Is the Best Single Marker in Assessing Unstable Angina Pectoris. *Cardiol Res Pract,* 2011, 175363. doi: 10.4061/2011/175363

El Harchaoui, K., van der Steg, W. A., Stroes, E. S. G., Kuivenhoven, J. A., Otvos, J. D., Wareham, N. J., . . . Boekholdt, S. M. (2007). Value of Low-Density Lipoprotein Particle Number and Size as Predictors of Coronary Artery Disease in Apparently Healthy Men and Women: The EPIC-Norfolk Prospective Population Study. *J Am Coll Cardiol,* 49(5), 547–553. doi: http://dx.doi.org/10.1016/j.jacc.2006.09.043

The Emerging Risk Factors Collaboration. (2009). Lipoprotein(a) concentration and the risk of coronary heart disease, stroke, and nonvascular mortality. *JAMA,* 302(4), 412–423.

Gotto, A. M., Whitney, E., Stein, E. A., Shapiro, D. R., Clearfield, M., Weis, S., . . . de Cani, J. S. (2000). Relation Between Baseline and On-Treatment Lipid Parameters and First Acute Major Coronary Events in the Air Force/Texas Coronary Atherosclerosis Prevention Study (AFCAPS/TexCAPS). *Circulation,* 101(5), 477–484. doi: 10.1161/01.cir.101.5.477

HEALTH, E. P. O. I. G. F. C., CHILDREN, R. R. I., & ADOLESCENTS. (2011). Expert Panel on Integrated Guidelines for Cardiovascular Health and Risk Reduction in Children and Adolescents: Summary Report. *Pediatrics,* 128(Supplement 5), S213–S256. doi: 10.1542/peds.2009-2107C

Hermans, M. P., Ahn, S. A., & Rousseau, M. F. (2012). The atherogenic dyslipidemia ratio [log(TG)/HDL-C] is associated with residual vascular risk, beta-cell function loss and microangiopathy in type 2 diabetes females. *Lipids Health Dis,* 11, 132. doi: 10.1186/1476-511X-11-132

Ingelsson, E., Schaefer, E. J., Contois, J. H., et al. (2007). Clinical utility of different lipid measures for prediction of coronary heart disease in men and women. *JAMA,* 298(7), 776–785. doi: 10.1001/jama.298.7.776

Kamstrup, P. R., Tybjærg-Hansen, A., Steffensen, R., & Nordestgaard, B. G. (2009). Genetically elevated lipoprotein(a) and increased risk of myocardial infarction. *JAMA,* 301(22), 2331–2339. doi: 10.1001/jama.2009.801

Kantor, M. A., Cullinane, E. M., Sady, S. P., Herbert, P. N., & Thompson, P. D. (1987). Exercise acutely increases high density lipoprotein-cholesterol and lipoprotein lipase activity in trained and untrained men. *Metabolism,* 36(2), 188–192. doi: http://dx.doi.org/10.1016/0026-0495(87)90016-3

Kit, B. K., Carroll, M. D., Lacher, D. A., Sorlie, P. D., DeJesus, J. M., & Ogden, C. L. (2012). Trends in serum lipids among us youths aged 6 to 19 years, 1988-2010. *JAMA,* 308(6), 591–600. doi: 10.1001/jama.2012.9136

Kronenberg, F., & Utermann, G. (2013). Lipoprotein(a): resurrected by genetics. *J Intern Med,* 273(1), 6–30. doi: 10.1111/j.1365-2796.2012.02592.x

Marcovina, S. M. (2003). Report of the National Heart, Lung, and Blood Institute Workshop on Lipoprotein(a) and Cardiovascular Disease: Recent Advances and Future Directions. *Clin Chem,* 49(11), 1785–1796. doi: 10.1373/clinchem.2003.023689

Mora, S., Otvos, J. D., Rifai, N., Rosenson, R. S., Buring, J. E., & Ridker, P. M. (2009). Lipoprotein Particle Profiles by Nuclear Magnetic Resonance Compared With Standard Lipids and Apolipoproteins in Predicting Incident Cardiovascular Disease in Women. *Circulation,* 119(7), 931–939. doi: 10.1161/circulationaha.108.816181

Nasr, N., Ruidavets, J. B., Farghali, A., Guidolin, B., Perret, B., & Larrue, V. (2011). Lipoprotein (a) and carotid atherosclerosis in young patients with stroke. *Stroke,* 42(12), 3616–3618. doi: 10.1161/STROKEAHA.111.624684

Nestel, P. J., Barnes, E. H., Tonkin, A. M., Simes, J., Fournier, M., White, H. D., . . . Sullivan, D. R. (2013). Plasma Lipoprotein(a) Concentration Predicts Future Coronary and Cardiovascular Events in Patients With Stable Coronary Heart Disease. *Arterioscler Thromb Vasc Bio.* doi: 10.1161/atvbaha.113.302479

Nissen, S. E., Nicholls, S. J., Sipahi, I., et al. (2006). Effect of very high-intensity statin therapy on regression of coronary atherosclerosis: The asteroid trial. *JAMA,* 295(13), 1556–1565. doi: 10.1001/jama.295.13.jpc60002

Nordestgaard, B. G., Chapman, M. J., Ray, K., Borén, J., Andreotti, F., Watts, G. F., . . . Panel, f. t. E. A. S. C. (2010). Lipoprotein(a) as a cardiovascular risk factor: current status. *Eur Heart J.* doi: 10.1093/eurheartj/ehq386

O'Donnell, M. J., Xavier, D., Liu, L., Zhang, H., Chin, S. L., Rao-Melacini, P., . . . Yusuf, S. Risk factors for ischaemic and intracerebral haemorrhagic stroke in 22 countries (the INTERSTROKE study): a case-control study. *The Lancet,* 376(9735), 112–123. doi: http://dx.doi.org/10.1016/S0140-6736(10)60834-3

Park, Y., Subar, A. F., Hollenbeck, A., & Schatzkin, A. (2011). Dietary fiber intake and mortality in the nih-aarp diet and health study. *Arch Intern Med,* 171(12), 1061–1068. doi: 10.1001/archinternmed.2011.18

Pfrieger, F. W. (2003). Role of cholesterol in synapse formation and function. *Biochimica et Biophysica Acta (BBA) Biomembranes,* 1610(2), 271–280. doi: http://dx.doi.org/10.1016/S0005-2736(03)00024-5

Ridker, P. M. (2012). Lipoprotein(a), Ethnicity, and Cardiovascular Risk: Erasing a Paradox and Filling a Clinical Gap. *Circulation,* 125(2), 207–209. doi: 10.1161/circulationaha.111.077354

Ritchie, S. K., Murphy, E. C., Ice, C., Cottrell, L. A., Minor, V., Elliott, E., & Neal, W. (2010). Universal versus targeted blood cholesterol screening among youth: The CARDIAC project. *Pediatrics,* 126(2), 260–265. doi: 10.1542/peds.2009-2546

Riwanto, M., Rohrer, L., Roschitzki, B., Besler, C., Mocharla, P., Mueller, M., . . . Landmesser, U. (2013). Altered activation of endothelial anti- and proapoptotic pathways by high-density lipoprotein from patients with coronary artery disease: role of high-density lipoprotein-proteome remodeling. *Circulation,* 127(8), 891–904. doi: 10.1161/CIRCULATIONAHA.112.108753

Roth, G. A., Fihn, S. D., Mokdad, A. H., Aekplakorn, W., Hasegawa, T., & Lim, S. S. (2011). High total serum cholesterol, medication coverage and therapeutic control: an analysis of national health examination survey data from eight countries. *Bulletin of the World Health Organization,* 89(2), 92–101. doi: 10.2471/BLT.10.079947

Sachdeva, A., Cannon, C. P., Deedwania, P. C., Labresh, K. A., Smith, S. C., Jr., Dai, D., . . . Fonarow, G. C. (2009). Lipid levels in patients hospitalized with coronary artery disease:

an analysis of 136,905 hospitalizations in Get With The Guidelines. *Am Heart J,* 157(1), 111–117 e112. doi: 10.1016/j.ahj.2008.08.010

Shepardson, N. E., Shankar, G. M., & Selkoe, D. J. (2011). Cholesterol level and statin use in Alzheimer disease: II. Review of human trials and recommendations. *Arch Neurol,* 68(11), 1385–1392. doi: 10.1001/archneurol.2011.242

Shin, J. Y., Suls, J., & Martin, R. (2008). Are cholesterol and depression inversely related? A meta-analysis of the association between two cardiac risk factors. *Ann Behav Med,* 36(1), 33–43. doi: 10.1007/s12160-008-9045-8

Singh-Manoux, A., Gimeno, D., Kivimaki, M., Brunner, E., & Marmot, M. G. (2008). Low HDL Cholesterol Is a Risk Factor for Deficit and Decline in Memory in Midlife: The Whitehall II Study. *Arterioscler Thromb Vasc Bio,* 28(8), 1556–1562. doi: 10.1161/atvbaha.108.163998

Suk Danik, J., Rifai, N., Buring, J. E., & Ridker, P. (2006). Lipoprotein(a), measured with an assay independent of apolipoprotein(a) isoform size, and risk of future cardiovascular events among initially healthy women. *JAMA,* 296(11), 1363–1370. doi: 10.1001/jama.296.11.1363

Superko, H. R., Pendyala, L., Williams, P. T., Momary, K. M., King, S. B., 3rd, & Garrett, B. C. (2012). High-density lipoprotein subclasses and their relationship to cardiovascular disease. *J Clin Lipidol,* 6(6), 496–523. doi: 10.1016/j.jacl.2012.03.001

Threapleton, D. E., Greenwood, D. C., Evans, C. E. L., Cleghorn, C. L., Nykjaer, C., Wood-head, C., . . . Burley, V. J. (2013). Dietary Fiber Intake and Risk of First Stroke: A Systematic Review and Meta-Analysis. *Stroke,* 44(5), 1360–1368. doi: 10.1161/strokeaha.111.000151

Tian, L., & Fu, M. (2010). The relationship between high density lipoprotein subclass profile and plasma lipids concentrations. *Lipids Health Dis,* 9, 118. doi: 10.1186/1476-511X-9-118

Tirschwell, D. L., Smith, N. L., Heckbert, S. R., Lemaitre, R. N., Longstreth, W. T., Jr., & Psaty, B. M. (2004). Association of cholesterol with stroke risk varies in stroke subtypes and patient subgroups. *Neurology,* 63(10), 1868–1875.

Tsimikas, S., Brilakis, E. S., Miller, E. R., McConnell, J. P., Lennon, R. J., Kornman, K. S., . . . Berger, P. B. (2005). Oxidized Phospholipids, Lp(a) Lipoprotein, and Coronary Artery Disease. *N Engl J Med,* 353(1), 46–57. doi:10.1056/NEJMoa043175

van der Ploeg, H. P., Chey, T., Korda, R. J., Banks, E., & Bauman, A. (2012). Sitting time and all-cause mortality risk in 222 497 australian adults. *Arch Intern Med,* 172(6), 494–500. doi: 10.1001/archinternmed.2011.2174

Varbo, A., Benn, M., Tybjaerg-Hansen, A., & Nordestgaard, B. G. (2013). Elevated Remnant Cholesterol Causes Both Low-Grade Inflammation and Ischemic Heart Disease, While Elevated Low-Density Lipoprotein Cholesterol Causes Ischemic Heart Disease without Inflammation. *Circulation.* doi: 10.1161/circulationaha.113.003008

Virani, S. S., Brautbar, A., Davis, B. C., Nambi, V., Hoogeveen, R. C., Sharrett, A. R., . . . Ballantyne, C. M. (2012). Associations Between Lipoprotein(a) Levels and Cardiovascular Outcomes in Black and White Subjects: The Atherosclerosis Risk in Communities (ARIC) Study. *Circulation,* 125(2), 241–249. doi: 10.1161/circulationaha.111.045120

Voight, B. F., Peloso, G. M., Orho-Melander, M., Frikke-Schmidt, R., Barbalic, M., Jensen, M. K., . . . Kathiresan, S. (2012). Plasma HDL cholesterol and risk of myocardial infarction: a mendelian randomisation study. *The Lancet,* 380(9841), 572–580. doi: 10.1016/s0140-6736(12)60312-2

Walldius, G., Aastveit, A. H., & Jungner, I. (2006). Stroke mortality and the apoB/apoA-I ratio: results of the AMORIS prospective study. *J Intern Med,* 259(3), 259–266. doi: 10.1111/j.1365-2796.2005.01610.x

Williams, P. T., & Feldman, D. E. (2011). Prospective study of coronary heart disease vs. HDL2, HDL3, and other lipoproteins in Gofman's Livermore Cohort. *Atherosclerosis, 214*(1), 196–202. doi: 10.1016/j.atherosclerosis.2010.10.024

Yusuf, S., Hawken, S., Ôunpuu, S., Dans, T., Avezum, A., Lanas, F., . . . Lisheng, L. (2004). Effect of potentially modifiable risk factors associated with myocardial infarction in 52 countries (the INTERHEART study): case-control study. *The Lancet, 364*(9438), 937–952. doi: 10.1016/s0140-6736(04)17018-9

Zhang, Y., Tuomilehto, J., Jousilahti, P., Wang, Y., Antikainen, R., & Hu, G. (2012). Total and high-density lipoprotein cholesterol and stroke risk. *Stroke, 43*(7), 1768–1774. doi: 10.1161/STROKEAHA.111.646778

Chapter Nine

Abdul-Ghani, M. A., Stern, M. P., Lyssenko, V., Tuomi, T., Groop, L., & Defronzo, R. A. (2010). Minimal contribution of fasting hyperglycemia to the incidence of type 2 diabetes in subjects with normal 2-h plasma glucose. *Diabetes Care, 33*(3), 557–561. doi: 10.2337/dc09-1145

American Diabetes, A. (2013). Standards of medical care in diabetes--2013. *Diabetes Care,* 36 Suppl 1, S11–66. doi: 10.2337/dc13-S011

Bravata, D. M., Smith-Spangler, C., Sundaram, V., et al. (2007). Using pedometers to increase physical activity and improve health: A systematic review. *JAMA, 298*(19), 2296–2304. doi: 10.1001/jama.298.19.2296

Cappuccio, F. P., D'Elia, L., Strazzullo, P., & Miller, M. A. (2010). Quantity and Quality of Sleep and Incidence of Type 2 Diabetes: A systematic review and meta-analysis. *Diabetes Care, 33*(2), 414–420. doi: 10.2337/dc09-1124

Catalano, P. M., Kirwan, J. P., Haugel-de Mouzon, S., & King, J. (2003). Gestational Diabetes and Insulin Resistance: Role in Short- and Long-Term Implications for Mother and Fetus. *J Nutr, 133*(5), 1674S–1683S.

Coutinho, T., Goel, K., Correa de Sa, D., Carter, R. E., Hodge, D. O., Kragelund, C., . . . Lopez-Jimenez, F. (2013). Combining body mass index with measures of central obesity in the assessment of mortality in subjects with coronary disease: role of "normal weight central obesity." *J Am Coll Cardiol, 61*(5), 553–560. doi: 10.1016/j.jacc.2012.10.035

DeFronzo, R. A. (2009). From the Triumvirate to the Ominous Octet: A New Paradigm for the Treatment of Type 2 Diabetes Mellitus. *Diabetes, 58*(4), 773–795. doi: 10.2337/db09-9028

Diabetes Prevention Program Research Group. Reduction in the Incidence of Type 2 Diabetes with Lifestyle Intervention or Metformin. (2002). *N Engl J Med, 346*(6), 393–403. doi: 10.1056/NEJMoa012512

Gami, A. S., Witt, B. J., Howard, D. E., Erwin, P. J., Gami, L. A., Somers, V. K., & Montori, V. M. (2007). Metabolic syndrome and risk of incident cardiovascular events and death: a systematic review and meta-analysis of longitudinal studies. *J Am Coll Cardiol, 49*(4), 403–414. doi: 10.1016/j.jacc.2006.09.032

Glucose tolerance and mortality: comparison of WHO and American Diabetic Association diagnostic criteria. (1999). *The Lancet, 354*(9179), 617–621. doi: http://dx.doi.org/10.1016/S0140-6736(98)12131-1

Grundy, S. M., Brewer, H. B., Cleeman, J. I., Smith, S. C., Lenfant, C., & Participants, f. t. C. (2004). Definition of Metabolic Syndrome: Report of the National Heart, Lung, and

Blood Institute/American Heart Association Conference on Scientific Issues Related to Definition. *Circulation,* 109(3), 433–438. doi: 10.1161/01.cir.0000111245.75752.c6

Ioannou, G. N., Bryson, C. L., & Boyko, E. J. (2007). Prevalence and trends of insulin resistance, impaired fasting glucose, and diabetes. *J Diabetes Complications,* 21(6), 363–370. doi: 10.1016/j.jdiacomp.2006.07.005

Kim, T. N., Kim, S., Yang, S. J., Yoo, H. J., Seo, J. A., Kim, S. G., . . . Choi, K. M. (2010). Vascular Inflammation in Patients With Impaired Glucose Tolerance and Type 2 Diabetes: Analysis With 18F-Fluorodeoxyglucose Positron Emission Tomography. *Circulation: Cardiovascular Imaging,* 3(2), 142–148. doi: 10.1161/circimaging.109.888909

Lalla, E., Kunzel, C., Burkett, S., Cheng, B., & Lamster, I. B. (2011). Identification of unrecognized diabetes and pre-diabetes in a dental setting. *J Dent Res,* 90(7), 855–860. doi: 10.1177/0022034511407069

Li, C., Ford, E. S., Meng, Y. X., Mokdad, A. H., & Reaven, G. M. (2008). Does the association of the triglyceride to high-density lipoprotein cholesterol ratio with fasting serum insulin differ by race/ethnicity? *Cardiovasc Diabetol,* 7, 4. doi: 10.1186/1475-2840-7-4

Matsuoka, L. Y., Wortsman, J., Gavin Iii, J. R., Kupchella, C. E., & Dietrich, J. G. (1986). Acanthosis nigricans, hypothyroidism, and insulin resistance. *Am J Med,* 81(1), 58–62. doi: http://dx.doi.org/10.1016/0002-9343(86)90182-8

McLaughlin, T., Reaven, G., Abbasi, F., Lamendola, C., Saad, M., Waters, D., . . . Krauss, R. M. (2005). Is There a Simple Way to Identify Insulin-Resistant Individuals at Increased Risk of Cardiovascular Disease? *Am J Cardiol,* 96(3), 399–404. doi: http://dx.doi.org/10.1016/j.amjcard.2005.03.085

Mozaffarian, D., Marfisi, R., Levantesi, G., Silletta, M. G., Tavazzi, L., Tognoni, G., . . . Marchioli, R. Incidence of new-onset diabetes and impaired fasting glucose in patients with recent myocardial infarction and the effect of clinical and lifestyle risk factors. *The Lancet,* 370(9588), 667–675. doi: http://dx.doi.org/10.1016/S0140-6736(07)61343-9

Nash, D. T. (2002). Insulin resistance, adma levels, and cardiovascular disease. *JAMA,* 287(11), 1451–1452. doi: 10.1001/jama.287.11.1451

Okosieme, O. E., Peter, R., Usman, M., Bolusani, H., Suruliram, P., George, L., & Evans, L. M. (2008). Can Admission and Fasting Glucose Reliably Identify Undiagnosed Diabetes in Patients With Acute Coronary Syndrome? *Diabetes Care,* 31(10), 1955–1959. doi: 10.2337/dc08-0197

Ong, K. L., Cheung, B. M. Y., Wong, L. Y. F., Wat, N. M. S., Tan, K. C. B., & Lam, K. S. L. (2008). Prevalence, Treatment, and Control of Diagnosed Diabetes in the U.S. National Health and Nutrition Examination Survey 1999–2004. *Annals of Epidemiology,* 18(3), 222–229. doi: http://dx.doi.org/10.1016/j.annepidem.2007.10.007

Parretti, E., Lapolla, A., Dalfrà, M., Pacini, G., Mari, A., Cioni, R., . . . Mello, G. (2006). Preeclampsia in Lean Normotensive Normotolerant Pregnant Women Can Be Predicted by Simple Insulin Sensitivity Indexes. *Hypertension,* 47(3), 449–453. doi: 10.1161/01.HYP.0000205122.47333.7f

Pessi, T., Karhunen, V., Karjalainen, P. P., Ylitalo, A., Airaksinen, J. K., Niemi, M., . . . Mikkelsson, J. (2013). Bacterial Signatures in Thrombus Aspirates of Patients With Myocardial Infarction. *Circulation,* 127(11), 1219–1228. doi: 10.1161/circulationaha.112.001254

Petrie, J. R., Malik, M. O., Balkau, B., Perry, C. G., Højlund, K., Pataky, Z., . . . Natali, A. (2013). Euglycemic Clamp Insulin Sensitivity and Longitudinal Systolic Blood Pressure: Role of Sex. *Hypertension.* doi: 10.1161/hypertensionaha.111.00439

Prior, J. O., Quiñones, M. J., Hernandez-Pampaloni, M., Facta, A. D., Schindler, T. H., Sayre, J. W., . . . Schelbert, H. R. (2005). Coronary Circulatory Dysfunction in Insulin Resistance, Impaired Glucose Tolerance, and Type 2 Diabetes Mellitus. *Circulation,* 111(18), 2291–2298. doi: 10.1161/01.cir.0000164232.62768.51

Qi, Q., Li, Y., Chomistek, A. K., Kang, J. H., Curhan, G. C., Pasquale, L. R., . . . Qi, L. (2012). Television watching, leisure time physical activity, and the genetic predisposition in relation to body mass index in women and men. *Circulation,* 126(15), 1821–1827. doi: 10.1161/CIRCULATIONAHA.112.098061

Rask-Madsen, C., Li, Q., Freund, B., Feather, D., Abramov, R., Wu, I. H., . . . King, G. L. (2010). Loss of insulin signaling in vascular endothelial cells accelerates atherosclerosis in apolipoprotein E null mice. *Cell Metab,* 11(5), 379–389. doi: 10.1016/j.cmet.2010.03.013

Sam, S., Coviello, A. D., Sung, Y.-A., Legro, R. S., & Dunaif, A. (2008). Metabolic Phenotype in the Brothers of Women with Polycystic Ovary Syndrome. *Diabetes Care,* 31(6), 1237–1241. doi: 10.2337/dc07-2190

Sawada, S. S., Lee, I.-M., Naito, H., Noguchi, J., Tsukamoto, K., Muto, T., . . . Blair, S. N. (2010). Long-Term Trends in Cardiorespiratory Fitness and the Incidence of Type 2 Diabetes. *Diabetes Care,* 33(6), 1353–1357. doi: 10.2337/dc09-1654

Selvin, E., Steffes, M. W., Zhu, H., Matsushita, K., Wagenknecht, L., Pankow, J., . . . Brancati, F. L. (2010). Glycated hemoglobin, diabetes, and cardiovascular risk in nondiabetic adults. *N Engl J Med,* 362(9), 800–811. doi: 10.1056/NEJMoa0908359

Stamatakis, E., Hamer, M., & Dunstan, D. W. (2011). Screen-Based Entertainment Time, All-Cause Mortality, and Cardiovascular Events: Population-Based Study With Ongoing Mortality and Hospital Events Follow-Up. *J Am Coll Cardiol,* 57(3), 292–299. doi: http://dx.doi.org/10.1016/j.jacc.2010.05.065

Varthakavi, P. K., Patel, K. L., Wadhwa, S. L., Khopkar, U., Sengupta, R. A., Merchant, P. C., . . . Nihalani, K. D. (2001). A study of insulin resistance in subjects with acanthosis nigricans. *J Assoc Physicians India,* 49, 705–712.

Vella, C. A., Burgos, X., Ellis, C. J., Zubia, R. Y., Ontiveros, D., Reyes, H., & Lozano, C. (2013). Associations of Insulin Resistance With Cardiovascular Risk Factors and Inflammatory Cytokines in Normal-Weight Hispanic Women. *Diabetes Care,* 36(5), 1377–1383. doi: 10.2337/dc12-1550

Wang, J.-S., Lee, I.-T., Lee, W.-J., Lin, S.-Y., Fu, C.-P., Ting, C.-T., . . . Sheu, W. H.-H. (2013). Performance of HbA1c and Fasting Plasma Glucose in Screening for Diabetes in Patients Undergoing Coronary Angiography. *Diabetes Care,* 36(5), 1138–1140. doi: 10.2337/dc12-1434

Wennberg, P., Gustafsson, P. E., Dunstan, D. W., Wennberg, M., & Hammarström, A. (2013). Television Viewing and Low Leisure-Time Physical Activity in Adolescence Independently Predict the Metabolic Syndrome in Mid-Adulthood. *Diabetes Care,* 36(7), 2090–2097. doi: 10.2337/dc12-1948

Whaley-Connell, A., & Sowers, J. R. (2009). Hypertension and Insulin Resistance. *Hypertension,* 54(3), 462–464. doi: 10.1161/hypertensionaha.109.134460

Xu, M., Qi, Q., Liang, J., Bray, G. A., Hu, F. B., Sacks, F. M., & Qi, L. (2013). Genetic determinant for amino acid metabolites and changes in body weight and insulin resistance in response to weight-loss diets: the preventing overweight using novel dietary strategies (POUNDS LOST) trial. *Circulation,* 127(12), 1283–1289. doi: 10.1161/CIRCULATIONAHA.112.000586

Chapter Ten

Arsenault, B. J., Boekholdt, S. M., Hovingh, G. K., Hyde, C. L., DeMicco, D. A., Chatterjee, A., . . . Investigators, I. (2012). The 719Arg variant of KIF6 and cardiovascular outcomes in statin-treated, stable coronary patients of the treating to new targets and incremental decrease in end points through aggressive lipid-lowering prospective studies. *Circ Cardiovasc Genet,* 5(1), 51–57. doi: 10.1161/CIRCGENETICS.111.960252

Asbury, C. L., Fehr, A. N., & Block, S. M. (2003). Kinesin moves by an asymmetric hand-over-hand mechanism. *Science,* 302(5653), 2130–2134. doi: 10.1126/science.1092985

Ashley, E. A., Hershberger, R. E., Caleshu, C., Ellinor, P. T., Garcia, J. G., Herrington, D. M., . . . American Heart Association Advocacy Coordinating, C. (2012). Genetics and cardiovascular disease: a policy statement from the American Heart Association. *Circulation,* 126(1), 142–157. doi: 10.1161/CIR.0b013e31825b07f8

Assimes, T. L., Holm, H., Kathiresan, S., Reilly, M. P., Thorleifsson, G., Voight, B. F., . . . Quertermous, T. (2010). Lack of association between the Trp719Arg polymorphism in kinesin-like protein-6 and coronary artery disease in 19 case-control studies. *J Am Coll Cardiol,* 56(19), 1552–1563. doi: 10.1016/j.jacc.2010.06.022

Baptista, R., Rebelo, M., Decq-Mota, J., Dias, P., Monteiro, P., Providencia, L. A., & Silva, J. M. (2011). Apolipoprotein E epsilon-4 polymorphism is associated with younger age at referral to a lipidology clinic and a poorer response to lipid-lowering therapy. *Lipids Health Dis,* 10, 48. doi: 10.1186/1476-511X-10-48

Bevilacqua, M. P., Pober, J. S., Wheeler, M. E., Cotran, R. S., & Gimbrone, M. A., Jr. (1985). Interleukin 1 acts on cultured human vascular endothelium to increase the adhesion of polymorphonuclear leukocytes, monocytes, and related leukocyte cell lines. *J Clin Invest,* 76(5), 2003–2011. doi: 10.1172/jci112200

Bjelakovic, G., Nikolova, D., & Gluud, C. (2013). Antioxidant supplements to prevent mortality. *JAMA,* 310(11), 1178–1179. doi: 10.1001/jama.2013.277028

Blum, S., Vardi, M., Brown, J. B., Russell, A., Milman, U., Shapira, C., . . . Levy, A. P. (2010). Vitamin E reduces cardiovascular disease in individuals with diabetes mellitus and the haptoglobin 2-2 genotype. *Pharmacogenomics,* 11(5), 675–684. doi: 10.2217/pgs.10.17

Brouwers, H. B., Biffi, A., McNamara, K. A., Ayres, A. M., Valant, V., Schwab, K., . . . Goldstein, J. N. (2012). Apolipoprotein E genotype is associated with CT angiography spot sign in lobar intracerebral hemorrhage. *Stroke,* 43(8), 2120–2125. doi: 10.1161/STROKEAHA.112.659094

Craik, F. I., Bialystok, E., & Freedman, M. (2010). Delaying the onset of Alzheimer disease: bilingualism as a form of cognitive reserve. *Neurology,* 75(19), 1726–1729. doi: 10.1212/WNL.0b013e3181fc2a1c

Dandona, S., Stewart, A. F., Chen, L., Williams, K., So, D., O'Brien, E., . . . Roberts, R. (2010). Gene dosage of the common variant 9p21 predicts severity of coronary artery disease. *J Am Coll Cardiol,* 56(6), 479–486. doi: 10.1016/j.jacc.2009.10.092

Davignon, J., Gregg, R. E., & Sing, C. F. (1988). Apolipoprotein E polymorphism and atherosclerosis. *Arterioscler Thromb Vasc Bio,* 8(1), 1–21. doi: 10.1161/01.atv.8.1.1

Desvarieux, M., Demmer, R. T., Jacobs, D. R., Jr., Rundek, T., Boden-Albala, B., Sacco, R. L., & Papapanou, P. N. (2010). Periodontal bacteria and hypertension: the oral infections and vascular disease epidemiology study (INVEST). *J Hypertens,* 28(7), 1413–1421. doi: 10.1097/HJH.0b013e328338cd36

Djousse, L., Pankow, J. S., Arnett, D. K., Eckfeldt, J. H., Myers, R. H., & Ellison, R. C. (2004). Apolipoprotein E polymorphism modifies the alcohol-HDL association observed in the National Heart, Lung, and Blood Institute Family Heart Study. *Am J Clin Nutr,* 80(6), 1639–1644.

Doria, A., Wojcik, J., Xu, R., Gervino, E. V., Hauser, T. H., Johnstone, M. T., . . . Warram, J. H. (2008). Interaction between poor glycemic control and 9p21 locus on risk of coronary artery disease in type 2 diabetes. *JAMA,* 300(20), 2389–2397. doi: 10.1001/jama.2008.649

Duff, G. W. (2006). Evidence for genetic variation as a factor in maintaining health. *Am J Clin Nutr,* 83(2), 431s–435s.

Dutta, A., Henley, W., Lang, I. A., Murray, A., Guralnik, J., Wallace, R. B., & Melzer, D. (2011). The coronary artery disease-associated 9p21 variant and later life 20-year survival to cohort extinction. *Circ Cardiovasc Genet,* 4(5), 542–548. doi: 10.1161/CIRCGENETICS.111.960146

Eichner, J. E., Dunn, S. T., Perveen, G., Thompson, D. M., Stewart, K. E., & Stroehla, B. C. (2002). Apolipoprotein E Polymorphism and Cardiovascular Disease: A Huge Review. *Am J Epidemiol,* 155(6), 487–495. doi: 10.1093/aje/155.6.487

Ertel, K. A., Glymour, M. M., & Berkman, L. F. (2008). Effects of social integration on preserving memory function in a nationally representative US elderly population. *Am J Public Health,* 98(7), 1215–1220. doi: 10.2105/ajph.2007.113654

Fan, M., Dandona, S., McPherson, R., Allayee, H., Hazen, S. L., Wells, G. A., . . . Stewart, A. F. R. (2013). Two Chromosome 9p21 Haplotype Blocks Distinguish Between Coronary Artery Disease and Myocardial Infarction Risk. *Circulation: Cardiovascular Genetics.* doi: 10.1161/circgenetics.113.000104

Fernandez-Cadenas, I., Del Rio-Espinola, A., Giralt, D., Domingues-Montanari, S., Quiroga, A., Mendioroz, M., . . . Montaner, J. (2012). IL1B and VWF variants are associated with fibrinolytic early recanalization in patients with ischemic stroke. *Stroke,* 43(10), 2659–2665. doi: 10.1161/STROKEAHA.112.657007

Ferreira, A. P., Ferreira, C. B., Brito, C. J., Souza, V. C., Córdova, C., Nóbrega, O. T., & França, N. M. (2013). The effect of aerobic exercise intensity on attenuation of postprandial lipemia is dependent on apolipoprotein E genotype. *Atherosclerosis,* 229(1), 139–144. doi: http://dx.doi.org/10.1016/j.atherosclerosis.2013.03.027

Harismendy, O., Notani, D., Song, X., Rahim, N. G., Tanasa, B., Heintzman, N., . . . Frazer, K. A. (2011). 9p21 DNA variants associated with coronary artery disease impair interferon-y signalling response. *Nature,* 470(7333), 264–268. doi: 10.1038/nature09753

Helgadottir, A., Thorleifsson, G., Magnusson, K. P., Gretarsdottir, S., Steinthorsdottir, V., Manolescu, A., . . . Stefansson, K. (2008). The same sequence variant on 9p21 associates with myocardial infarction, abdominal aortic aneurysm and intracranial aneurysm. *Nat Genet,* 40(2), 217–224. doi: 10.1038/ng.72

Hopewell, J. C., Parish, S., Clarke, R., Armitage, J., Bowman, L., Hager, J., . . . Group, M. B. H. P. S. C. (2011). No impact of KIF6 genotype on vascular risk and statin response among 18,348 randomized patients in the heart protection study. *J Am Coll Cardiol,* 57(20), 2000–2007. doi: 10.1016/j.jacc.2011.02.015

Hubacek, J. A., Peasey, A., Pikhart, H., Stavek, P., Kubinova, R., Marmot, M., & Bobak, M. (2010). APOE polymorphism and its effect on plasma C-reactive protein levels in a large general population sample. *Hum Immunol,* 71(3), 304–308. doi: 10.1016/j.humimm.2010.01.008

Huikuri, H. V., Castellanos, A., & Myerburg, R. J. (2001). Sudden Death Due to Cardiac Arrhythmias. *N Engl J Med,* 345(20), 1473–1482. doi: 10.1056/NEJMra000650

Iakoubova, O. A., Sabatine, M. S., Rowland, C. M., Tong, C. H., Catanese, J. J., Ranade, K., . . . Braunwald, E. (2008). Polymorphism in KIF6 gene and benefit from statins after acute coronary syndromes: results from the PROVE IT-TIMI 22 study. *J Am Coll Cardiol,* 51(4), 449–455. doi: 10.1016/j.jacc.2007.10.017

Iakoubova, O. A., Tong, C. H., Rowland, C. M., Kirchgessner, T. G., Young, B. A., Arellano, A. R., . . . Sacks, F. M. (2008). Association of the Trp719Arg Polymorphism in Kinesin-Like Protein 6 With Myocardial Infarction and Coronary Heart Disease in 2 Prospective Trials: The CARE and WOSCOPS Trials. *J Am Coll Cardiol,* 51(4), 435–443. doi: http://dx.doi.org/10.1016/j.jacc.2007.05.057

Johnston, W. F., Salmon, M., Su, G., Lu, G., Stone, M. L., Zhao, Y., . . . Ailawadi, G. (2013). Genetic and pharmacologic disruption of interleukin-1beta signaling inhibits experimental aortic aneurysm formation. *Arterioscler Thromb Vasc Biol,* 33(2), 294–304. doi: 10.1161/ATVBAHA.112.300432

Kalet-Litman, S., Moreno, P. R., & Levy, A. P. (2010). The haptoglobin 2-2 genotype is associated with increased redox active hemoglobin derived iron in the atherosclerotic plaque. *Atherosclerosis,* 209(1), 28–31. doi: 10.1016/j.atherosclerosis.2009.09.002

Kolovou, G., Damaskos, D., Anagnostopoulou, K., & Cokkinos, D. V. (2009). Apolipoprotein E gene polymorphism and gender. *Ann Clin Lab Sci,* 39(2), 120–133.

Levy, A. P., Gerstein, H. C., Miller-Lotan, R., Ratner, R., McQueen, M., Lonn, E., & Pogue, J. (2004). The Effect of Vitamin E Supplementation on Cardiovascular Risk in Diabetic Individuals With Different Haptoglobin Phenotypes. *Diabetes Care,* 27(11), 2767. doi: 10.2337/diacare.27.11.2767

Li, Y., Iakoubova, O. A., Shiffman, D., Devlin, J. J., Forrester, J. S., & Superko, H. R. (2010). KIF6 Polymorphism as a Predictor of Risk of Coronary Events and of Clinical Event Reduction by Statin Therapy. *Am J Cardiol,* 106(7), 994–998. doi: http://dx.doi.org/10.1016/j.amjcard.2010.05.033

Lieb, W., & Vasan, R. S. (2013). Genetics of Coronary Artery Disease. *Circulation,* 128(10), 1131–1138. doi: 10.1161/circulationaha.113.005350

Milman, U., Blum, S., Shapira, C., Aronson, D., Miller-Lotan, R., Anbinder, Y., . . . Levy, A. P. (2008). Vitamin E supplementation reduces cardiovascular events in a subgroup of middle-aged individuals with both type 2 diabetes mellitus and the haptoglobin 2-2 genotype: a prospective double-blinded clinical trial. *Arterioscler Thromb Vasc Biol,* 28(2), 341–347. doi: 10.1161/ATVBAHA.107.153965

Moreno, J. A., Perez-Jimenez, F., Marin, C., Gomez, P., Perez-Martinez, P., Moreno, R., . . . Lopez-Miranda, J. (2004). The effect of dietary fat on LDL size is influenced by apolipoprotein E genotype in healthy subjects. *J Nutr,* 134(10), 2517–2522.

Olofsson, P. S., Sheikine, Y., Jatta, K., Ghaderi, M., Samnegard, A., Eriksson, P., & Sirsjo, A. (2009). A functional interleukin-1 receptor antagonist polymorphism influences atherosclerosis development. The interleukin-1beta:interleukin-1 receptor antagonist balance in atherosclerosis. *Circ J,* 73(8), 1531–1536.

Olsson, S., Holmegaard, L., Jood, K., Sjogren, M., Engstrom, G., Lovkvist, H., . . . Jern, C. (2012). Genetic variation within the interleukin-1 gene cluster and ischemic stroke. *Stroke,* 43(9), 2278–2282. doi: 10.1161/STROKEAHA.111.647446

OralDNA: www.oraldna.com

Orth, M., Weng, W., Funke, H., Steinmetz, A., Assmann, G., Nauck, M., . . . Luley, C. (1999). Effects of a Frequent Apolipoprotein E Isoform, ApoE4Freiburg (Leu28-Pro), on

Lipoproteins and the Prevalence of Coronary Artery Disease in Whites. *Arterioscler Thromb Vasc Bio,* 19(5), 1306–1315. doi: 10.1161/01.atv.19.5.1306

Palomaki, G. E., Melillo, S., & Bradley, L. A. (2010). Association between 9p21 genomic markers and heart disease: A meta-analysis. *JAMA,* 303(7), 648–656. doi: 10.1001/jama.2010.118

Reitz, C., Jun, G., Naj, A., et al. (2013). Variants in the atp-binding cassette transporter (abca7), apolipoprotein e 4, and the risk of late-onset alzheimer disease in african americans. *JAMA,* 309(14), 1483–1492. doi: 10.1001/jama.2013.2973

Sattelmair, J., Pertman, J., Ding, E. L., Kohl, H. W., 3rd, Haskell, W., & Lee, I. M. (2011). Dose response between physical activity and risk of coronary heart disease: a meta-analysis. *Circulation,* 124(7), 789–795. doi: 10.1161/CIRCULATIONAHA.110.010710

Sattelmair, et al., 2011; Sever et al., (2003) "GINA ACT." *National Institute of Health.* http://report.nih.gov/nihfactsheets/ViewFactSheet.aspx?csid = 81

Scarmeas, N., Luchsinger, J. A., Schupf, N., Brickman, A. M., Cosentino, S., Tang, M. X., & Stern, Y. (2009). Physical activity, diet, and risk of Alzheimer disease. *JAMA,* 302(6), 627–637. doi: 10.1001/jama.2009.1144

Sever, P. S., Dahlöf, B., Poulter, N. R., Wedel, H., Beevers, G., Caulfield, M., . . . Östergren, J. (2003). Prevention of coronary and stroke events with atorvastatin in hypertensive patients who have average or lower-than-average cholesterol concentrations, in the Anglo-Scandinavian Cardiac Outcomes Trial—Lipid Lowering Arm (ASCOT-LLA): a multicentre randomised controlled trial. *The Lancet,* 361(9364), 1149–1158. doi: http://dx.doi.org/10.1016/S0140-6736(03)12948-0

Shiffman, D., Sabatine, M. S., Louie, J. Z., Kirchgessner, T. G., Iakoubova, O. A., Campos, H., . . . Sacks, F. M. (2010). Effect of pravastatin therapy on coronary events in carriers of the KIF6 719Arg allele from the cholesterol and recurrent events trial. *Am J Cardiol,* 105(9), 1300–1305. doi: 10.1016/j.amjcard.2009.12.049

Solomon, A., Kivipelto, M., Wolozin, B., Zhou, J., & Whitmer, R. A. (2009). Midlife serum cholesterol and increased risk of Alzheimer's and vascular dementia three decades later. *Dement Geriatr Cogn Disord,* 28(1), 75–80. doi: 10.1159/000231980

Stewart, A. F., Dandona, S., Chen, L., Assogba, O., Belanger, M., Ewart, G., . . . Roberts, R. (2009). Kinesin family member 6 variant Trp719Arg does not associate with angiographically defined coronary artery disease in the Ottawa Heart Genomics Study. *J Am Coll Cardiol,* 53(16), 1471–1472. doi: 10.1016/j.jacc.2008.12.051

Tang, M., Stern, Y., Marder, K., et al. (1998). The apoe-4 allele and the risk of alzheimer disease among african americans, whites, and hispanics. *JAMA,* 279(10), 751–755. doi: 10.1001/jama.279.10.751

Van Tassell, B. W., Toldo, S., Mezzaroma, E., & Abbate, A. (2013). Targeting interleukin-1 in heart disease. *Circulation,* 128(17), 1910–1923. doi: 10.1161/circulationaha.113.003199

Vardi, M., Blum, S., & Levy, A. P. (2012). Haptoglobin genotype and cardiovascular outcomes in diabetes mellitus - natural history of the disease and the effect of vitamin E treatment. Meta-analysis of the medical literature. *Eur J Intern Med,* 23(7), 628–632. doi: 10.1016/j.ejim.2012.04.009

Versmissen, J., Oosterveer, D. M., Hoekstra, M., Out, R., Berbée, J. F. P., Blommesteijn-Touw, A. C., . . . Sijbrands, E. J. G. (2011). Apolipoprotein Isoform E4 Does Not Increase Coronary Heart Disease Risk in Carriers of Low-Density Lipoprotein Receptor Mutations. *Circulation: Cardiovascular Genetics,* 4(6), 655–660. doi: 10.1161/circgenetics.111.959858

Ward, H., Mitrou, P. N., Bowman, R., Luben, R., Wareham, N. J., Khaw, K. T., & Bingham, S. (2009). APOE genotype, lipids, and coronary heart disease risk: a prospective population study. *Arch Intern Med,* 169(15), 1424–1429. doi: 10.1001/archinternmed.2009.234

Wilson, P. F., Myers, R. H., Larson, M. G., Ordovas, J. M., Wolf, P. A., & Schaefer, E. J. (1994). Apolipoprotein e alleles, dyslipidemia, and coronary heart disease: The framingham offspring study. *JAMA,* 272(21), 1666–1671. doi: 10.1001/jama.1994.03520210050031

Wilson, R. S., Mendes de Leon, C. F., Barnes, L. L., et al. (2002). Participation in cognitively stimulating activities and risk of incident alzheimer disease. *JAMA,* 287(6), 742–748. doi: 10.1001/jama.287.6.742

Yue, L., Bian, J. T., Grizelj, I., Cavka, A., Phillips, S. A., Makino, A., & Mazzone, T. (2012). Apolipoprotein E enhances endothelial-NO production by modulating caveolin 1 interaction with endothelial NO synthase. *Hypertension,* 60(4), 1040–1046. doi: 10.1161/HYPERTENSIONAHA.112.196667

Zhang, W., Chen, Y., Liu, P., Chen, J., Song, L., Tang, Y., . . . Hui, R. (2012). Variants on Chromosome 9p21.3 Correlated With ANRIL Expression Contribute to Stroke Risk and Recurrence in a Large Prospective Stroke Population. *Stroke,* 43(1), 14–21. doi: 10.1161/strokeaha.111.625442

Chapter Eleven

The ACCORD Study Group. Effects of Intensive Blood-Pressure Control in Type 2 Diabetes Mellitus. (2010). *N Engl J Med,* 362(17), 1575–1585. doi:10.1056/NEJMoa1001286

Alderman, M. H. (2004). JNC 7: brief summary and critique. *Clin Exp Hypertens,* 26(7–8), 753–761.

American Diabetes, A. (2013). Standards of medical care in diabetes–2013. *Diabetes Care,* 36 Suppl 1, S11–66. doi: 10.2337/dc13-S011

Bale, B. (2010). Optimizing hypertension management in underserved rural populations. *J Natl Med Assoc,* 102(1), 10–17.

Bangalore, S., Kumar, S., Lobach, I., & Messerli, F. H. (2011). Blood Pressure Targets in Subjects With Type 2 Diabetes Mellitus/Impaired Fasting Glucose: Observations From Traditional and Bayesian Random-Effects Meta-Analyses of Randomized Trials. *Circulation,* 123(24), 2799–2810. doi: 10.1161/circulationaha.110.016337

Beckett, N. S., Peters, R., Fletcher, A. E., Staessen, J. A., Liu, L., Dumitrascu, D., . . . Bulpitt, C. J. (2008). Treatment of Hypertension in Patients 80 Years of Age or Older. *N Engl J Med,* 358(18), 1887–1898. doi: 10.1056/NEJMoa0801369

Betti, I., Castelli, G., Barchielli, A., Beligni, C., Boscherini, V., De Luca, L., . . . Zuppiroli, A. (2009). The Role of N-terminal PRO-Brain Natriuretic Peptide and Echocardiography for Screening Asymptomatic Left Ventricular Dysfunction in a Population at High Risk for Heart Failure: The PROBE-HF Study. *Journal of Cardiac Failure,* 15(5), 377–384. doi: http://dx.doi.org/10.1016/j.cardfail.2008.12.002

Borden, W. B., Redberg, R. F., Mushlin, A. I., Dai, D., Kaltenbach, L. A., & Spertus, J. A. (2011). Patterns and intensity of medical therapy in patients undergoing percutaneous coronary intervention. *JAMA,* 305(18), 1882–1889. doi: 10.1001/jama.2011.601

Chow, C. K., Teo, K. K., Rangarajan, S., Islam, S., Gupta, R., Avezum, A., . . . investigators, P. S. (2013). Prevalence, awareness, treatment, and control of hypertension in rural and urban communities in high-, middle-, and low-income countries. *JAMA,* 310(9), 959–968. doi: 10.1001/jama.2013.184182

Colan, S. D., Lipshultz, S. E., Lowe, A. M., Sleeper, L. A., Messere, J., Cox, G. F., . . . Towbin, J. A. (2007). Epidemiology and cause-specific outcome of hypertrophic cardiomyopathy in children: findings from the Pediatric Cardiomyopathy Registry. *Circulation, 115*(6), 773–781. doi: 10.1161/CIRCULATIONAHA.106.621185

Ford, E. S., Schulze, M. B., Bergmann, M. M., Thamer, C., Joost, H.-G., & Boeing, H. (2008). Liver Enzymes and Incident Diabetes: Findings from the European Prospective Investigation Into Cancer and Nutrition (EPIC)-Potsdam Study. *Diabetes Care, 31*(6), 1138–1143. doi: 10.2337/dc07-2159

Gray, L., Lee, I. M., Sesso, H. D., & Batty, G. D. (2011). Blood Pressure in Early Adulthood, Hypertension in Middle Age, and Future Cardiovascular Disease Mortality: HAHS (Harvard Alumni Health Study). *J Am Coll Cardiol, 58*(23), 2396–2403. doi: http://dx.doi.org/10.1016/j.jacc.2011.07.045

Hsu, C., McCulloch, C. E., Darbinian, J., Go, A. S., & Iribarren, C. (2005). Elevated blood pressure and risk of end-stage renal disease in subjects without baseline kidney disease. *Arch Intern Med, 165*(8), 923–928. doi: 10.1001/archinte.165.8.923

Jouven, X., Empana, J.-P., Schwartz, P. J., Desnos, M., Courbon, D., & Ducimetière, P. (2005). Heart-Rate Profile during Exercise as a Predictor of Sudden Death. *N Engl J Med, 352*(19), 1951–1958. doi: 10.1056/NEJMoa043012

Kamstrup, P. R., Tybjærg-Hansen, A., Steffensen, R., & Nordestgaard, B. G. (2009). Genetically elevated lipoprotein(a) and increased risk of myocardial infarction. *JAMA, 301*(22), 2331–2339. doi: 10.1001/jama.2009.801

Khalique, O., Aronow, W. S., Ahn, C., Mazar, M., Schair, B., Shao, J., & Channamsetty, V. (2007). Relation of Moderate or Severe Reduction in Glomerular Filtration Rate to Number of Coronary Arteries Narrowed > 50% in Patients Undergoing Coronary Angiography for Suspected Coronary Artery Disease. *Am J Cardiol, 100*(3), 415–416. doi: http://dx.doi.org/10.1016/j.amjcard.2007.03.038

Kragelund, C., Grønning, B., Køber, L., Hildebrandt, P., & Steffensen, R. (2005). N-Terminal Pro–B-Type Natriuretic Peptide and Long-Term Mortality in Stable Coronary Heart Disease. *N Engl J Med, 352*(7), 666–675. doi: 10.1056/NEJMoa042330

Law, M. R., Morris, J. K., & Wald, N. J. (2009). Use of blood pressure lowering drugs in the prevention of cardiovascular disease: meta-analysis of 147 randomised trials in the context of expectations from prospective epidemiological studies. *Bmj, 338*, b1665. doi: 10.1136/bmj.b1665

Lawes, C. M. M., Hoorn, S. V., & Rodgers, A. (2001). Global burden of blood-pressure-related disease, 2001. *The Lancet, 371*(9623), 1513–1518. doi: http://dx.doi.org/10.1016/S0140-6736(08)60655-8

Lee, M., Saver, J. L., Chang, B., Chang, K. H., Hao, Q., & Ovbiagele, B. (2011). Presence of baseline prehypertension and risk of incident stroke: a meta-analysis. *Neurology, 77*(14), 1330–1337. doi: 10.1212/WNL.0b013e3182315234

Lewington, S., Clarke, R., Qizilbash, N., Peto, R., & Collins, R. (2002). Age-specific relevance of usual blood pressure to vascular mortality: a meta-analysis of individual data for one million adults in 61 prospective studies. *The Lancet, 360*(9349), 1903–1913.

Loredo, J. S., Ancoli-Israel, S., & Dimsdale, J. E. (2001). Sleep quality and blood pressure dipping in obstructive sleep apnea*. *American Journal of Hypertension, 14*(9), 887–892. doi: 10.1016/s0895-7061(01)02143-4

Luepker, R. V., Steffen, L. M., Jacobs, D. R., Jr., Zhou, X., & Blackburn, H. (2012). Trends in blood pressure and hypertension detection, treatment, and control 1980 to 2009:

the Minnesota Heart Survey. *Circulation,* 126(15), 1852–1857. doi: 10.1161/CIRCULATIONAHA.112.098517

Maher, V. G., Brown, B., Marcovina, S. M., Hillger, L. A., Zhao, X., & Albers, J. J. (1995). Effects of lowering elevated ldl cholesterol on the cardiovascular risk of lipoprotein(a). *JAMA,* 274(22), 1771–1774. doi: 10.1001/jama.1995.03530220037029

Mason, C. M., & Doneen, A. L. (2012). Niacin—a critical component to the management of atherosclerosis: contemporary management of dyslipidemia to prevent, reduce, or reverse atherosclerotic cardiovascular disease. *J Cardiovasc Nurs,* 27(4), 303–316. doi: 10.1097/JCN.0b013e31821bf93f

McBrien, K., Rabi, D. M., Campbell, N., Barnieh, L., Clement, F., Hemmelgarn, B. R., . . . Manns, B. J. (2012). Intensive and Standard Blood Pressure Targets in Patients With Type 2 Diabetes Mellitus: Systematic Review and Meta-analysis. *Arch Intern Med,* 172(17), 1296–1303. doi: 10.1001/archinternmed.2012.3147

Messerli, F. H., Mancia, G., Conti, C. R., Hewkin, A. C., Kupfer, S., Champion, A., . . . Pepine, C. J. (2006). Dogma disputed: can aggressively lowering blood pressure in hypertensive patients with coronary artery disease be dangerous? *Ann Intern Med,* 144(12), 884–893.

O'Donnell, M. J., Xavier, D., Liu, L., Zhang, H., Chin, S. L., Rao-Melacini, P., . . . Yusuf, S. Risk factors for ischaemic and intracerebral haemorrhagic stroke in 22 countries (the INTERSTROKE study): a case-control study. *The Lancet,* 376(9735), 112–123. doi: http://dx.doi.org/10.1016/S0140-6736(10)60834-3

Pletcher, M. J., Sibley, C. T., Pignone, M., Vittinghoff, E., & Greenland, P. (2013). Interpretation of the Coronary Artery Calcium Score in Combination With Conventional Cardiovascular Risk Factors: The Multi-Ethnic Study of Atherosclerosis (MESA). *Circulation,* 128(10), 1076–1084. doi: 10.1161/circulationaha.113.002598

Qureshi, A. I., Suri, M. F. K., Kirmani, J. F., Divani, A. A., & Mohammad, Y. (2005). Is Prehypertension a Risk Factor for Cardiovascular Diseases? *Stroke,* 36(9), 1859–1863. doi: 10.1161/01.STR.0000177495.45580.f1

Rodondi, N., den Elzen, W. J., Bauer, D. C., et al. (2010). Subclinical hypothyroidism and the risk of coronary heart disease and mortality. *JAMA,* 304(12), 1365–1374. doi: 10.1001/jama.2010.1361

Sharabi, Y., Scope, A., Chorney, N., Grotto, I., & Dagan, Y. (2003). Diastolic blood pressure is the first to rise in association with early subclinical obstructive sleep apnea: lessons from periodic examination screening. *American Journal of Hypertension,* 16(3), 236–239. doi: 10.1016/s0895-7061(02)03250-8

Shlipak, M. G., Sarnak, M. J., Katz, R., Fried, L. F., Seliger, S. L., Newman, A. B., . . . Stehman-Breen, C. (2005). Cystatin C and the Risk of Death and Cardiovascular Events among Elderly Persons. *N Engl J Med,* 352(20), 2049–2060. doi: 10.1056/NEJMoa043161

Teo, K., Chow, C. K., Vaz, M., Rangarajan, S., & Yusuf, S. (2009). The Prospective Urban Rural Epidemiology (PURE) study: Examining the impact of societal influences on chronic noncommunicable diseases in low-, middle-, and high-income countries. *Am Heart J,* 158(1), 1–7.e1. doi: http://dx.doi.org/10.1016/j.ahj.2009.04.019

Tricoci, P., Allen, J. M., Kramer, J. M., Califf, R. M., & Smith, S. C. (2009). Scientific evidence underlying the acc/aha clinical practice guidelines. *JAMA,* 301(8), 831–841. doi: 10.1001/jama.2009.205

Verdecchia, P., Gentile, G., Angeli, F., Mazzotta, G., Mancia, G., & Reboldi, G. (2010). Influence of blood pressure reduction on composite cardiovascular endpoints in clinical trials. *J Hypertens,* 28(7), 1356–1365. doi: 10.1097/HJH.0b013e328338e2bb

Wang, T. J., Wollert, K. C., Larson, M. G., Coglianese, E., McCabe, E. L., Cheng, S., . . . Januzzi, J. L. (2012). Prognostic utility of novel biomarkers of cardiovascular stress: the Framingham Heart Study. *Circulation,* 126(13), 1596–1604. doi: 10.1161/CIRCULATIONAHA.112.129437

Chapter Twelve

Adams, C. A., Leary, M. R. (2007). Promoting Self–Compassionate Attitudes Toward Eating Among Restrictive and Guilty Eaters. *Journal of Social and Clinical Psychology,* 26(10), 2007, 1120–1144.

Allen, N. E., Beral, V., Casabonne, D., Kan, S. W., Reeves, G. K., Brown, A., . . . Million Women Study, C. (2009). Moderate alcohol intake and cancer incidence in women. *J Natl Cancer Inst,* 101(5), 296–305. doi: 10.1093/jnci/djn514

Ardern, C. I., Katzmarzyk, P. T., Janssen, I., Church, T. S., & Blair, S. N. (2005). Revised Adult Treatment Panel III Guidelines and Cardiovascular Disease Mortality in Men Attending a Preventive Medical Clinic. *Circulation,* 112(10), 1478–1485. doi: 10.1161/circulationaha.105.548198

Azadbakht, L., Haghighatdoost, F., Karimi, G., & Esmaillzadeh, A. (2013). Effect of consuming salad and yogurt as preload on body weight management and cardiovascular risk factors: a randomized clinical trial. *Int J Food Sci Nutr,* 64(4), 392–399. doi: 10.3109/09637486.2012.753039

Berrington de Gonzalez, A., Hartge, P., Cerhan, J. R., Flint, A. J., Hannan, L., MacInnis, R. J., . . . Thun, M. J. (2010). Body-Mass Index and Mortality among 1.46 Million White Adults. *N Engl J Med,* 363(23), 2211–2219. doi: 10.1056/NEJMoa1000367

Bleich, S., Wilhelm, J., Graesel, E., Degner, D., Sperling, W., Rossner, V., . . . Kornhuber, J. (2003). Apolipoprotein E epsilon 4 is associated with hippocampal volume reduction in females with alcoholism. *J Neural Transm,* 110(4), 401–411. doi: 10.1007/s00702-002-0789-1

Bravata, D. M., Smith-Spangler, C., Sundaram, V., et al. (2007). Using pedometers to increase physical activity and improve health: A systematic review. *JAMA,* 298(19), 2296–2304. doi: 10.1001/jama.298.19.2296

Buijsse, B., Weikert, C., Drogan, D., Bergmann, M., & Boeing, H. (2010). Chocolate consumption in relation to blood pressure and risk of cardiovascular disease in German adults. *Eur Heart J,* 31(13), 1616–1623. doi: 10.1093/eurheartj/ehq068

Butryn, M. L., Phelan, S., Hill, J. O., & Wing, R. R. (2007). Consistent self-monitoring of weight: a key component of successful weight loss maintenance. *Obesity (Silver Spring),* 15(12), 3091–3096. doi: 10.1038/oby.2007.368

Carraca, E. V., Silva, M. N., Markland, D., Vieira, P. N., Minderico, C. S., Sardinha, L. B., & Teixeira, P. J. (2011). Body image change and improved eating self-regulation in a weight management intervention in women. *Int J Behav Nutr Phys Act,* 8, 75. doi: 10.1186/1479-5868-8-75

Catenacci, V. A., Ogden, L. G., Stuht, J., Phelan, S., Wing, R. R., Hill, J. O., & Wyatt, H. R. (2008). Physical activity patterns in the National Weight Control Registry. *Obesity (Silver Spring),* 16(1), 153–161. doi: 10.1038/oby.2007.6

Chiuve, S. E., Rexrode, K. M., Spiegelman, D., Logroscino, G., Manson, J. E., & Rimm, E. B. (2008). Primary prevention of stroke by healthy lifestyle. *Circulation,* 118(9), 947–954. doi: 10.1161/CIRCULATIONAHA.108.781062

Chow, C. K., Jolly, S., Rao-Melacini, P., Fox, K. A. A., Anand, S. S., & Yusuf, S. (2010). Association of Diet, Exercise, and Smoking Modification With Risk of Early Cardiovascular Events After Acute Coronary Syndromes. *Circulation,* 121(6), 750–758. doi: 10.1161/circulationaha.109.891523

Corella, D., Carrasco, P., Sorlí, J. V., Estruch, R., Rico-Sanz, J., Martínez-González, M. Á., . . . Ordovás, J. M. (2013). Mediterranean Diet Reduces the Adverse Effect of the TCF7L2-rs7903146 Polymorphism on Cardiovascular Risk Factors and Stroke Incidence: A randomized controlled trial in a high-cardiovascular-risk population. *Diabetes Care.* doi: 10.2337/dc13-0955

Corella, D., Tucker, K., Lahoz, C., Coltell, O., Cupples, L. A., Wilson, P. W., . . . Ordovas, J. M. (2001). Alcohol drinking determines the effect of the APOE locus on LDL-cholesterol concentrations in men: the Framingham Offspring Study. *Am J Clin Nutr,* 73(4), 736–745.

Daeninck, E., & Miller, M. (2006). What can the National Weight Control Registry teach us? *Curr Diab Rep,* 6(5), 401–404.

Deckelbaum, R. J., Fisher, E. A., Winston, M., Kumanyika, S., Lauer, R. M., Pi-Sunyer, F. X., . . . Weinstein, I. B. (1999). Summary of a Scientific Conference on Preventive Nutrition: Pediatrics to Geriatrics. *Circulation,* 100(4), 450–456. doi: 10.1161/01.cir.100.4.450

Djousse, L., Pankow, J. S., Arnett, D. K., Eckfeldt, J. H., Myers, R. H., & Ellison, R. C. (2004). Apolipoprotein E polymorphism modifies the alcohol-HDL association observed in the National Heart, Lung, and Blood Institute Family Heart Study. *Am J Clin Nutr,* 80(6), 1639–1644.

Eaker, E. D., Pinsky, J., & Castelli, W. P. (1992). Myocardial infarction and coronary death among women: psychosocial predictors from a 20-year follow-up of women in the Framingham Study. *Am J Epidemiol,* 135(8), 854–864.

Eichner, J. E., Dunn, S. T., Perveen, G., Thompson, D. M., Stewart, K. E., & Stroehla, B. C. (2002). Apolipoprotein E Polymorphism and Cardiovascular Disease: A Huge Review. *Am J Epidemiol,* 155(6), 487–495. doi: 10.1093/aje/155.6.487

Erkkilä, A. T., Sarkkinen, E. S., Lindi, V., Lehto, S., Laakso, M., & Uusitupa, M. I. (2001). APOE polymorphism and the hypertriglyceridemic effect of dietary sucrose. *Am J Clin Nutr,* 73(4), 746–752.

Estruch, R., Ros, E., Salas-Salvado, J., Covas, M. I., Corella, D., Aros, F., . . . Investigators, P. S. (2013). Primary prevention of cardiovascular disease with a Mediterranean diet. *N Engl J Med,* 368(14), 1279–1290. doi: 10.1056/NEJMoa1200303

Ford, E. S., Greenlund, K. J., & Hong, Y. (2012). Ideal Cardiovascular Health and Mortality From All Causes and Diseases of the Circulatory System Among Adults in the United States. *Circulation,* 125(8), 987–995. doi: 10.1161/circulationaha.111.049122

Gardner, C. D., Kiazand, A., Alhassan, S., et al. (2007). Comparison of the atkins, zone, ornish, and learn diets for change in weight and related risk factors among overweight premenopausal women: The a to z weight loss study: a randomized trial. *JAMA,* 297(9), 969–977. doi: 10.1001/jama.297.9.969

Givi, M. (2013). Durability of effect of massage therapy on blood pressure. *Int J Prev Med,* 4(5), 511–516.

Gómez-Coronado, D., Álvarez, J. J., Entrala, A., Olmos, J. M. a., Herrera, E., & Lasunción, M. Á. (1999). Apolipoprotein E polymorphism in men and women from a Spanish population: allele frequencies and influence on plasma lipids and apolipoproteins. *Atherosclerosis,* 147(1), 167–176. doi: http://dx.doi.org/10.1016/S0021-9150(99)00168-9

Gray, L., Lee, I., Sesso, H. D., & Batty, G. (2011). Body weight in early and mid-adulthood in relation to subsequent coronary heart disease mortality: 80-year follow-up in the harvard alumni study. *Arch Intern Med,* 171(19), 1768–1770. doi: 10.1001/archinternmed.2011.486

Gump, B. B., & Matthews, K. A. (2000). Are Vacations Good for Your Health? The 9-Year Mortality Experience After the Multiple Risk Factor Intervention Trial. *Psychosomatic Medicine,* 62(5), 608–612.

Hagberg, J. M., Wilund, K. R., & Ferrell, R. E. (2000). APO E gene and gene-environment effects on plasma lipoprotein-lipid levels. *Physiol Genomics,* 4(2), 101–108.

Hall, S. A., Shackelton, R., Rosen, R. C., & Araujo, A. B. (2010). Sexual activity, erectile dysfunction, and incident cardiovascular events. *Am J Cardiol,* 105(2), 192–197. doi: 10.1016/j.amjcard.2009.08.671

Hankinson, A. L., Daviglus, M. L., Bouchard, C., et al. (2010). Maintaining a high physical activity level over 20 years and weight gain. *JAMA,* 304(23), 2603–2610. doi: 10.1001/jama.2010.1843

Head, A., Kendall, M. J., Ferner, R., & Eagles, C. (1996). Acute effects of beta blockade and exercise on mood and anxiety. *British Journal of Sports Medicine,* 30(3), 238–242. doi: 10.1136/bjsm.30.3.238

Ishiwata, K., Homma, Y., Ishikawa, T., Nakamura, H., & Handa, S. (2002). Influence of apolipoprotein E phenotype on metabolism of lipids and apolipoproteins after plant stanol ester ingestion in japanese subjects. *Nutrition,* 18(7–8), 561–565. doi: http://dx.doi.org/10.1016/S0899-9007(02)00803-1

Jenkins, D., Kendall, C., Marchie, A., Faulkner, D., Wong, J., de Souza, R., . . . Connelly, P. (2003). Effects of a dietary portfolio of cholesterol-lowering foods vs lovastatin on serum lipids and C-reactive protein. *JAMA,* 290, 502–510.

Jenkins, D. J., Hegele, R. A., Jenkins, A. L., Connelly, P. W., Hallak, K., Bracci, P., . . . et al. (1993). The apolipoprotein E gene and the serum low-density lipoprotein cholesterol response to dietary fiber. *Metabolism,* 42(5), 585–593.

Kataoka, S., Robbins, D. C., Cowan, L. D., Go, O., Yeh, J. L., Devereux, R. B., . . . Investigators, f. t. S. H. S. (1996). Apolipoprotein E Polymorphism in American Indians and Its Relation to Plasma Lipoproteins and Diabetes: The Strong Heart Study. *Arterioscler Thromb Vasc Bio,* 16(8), 918–925. doi: 10.1161/01.atv.16.8.918

Klem, M. L., Wing, R. R., McGuire, M. T., Seagle, H. M., & Hill, J. O. (1997). A descriptive study of individuals successful at long-term maintenance of substantial weight loss. *Am J Clin Nutr,* 66(2), 239–246.

Knoops, K. B., de Groot, L. M., Kromhout, D., et al. (2004). Mediterranean diet, lifestyle factors, and 10-year mortality in elderly european men and women: The hale project. *JAMA,* 292(12), 1433–1439. doi: 10.1001/jama.292.12.1433

Kolovou, G. D., & Anagnostopoulou, K. K. (2007). Apolipoprotein E polymorphism, age and coronary heart disease. *Ageing Res Rev,* 6(2), 94–108. doi: 10.1016/j.arr.2006.11.001

Kong, A., Beresford, S. A., Alfano, C. M., Foster-Schubert, K. E., Neuhouser, M. L., Johnson, D. B., . . . McTiernan, A. (2012). Self-monitoring and eating-related behaviors are associated with 12-month weight loss in postmenopausal overweight-to-obese women. *J Acad Nutr Diet,* 112(9), 1428–1435. doi: 10.1016/j.jand.2012.05.014

Krauss, R. M., Eckel, R. H., Howard, B., Appel, L. J., Daniels, S. R., Deckelbaum, R. J., . . . Bazzarre, T. L. (2000). AHA Dietary Guidelines: Revision 2000: A Statement for Healthcare Professionals From the Nutrition Committee of the American Heart Association. *Circulation,* 102(18), 2284–2299. doi: 10.1161/01.cir.102.18.2284

Kriska, A. M. (2003). Physical Activity, Obesity, and the Incidence of Type 2 Diabetes in a High-Risk Population. *Am J Epidemiol,* 158(7), 669–675. doi: 10.1093/aje/kwg191

Lee, I. M., & Paffenbarger, R. S. (1998). Physical Activity and Stroke Incidence : The Harvard Alumni Health Study. *Stroke,* 29(10), 2049–2054. doi: 10.1161/01.str.29.10.2049

Lehtinen, S., Lehtimäki, T., Sisto, T., Salenius, J.-P., Nikkilä, M., Jokela, H., . . . Ehnholm, C. (1995). Apolipoprotein E polymorphism, serum lipids, myocardial infarction and severity of angiographically verified coronary artery disease in men and women. *Atherosclerosis,* 114(1), 83–91. doi: http://dx.doi.org/10.1016/0021-9150(94)05469-Y

Lloyd-Jones, D. M., Hong, Y., Labarthe, D., Mozaffarian, D., Appel, L. J., Van Horn, L., . . . Committee, S. (2010). Defining and Setting National Goals for Cardiovascular Health Promotion and Disease Reduction: The American Heart Association's Strategic Impact Goal Through 2020 and Beyond. *Circulation,* 121(4), 586–613. doi: 10.1161/circulationaha.109.192703

Loktionov, A., Bingham, S. A., Vorster, H., Jerling, J. C., Runswick, S. A., & Cummings, J. H. (1998). Apolipoprotein E genotype modulates the effect of black tea drinking on blood lipids and blood coagulation factors: a pilot study. *Br J Nutr,* 79(2), 133–139.

Lussier-Cacan, S., Bolduc, A., Xhignesse, M., Niyonsenga, T., & Sing, C. F. (2002). Impact of Alcohol Intake on Measures of Lipid Metabolism Depends on Context Defined by Gender, Body Mass Index, Cigarette Smoking, and Apolipoprotein E Genotype. *Arterioscler Thromb Vasc Bio,* 22(5), 824–831. doi: 10.1161/01.atv.0000014589.22121.6c

Ma, Y. (2003). Association between Eating Patterns and Obesity in a Free-living US Adult Population. *Am J Epidemiol,* 158(1), 85–92. doi: 10.1093/aje/kwg117

Manson, J. E., Hu, F. B., Rich-Edwards, J. W., Colditz, G. A., Stampfer, M. J., Willett, W. C., . . . Hennekens, C. H. (1999). A Prospective Study of Walking as Compared with Vigorous Exercise in the Prevention of Coronary Heart Disease in Women. *N Engl J Med,* 341(9), 650–658. doi: 10.1056/NEJM199908263410904

Marques-Vidal, P., Bongard, V., Ruidavets, J. B., Fauvel, J., Hanaire-Broutin, H., Perret, B., & Ferrieres, J. (2003). Obesity and alcohol modulate the effect of apolipoprotein E polymorphism on lipids and insulin. *Obes Res,* 11(10), 1200–1206. doi: 10.1038/oby.2003.165

Masson, L. F., McNeill, G., & Avenell, A. (2003). Genetic variation and the lipid response to dietary intervention: a systematic review. *Am J Clin Nutr,* 77(5), 1098–1111.

McDonnell, M. N., Hillier, S. L., Hooker, S. P., Le, A., Judd, S. E., & Howard, V. J. (2013). Physical Activity Frequency and Risk of Incident Stroke in a National US Study of Blacks and Whites. *Stroke.* doi: 10.1161/strokeaha.113.001538

McGuire, M. T., Wing, R. R., Klem, M. L., & Hill, J. O. (1999). Behavioral strategies of individuals who have maintained long-term weight losses. *Obes Res,* 7(4), 334–341.

McGuire, M. T., Wing, R. R., Klem, M. L., Seagle, H. M., & Hill, J. O. (1998). Long-term maintenance of weight loss: do people who lose weight through various weight loss methods use different behaviors to maintain their weight? *Int J Obes Relat Metab Disord,* 22(6), 572–577.

Minihane, A. M., Khan, S., Leigh-Firbank, E. C., Talmud, P., Wright, J. W., Murphy, M. C., . . . Williams, C. M. (2000). ApoE Polymorphism and Fish Oil Supplementation in Subjects

With an Atherogenic Lipoprotein Phenotype. *Arterioscler Thromb Vasc Bio, 20*(8), 1990–1997. doi: 10.1161/01.atv.20.8.1990

Moreno, J. A., Perez-Jimenez, F., Marin, C., Gomez, P., Perez-Martinez, P., Moreno, R., . . . Lopez-Miranda, J. (2004). The effect of dietary fat on LDL size is influenced by apolipo-protein E genotype in healthy subjects. *J Nutr, 134*(10), 2517–2522.

Mukamal, K. J., Chen, C. M., Rao, S. R., & Breslow, R. A. (2010). Alcohol consumption and cardiovascular mortality among U.S. adults, 1987 to 2002. *J Am Coll Cardiol, 55*(13), 1328–1335. doi: 10.1016/j.jacc.2009.10.056

Mukamal, K. J., Cushman, M., Mittleman, M. A., Tracy, R. P., & Siscovick, D. S. (2004). Alco-hol consumption and inflammatory markers in older adults: the Cardiovascular Health Study. *Atherosclerosis, 173*(1), 79–87. doi: 10.1016/j.atherosclerosis.2003.10.011

O'Keefe, J. H., Patil, H. R., Lavie, C. J., Magalski, A., Vogel, R. A., & McCullough, P. A. (2012). Potential adverse cardiovascular effects from excessive endurance exercise. *Mayo Clin Proc, 87*(6), 587–595. doi: 10.1016/j.mayocp.2012.04.005

Perez-Escamilla, R., Obbagy, J. E., Altman, J. M., Essery, E. V., McGrane, M. M., Wong, Y. P., . . . Williams, C. L. (2012). Dietary energy density and body weight in adults and chil-dren: a systematic review. *J Acad Nutr Diet, 112*(5), 671–684. doi: 10.1016/j.jand.2012.01.020

Phelan, S., Wyatt, H. R., Hill, J. O., & Wing, R. R. (2006). Are the eating and exercise habits of successful weight losers changing? *Obesity (Silver Spring), 14*(4), 710–716. doi: 10.1038/oby.2006.81

Rasmussen-Torvik, L. J., Shay, C. M., Abramson, J. G., Friedrich, C. A., Nettleton, J. A., Priz-ment, A. E., & Folsom, A. R. (2013). Ideal cardiovascular health is inversely associated with incident cancer: the atherosclerosis risk in communities study. *Circulation, 127*(12), 1270–1275. doi: 10.1161/CIRCULATIONAHA.112.001183

Raynor, D. A., Phelan, S., Hill, J. O., & Wing, R. R. (2006). Television viewing and long-term weight maintenance: results from the National Weight Control Registry. *Obesity (Silver Spring), 14*(10), 1816–1824. doi: 10.1038/oby.2006.209

Raynor, H. A., Jeffery, R. W., Phelan, S., Hill, J. O., & Wing, R. R. (2005). Amount of food group variety consumed in the diet and long-term weight loss maintenance. *Obes Res, 13*(5), 883–890. doi: 10.1038/oby.2005.102

Rimm, E. B., Klatsky, A., Grobbee, D., & Stampfer, M. J. (1996). Review of moderate alco-hol consumption and reduced risk of coronary heart disease: is the effect due to beer, wine, or spirits? *Bmj, 312*(7033), 731–736. doi: 10.1136/bmj.312.7033.731

Roe, L. S., Meengs, J. S., & Rolls, B. J. (2012). Salad and satiety. The effect of timing of salad consumption on meal energy intake. *Appetite, 58*(1), 242–248. doi: http://dx.doi.org/10.1016/j.appet.2011.10.003

Roger, V. L., Go, A. S., Lloyd-Jones, D. M., Benjamin, E. J., Berry, J. D., Borden, W. B., . . . Stroke Statistics, S. (2012). Heart disease and stroke statistics—2012 update: a report from the American Heart Association. *Circulation, 125*(1), e2–e220. doi: 10.1161/CIR.0b013e31823ac046

Rolls, B. J., Roe, L. S., & Meengs, J. S. (2004). Salad and satiety: Energy density and portion size of a first-course salad affect energy intake at lunch. *Journal of the American Dietetic Association, 104*(10), 1570–1576. doi: http://dx.doi.org/10.1016/j.jada.2004.07.001

Saidi, S., Slamia, L. B., Ammou, S. B., Mahjoub, T., & Almawi, W. Y. (2007). Association of Apolipoprotein E Gene Polymorphism With Ischemic Stroke Involving Large-Vessel Dis-ease and Its Relation to Serum Lipid Levels. *Journal of Stroke and Cerebrovascular Diseases, 16*(4), 160–166. doi: http://dx.doi.org/10.1016/j.jstrokecerebrovasdis.2007.03.001

Sattelmair, J., Pertman, J., Ding, E. L., Kohl, H. W., 3rd, Haskell, W., & Lee, I. M. (2011). Dose response between physical activity and risk of coronary heart disease: a meta-analysis. *Circulation,* 124(7), 789–795. doi: 10.1161/CIRCULATIONAHA.110.010710

Selvin, E., Paynter, N. P., & Erlinger, T. P. (2007). The effect of weight loss on c-reactive protein: A systematic review. *Arch Intern Med,* 167(1), 31–39. doi: 10.1001/archinte.167.1.31

Shick, S. M., Wing, R. R., Klem, M. L., McGuire, M. T., Hill, J. O., & Seagle, H. (1998). Persons successful at long-term weight loss and maintenance continue to consume a low-energy, low-fat diet. *J Am Diet Assoc,* 98(4), 408–413. doi: 10.1016/s0002-8223(98)00093-5

Slentz, C. A., Duscha, B. D., Johnson, J. L., et al. (2004). Effects of the amount of exercise on body weight, body composition, and measures of central obesity: Strride—a randomized controlled study. *Arch Intern Med,* 164(1), 31–39. doi: 10.1001/archinte.164.1.31

Thomas, J. G., & Wing, R. R. (2009). Maintenance of long-term weight loss. *Med Health R I,* 92(2), 53, 56–57.

Trappe, H. J. (2010). The effects of music on the cardiovascular system and cardiovascular health. *Heart,* 96(23), 1868–1871. doi: 10.1136/hrt.2010.209858

Tworoger, S. S., Yasui, Y., Vitiello, M. V., Schwartz, R. S., Ulrich, C. M., Aiello, E. J., . . . McTiernan, A. (2003). Effects of a yearlong moderate-intensity exercise and a stretching intervention on sleep quality in postmenopausal women. *Sleep,* 26(7), 830–836.

Vigna, G. B., Pansini, F., Bonaccorsi, G., Albertazzi, P., Donega, P., Zanotti, L., . . . Fellin, R. (2000). Plasma lipoproteins in soy-treated postmenopausal women: a double-blind, placebo-controlled trial. *Nutr Metab Cardiovasc Dis,* 10(6), 315–322.

Wen, C. P., Wai, J. P. M., Tsai, M. K., Yang, Y. C., Cheng, T. Y. D., Lee, M.-C., . . . Wu, X. (2011). Minimum amount of physical activity for reduced mortality and extended life expectancy: a prospective cohort study. *The Lancet,* 378(9798), 1244–1253. doi: http://dx.doi.org/10.1016/S0140-6736(11)60749-6

Wing, R. R., & Hill, J. O. (2001). Successful weight loss maintenance. *Annu Rev Nutr,* 21, 323–341. doi: 10.1146/annurev.nutr.21.1.323

Wolever, T. M., Hegele, R. A., Connelly, P. W., Ransom, T. P., Story, J. A., Furumoto, E. J., & Jenkins, D. J. (1997). Long-term effect of soluble-fiber foods on postprandial fat metabolism in dyslipidemic subjects with apo E3 and apo E4 genotypes. *Am J Clin Nutr,* 66(3), 584–590.

Wolk, R., Shamsuzzaman, A. S. M., & Somers, V. K. (2003). Obesity, Sleep Apnea, and Hypertension. *Hypertension,* 42(6), 1067–1074. doi: 10.1161/01.hyp.0000101686.98973.a3

Wyatt, H. R., Grunwald, G. K., Mosca, C. L., Klem, M. L., Wing, R. R., & Hill, J. O. (2002). Long-term weight loss and breakfast in subjects in the National Weight Control Registry. *Obes Res,* 10(2), 78–82. doi: 10.1038/oby.2002.13

Wyatt, H. R., Grunwald, G. K., Seagle, H. M., Klem, M. L., McGuire, M. T., Wing, R. R., & Hill, J. O. (1999). Resting energy expenditure in reduced-obese subjects in the National Weight Control Registry. *Am J Clin Nutr,* 69(6), 1189–1193.

Xu, C. F., Talmud, P. J., Angelico, F., Del Ben, M., Savill, J., & Humphries, S. E. (1991). Apolipoprotein E polymorphism and plasma lipid, lipoprotein, and apolipoprotein levels in Italian children. *Genet Epidemiol,* 8(6), 389–398. doi: 10.1002/gepi.1370080605

Yu, J. C., & Berger, P., 3rd. (2011). Sleep apnea and obesity. *S D Med,* Spec No, 28–34.

Chapter Thirteen

Aggarwal, S., Loomba, R., Arora, R., & Molnar, J. (2012). Sleep Patterns and Prevalence of Cardiovascular Outcomes—Analysis of National Health and Nutrition Examination Survey Database 2007–08. *J Am Coll Cardiol*, 59(13s1), E1748–E1748. doi: 10.1016/S0735-1097(12)61749-5

Ahmed, W., Khan, N., Glueck, C. J., Pandey, S., Wang, P., Goldenberg, N., . . . Khanal, S. (2009). Low serum 25 (OH) vitamin D levels (< 32 ng/mL) are associated with reversible myositis-myalgia in statin-treated patients. *Transl Res*, 153(1), 11–16. doi: 10.1016/j.trsl.2008.11.002

Allen, R. W., Schwartzman, E., Baker, W. L., Coleman, C. I., & Phung, O. J. (2013). Cinnamon use in type 2 diabetes: an updated systematic review and meta-analysis. Ann Fam Med, 11(5), 452–459. doi: 10.1370/afm.1517

Alshaarawy, O., Xiao, J., & Shankar, A. (2013). Association of serum cotinine levels and hypertension in never smokers. *Hypertension*, 61(2), 304–308. doi: 10.1161/HYPERTENSIONAHA.112.198218

Amer, M., & Qayyum, R. (2012). Relation Between Serum 25-Hydroxyvitamin D and C-Reactive Protein in Asymptomatic Adults (From the Continuous National Health and Nutrition Examination Survey 2001 to 2006). *Am J Cardiol*, 109(2), 226–230. doi: http://dx.doi.org/10.1016/j.amjcard.2011.08.032

Amsterdam, J. D., Li, Y., Soeller, I., Rockwell, K., Mao, J. J., & Shults, J. (2009). A randomized, double-blind, placebo-controlled trial of oral Matricaria recutita (chamomile) extract therapy for generalized anxiety disorder. *J Clin Psychopharmacol*, 29(4), 378–382. doi: 10.1097/JCP.0b013e3181ac935c

Bair, T., J. B. Muhlestein, H. T. May, et al. Supplementing Deficient Vitamin D levels is associated with reduced cardiovascular risk. *Journal of the American College of Cardiology*, 55(10a), A59.E564, 2010.

Bale, B. F., Doneen, A. L. (2013). Autophagy, Senescence, and Arterial Inflammation: Relationship to Arterial Health and Longevity. *Altern Ther Health Med*, 19(4), 8–10.

Barnoya, J., & Glantz, S. A. (2005). Cardiovascular Effects of Secondhand Smoke: Nearly as Large as Smoking. *Circulation*, 111(20), 2684–2698. doi: 10.1161/circulationaha.104.492215

Barton, P. D.; Connor, W. E. (2008). Abstract 3701: Vitamin D Deficiency is Associated With Myalgias in Hyperlipidemic Subjects Taking Statins. *Circulation*, 118, S_470. http://circ.ahajournals.org/cgi/content/meeting_abstract/118/18_MeetingAbstracts/S_470

Barua, R. S., & Ambrose, J. A. (2013). Mechanisms of Coronary Thrombosis in Cigarette Smoke Exposure. *Arterioscler Thromb Vasc Bio*, 33(7), 1460–1467. doi: 10.1161/atvbaha.112.300154

Bays, H. E., McKenney, J., Maki, K. C., Doyle, R. T., Carter, R. N., & Stein, E. (2010). Effects of prescription omega-3-acid ethyl esters on non--high-density lipoprotein cholesterol when coadministered with escalating doses of atorvastatin. *Mayo Clin Proc*, 85(2), 122–128. doi: 10.4065/mcp.2009.0397

Belch, J., MacCuish, A., Campbell, I., Cobbe, S., Taylor, R., Prescott, R., . . . MacWalter, R. (2008). The prevention of progression of arterial disease and diabetes (POPADAD) trial: factorial randomised placebo controlled trial of aspirin and antioxidants in patients with diabetes and asymptomatic peripheral arterial disease. *Bmj*, 337, a1840. doi: 10.1136/bmj.a1840

Bjelakovic, G., Nikolova, D., & Gluud, C. (2013). Antioxidant supplements to prevent mortality. *JAMA*, 310(11), 1178–1179. doi: 10.1001/jama.2013.277028

Bolland, M. J., Grey, A., Avenell, A., Gamble, G. D., & Reid, I. R. (2011). Calcium supplements with or without vitamin D and risk of cardiovascular events: reanalysis of the Women's Health Initiative limited access dataset and meta-analysis. *Bmj*, 342(1), d2040–d2040. doi: 10.1136/bmj.d2040

Bounhoure, J. P., Galinier, M., Didier, A., & Leophonte, P. (2005). Sleep apnea syndromes and cardiovascular disease. *Bull Acad Natl Med*, 189(3), 445–459; discussion 460–444.

Bravata, D. M., Ho, S.-Y., Meehan, T. P., Brass, L. M., & Concato, J. (2007). Readmission and Death After Hospitalization for Acute Ischemic Stroke: 5-Year Follow-Up in the Medicare Population. *Stroke*, 38(6), 1899–1904. doi: 10.1161/strokeaha.106.481465

Brown, A. L., Zhu, X., Rong, S., Shewale, S., Seo, J., Boudyguina, E., . . . Parks, J. S. (2012). Omega-3 fatty acids ameliorate atherosclerosis by favorably altering monocyte subsets and limiting monocyte recruitment to aortic lesions. *Arterioscler Thromb Vasc Biol*, 32(9), 2122–2130. doi: 10.1161/atvbaha.112.253435

Brown, B. G., Zhao, X.-Q., Chait, A., Fisher, L. D., Cheung, M. C., Morse, J. S., . . . Albers, J. J. (2001). Simvastatin and Niacin, Antioxidant Vitamins, or the Combination for the Prevention of Coronary Disease. *N Engl J Med*, 345(22), 1583–1592. doi: 10.1056/NEJMoa011090

Buijsse, B., Weikert, C., Drogan, D., Bergmann, M., & Boeing, H. (2010). Chocolate consumption in relation to blood pressure and risk of cardiovascular disease in German adults. *Eur Heart J*, 31(13), 1616–1623. doi: 10.1093/eurheartj/ehq068

Buitrago-Lopez, A., Sanderson, J., Johnson, L., Warnakula, S., Wood, A., Di Angelantonio, E., & Franco, O. H. (2011). Chocolate consumption and cardiometabolic disorders: systematic review and meta-analysis. *Bmj*, 343, d4488. doi: 10.1136/bmj.d4488

Buxton, O. M., Cain, S. W., O'Connor, S. P., Porter, J. H., Duffy, J. F., Wang, W., . . . Shea, S. A. (2012). Adverse metabolic consequences in humans of prolonged sleep restriction combined with circadian disruption. *Sci Transl Med*, 4(129), 129ra143. doi: 10.1126/scitranslmed.3003200

Cappuccio, F. P., D'Elia, L., Strazzullo, P., & Miller, M. A. (2010). Quantity and Quality of Sleep and Incidence of Type 2 Diabetes: A systematic review and meta-analysis. *Diabetes Care*, 33(2), 414–420. doi: 10.2337/dc09-1124

Caso, G., Kelly, P., McNurlan, M. A., & Lawson, W. E. (2007). Effect of coenzyme q10 on myopathic symptoms in patients treated with statins. *Am J Cardiol*, 99(10), 1409–1412. doi: 10.1016/j.amjcard.2006.12.063

Chlan L. L., W. C. R. H. A., et al. (2013). Effects of patient-directed music intervention on anxiety and sedative exposure in critically ill patients receiving mechanical ventilatory support: A randomized clinical trial. *JAMA*, 1–10. doi: 10.1001/jama.2013.5670

Cho, M. Y., Min, E. S., Hur, M. H., & Lee, M. S. (2013). Effects of aromatherapy on the anxiety, vital signs, and sleep quality of percutaneous coronary intervention patients in intensive care units. *Evid Based Complement Alternat Med*, 2013, 381381. doi: http://dx.doi.org/10.1155/2013/381381

Choi, A. M., Ryter, S. W., & Levine, B. (2013). Autophagy in human health and disease. *N Engl J Med*, 368(7), 651–662. doi: 10.1056/NEJMra1205406

Chowdhury, R., Stevens, S., Gorman, D., Pan, A., Warnakula, S., Chowdhury, S., . . . Franco, O. H. (2012). Association between fish consumption, long chain omega 3 fatty acids, and risk of cerebrovascular disease: systematic review and meta-analysis. *Bmj*, 345(oct30 3), e6698–e6698. doi: 10.1136/bmj.e6698

Ciubotaru, I., Lee, Y.-S., & Wander, R. C. (2003). Dietary fish oil decreases C-reactive protein, interleukin-6, and triacylglycerol to HDL-cholesterol ratio in postmenopausal women on HRT. *The Journal of Nutritional Biochemistry*, 14(9), 513–521. doi: http://dx.doi.org/10.1016/S0955-2863(03)00101-3

Crane, F. L. (2001). Biochemical functions of coenzyme Q10. *J Am Coll Nutr*, 20(6), 591–598.

Crowe, F. L., Roddam, A. W., Key, T. J., Appleby, P. N., Overvad, K., Jakobsen, M. U., . . . Collaborators, N.-H. S. (2011). Fruit and vegetable intake and mortality from ischaemic heart disease: results from the European Prospective Investigation into Cancer and Nutrition (EPIC)-Heart study. *Eur Heart J*. doi: 10.1093/eurheartj/ehq465

Davidson, M. H. (2008). Niacin use and cutaneous flushing: mechanisms and strategies for prevention. *Am J Cardiol*, 101(8A), 14B–19B. doi: 10.1016/j.amjcard.2008.02.028

Davidson, M. H., Stein, E. A., Bays, H. E., Maki, K. C., Doyle, R. T., Shalwitz, R. A., . . . Ginsberg, H. N. (2007). Efficacy and tolerability of adding prescription Omega-3 fatty acids 4 g/d to Simvastatin 40 mg/d in hypertriglyceridemic patients: An 8-week, randomized, double-blind, placebo-controlled study. *Clinical Therapeutics*, 29(7), 1354–1367. doi: http://dx.doi.org/10.1016/j.clinthera.2007.07.018

Davis, M. M., Taubert, K., Benin, A. L., Brown, D. W., Mensah, G. A., Baddour, L. M., . . . Krumholz, H. M. (2006). Influenza Vaccination as Secondary Prevention for Cardiovascular Disease: A Science Advisory From the American Heart Association/American College of Cardiology: Endorsed by the American Association of Cardiovascular and Pulmonary Rehabilitation, the American Association of Critical Care Nurses, the American Association of Heart Failure Nurses, the American Diabetes Association, the Association of Black Cardiologists, Inc., the Heart Failure Society of America, and the Preventive Cardiovascular Nurses Association: The American Academy of Nurse Practitioners supports the recommendations of this scientific advisory: This science advisory is consistent with the recommendations of the Centers for Disease Control and Prevention and the Advisory Committee on Immunization Practices. *Circulation*, 114(14), 1549–1553. doi: 10.1161/circulationaha.106.178242

Davis, P. A., & Yokoyama, W. (2011). Cinnamon intake lowers fasting blood glucose: meta-analysis. *J Med Food*, 14(9), 884–889. doi: 10.1089/jmf.2010.0180

de Koning, L., Malik, V. S., Kellogg, M. D., Rimm, E. B., Willett, W. C., & Hu, F. B. (2012). Sweetened Beverage Consumption, Incident Coronary Heart Disease, and Biomarkers of Risk in Men. *Circulation*, 125(14), 1735–1741. doi: 10.1161/circulationaha.111.067017

Deka, A., & Vita, J. A. (2011). Tea and cardiovascular disease. *Pharmacol Res*, 64(2), 136–145. doi: 10.1016/j.phrs.2011.03.009

Dhingra, R., Sullivan, L., Jacques, P. F., Wang, T. J., Fox, C. S., Meigs, J. B., . . . Vasan, R. S. (2007). Soft Drink Consumption and Risk of Developing Cardiometabolic Risk Factors and the Metabolic Syndrome in Middle-Aged Adults in the Community. *Circulation*, 116(5), 480–488. doi: 10.1161/circulationaha.107.689935

Durup, D., Jørgensen, H. L., Christensen, J., Schwarz, P., Heegaard, A. M., & Lind, B. (2012). A Reverse J-Shaped Association of All-Cause Mortality with Serum 25-Hydroxyvitamin D in General Practice, the CopD Study. *Journal of Clinical Endocrinology & Metabolism*. doi: 10.1210/jc.2012-1176

Elam, M. B., Hunninghake, D. B., Davis, K. B., et al. (2000). Effect of niacin on lipid and lipoprotein levels and glycemic control in patients with diabetes and peripheral arterial disease: The admit study: a randomized trial. *JAMA*, 284(10), 1263–1270. doi: 10.1001/jama.284.10.1263

Emmerich, J. (2008). FARIVE study—case-control study suggests for the first time that vaccination against influenza may reduce the risk of venous thromboembolism (VTE). American Heart Association 2008 Scientific Sessions.

Faught, B. E., Flouris, A. D., & Cairney, J. (2009). Epidemiological evidence associating secondhand smoke exposure with cardiovascular disease. *Inflamm Allergy Drug Targets*, 8(5), 321–327.

Fiore, M., Jaén, C. R., Baker, T. B., et al. A clinical practice guideline for treating tobacco use and dependence: 2008 update. A U.S. Public Health Service report. (2008). *Am J Prev Med*, 35(2), 158–176. doi: 10.1016/j.amepre.2008.04.009

Flammer, A. J., Hermann, F., Sudano, I., Spieker, L., Hermann, M., Cooper, K. A., . . . Corti, R. (2007). Dark Chocolate Improves Coronary Vasomotion and Reduces Platelet Reactivity. *Circulation*, 116(21), 2376–2382. doi: 10.1161/circulationaha.107.713867

Fry, W. F., Jr. (1992). The physiologic effects of humor, mirth, and laughter. *JAMA*, 267(13), 1857–1858.

Galluzzi, L., & Kroemer, G. (2012). Autophagy mediates the metabolic benefits of endurance training. *Circ Res*, 110(10), 1276–1278. doi: 10.1161/RES.0b013e318259e70b

Galvano, F., Li Volti, G., Malaguarnera, M., Avitabile, T., Antic, T., Vacante, M., & Malaguarnera, M. (2009). Effects of simvastatin and carnitine versus simvastatin on lipoprotein(a) and apoprotein(a) in type 2 diabetes mellitus. *Expert Opin Pharmacother*, 10(12), 1875–1882. doi: 10.1517/14656560903081745

Gardener, H., Rundek, T., Markert, M., Wright, C. B., Elkind, M. S., & Sacco, R. L. (2012). Diet soft drink consumption is associated with an increased risk of vascular events in the Northern Manhattan Study. *J Gen Intern Med*, 27(9), 1120–1126. doi: 10.1007/s11606-011-1968-2

Ghirlanda, G., Oradei, A., Manto, A., Lippa, S., Uccioli, L., Caputo, S., . . . Littarru, G. P. (1993). Evidence of plasma CoQ10-lowering effect by HMG-CoA reductase inhibitors: a double-blind, placebo-controlled study. *J Clin Pharmacol*, 33(3), 226–229.

Gilden, D. (2011). Efficacy of live zoster vaccine in preventing zoster and postherpetic neuralgia. *J Intern Med*, 269(5), 496–506. doi: 10.1111/j.1365-2796.2011.02359.x

Grassi, D., Desideri, G., Necozione, S., Ruggieri, F., Blumberg, J. B., Stornello, M., & Ferri, C. (2012). Protective effects of flavanol-rich dark chocolate on endothelial function and wave reflection during acute hyperglycemia. *Hypertension*, 60(3), 827–832. doi: 10.1161/HYPERTENSIONAHA.112.193995

Grundy, S. M., Vega, G., McGovern, M. E., et al. (2002). Efficacy, safety, and tolerability of once-daily niacin for the treatment of dyslipidemia associated with type 2 diabetes: Results of the assessment of diabetes control and evaluation of the efficacy of niaspan trial. *Arch Intern Med*, 162(14), 1568–1576. doi: 10.1001/archinte.162.14.1568

Guyton, J. R., & Simmons, P. D. (2009). Flushing and other dermatologic adverse events associated with extended-release niacin therapy. *J Clin Lipidol*, 3(2), 101–108. doi: 10.1016/j.jacl.2009.02.003

Hamilton, S. J., Chew, G. T., & Watts, G. F. (2009). Coenzyme Q10 improves endothelial dysfunction in statin-treated type 2 diabetic patients. *Diabetes Care*, 32(5), 810–812. doi: 10.2337/dc08-1736

Helmrich, S. P., Ragland, D. R., Leung, R. W., & Paffenbarger, R. S. (1991). Physical Activity and Reduced Occurrence of Non-Insulin-Dependent Diabetes Mellitus. *N Engl J Med*, 325(3), 147–152. doi: 10.1056/NEJM199107183250302

Hodgson, J. M., Watts, G. F., Playford, D. A., Burke, V., & Croft, K. D. (2002). Coenzyme Q10 improves blood pressure and glycaemic control: a controlled trial in subjects with type 2 diabetes. *Eur J Clin Nutr,* 56(11), 1137–1142. doi: 10.1038/sj.ejcn.1601464

Hossein-Nezhad, A., & Holick, M. F. (2013). Vitamin d for health: a global perspective. *Mayo Clin Proc,* 88(7), 720–755. doi: 10.1016/j.mayocp.2013.05.011

Iervasi, G., Molinaro, S., Landi, P., Taddei, M. C., Galli, E., Mariani, F., . . . Pingitore, A. (2007). Association between increased mortality and mild thyroid dysfunction in cardiac patients. *Arch Intern Med,* 167(14), 1526–1532. doi: 10.1001/archinte.167.14.1526

Javaheri, S., Parker, T. J., Wexler, L., Michaels, S. E., Stanberry, E., Nishyama, H., & Roselle, G. A. (1995). Occult sleep-disordered breathing in stable congestive heart failure. *Ann Intern Med,* 122(7), 487–492.

Jha, P., Ramasundarahettige, C., Landsman, V., Rostron, B., Thun, M., Anderson, R. N., . . . Peto, R. (2013). 21st-century hazards of smoking and benefits of cessation in the United States. *N Engl J Med,* 368(4), 341–350. doi: 10.1056/NEJMsa1211128

Judd, S. E., & Tangpricha, V. (2009). Vitamin D deficiency and risk for cardiovascular disease. *Am J Med Sci,* 338(1), 40–44. doi: 10.1097/MAJ.0b013e3181aaee91

Kang, J.-H., Ho, J.-D., Chen, Y.-H., & Lin, H.-C. (2009). Increased Risk of Stroke After a Herpes Zoster Attack: A Population-Based Follow-Up Study. *Stroke,* 40(11), 3443–3448. doi: 10.1161/strokeaha.109.562017

Kasasbeh, E., Chi, D. S., & Krishnaswamy, G. (2006). Inflammatory aspects of sleep apnea and their cardiovascular consequences. *South Med J,* 99(1), 58–67; quiz 68-59, 81.

Kayaniyil, S., Vieth, R., Retnakaran, R., Knight, J. A., Qi, Y., Gerstein, H. C., . . . Hanley, A. J. (2010). Association of Vitamin D With Insulin Resistance and ßCell Dysfunction in Subjects at Risk for Type 2 Diabetes. *Diabetes Care,* 33(6), 1379–1381. doi: 10.2337/dc09-2321

Kenfield, S. A., Stampfer, M. J., Rosner, B. A., & Colditz, G. A. (2008). Smoking and smoking cessation in relation to mortality in women. *JAMA,* 299(17), 2037–2047. doi: 10.1001/jama.299.17.2037

Khan, A., Safdar, M., Ali Khan, M. M., Khattak, K. N., & Anderson, R. A. (2003). Cinnamon Improves Glucose and Lipids of People With Type 2 Diabetes. *Diabetes Care,* 26(12), 3215–3218. doi: 10.2337/diacare.26.12.3215

Koeth, R. A., Wang, Z., Levison, B. S., Buffa, J. A., Org, E., Sheehy, B. T., . . . Hazen, S. L. (2013). Intestinal microbiota metabolism of l-carnitine, a nutrient in red meat, promotes atherosclerosis. *Nat Med,* 19(5), 576–585. doi: 10.1038/nm.3145

Kojima, G., Bell, C., Abbott, R. D., Launer, L., Chen, R., Motonaga, H., . . . Masaki, K. (2012). Low dietary vitamin D predicts 34-year incident stroke: the Honolulu Heart Program. *Stroke,* 43(8), 2163–2167. doi: 10.1161/STROKEAHA.112.651752

Kokubo, Y., Iso, H., Saito, I., Yamagishi, K., Yatsuya, H., Ishihara, J., . . . Tsugane, S. (2013). The impact of green tea and coffee consumption on the reduced risk of stroke incidence in Japanese population: the Japan public health center-based study cohort. *Stroke,* 44(5), 1369–1374. doi: 10.1161/STROKEAHA.111.677500

Lamontagne, F., Garant, M.-P., Carvalho, J.-C., Lanthier, L., Smieja, M., & Pilon, D. (2008). Pneumococcal vaccination and risk of myocardial infarction. *Canadian Medical Association Journal,* 179(8), 773–777. doi: 10.1503/cmaj.070221

Larsson, S. C., Virtamo, J., & Wolk, A. (2011). Chocolate Consumption and Risk of Stroke in Women. *J Am Coll Cardiol,* 58(17), 1828–1829. doi: http://dx.doi.org/10.1016/j.jacc.2011.07.023

Lavie, C. J., Lee, J. H., & Milani, R. V. (2011). Vitamin D and Cardiovascular Disease: Will It Live Up to its Hype? *J Am Coll Cardiol,* 58(15), 1547–1556. doi: http://dx.doi.org/10.1016/j.jacc.2011.07.008

Levine, G. N., Steinke, E. E., Bakaeen, F. G., Bozkurt, B., Cheitlin, M. D., Conti, J. B., . . . Outcomes, R. (2012). Sexual activity and cardiovascular disease: a scientific statement from the American Heart Association. *Circulation,* 125(8), 1058–1072. doi: 10.1161/CIR.0b013e3182447787

Li, K., Kaaks, R., Linseisen, J., & Rohrmann, S. (2012). Associations of dietary calcium intake and calcium supplementation with myocardial infarction and stroke risk and overall cardiovascular mortality in the Heidelberg cohort of the European Prospective Investigation into Cancer and Nutrition study (EPIC-Heidelberg). *Heart,* 98(12), 920–925. doi: 10.1136/heartjnl-2011-301345

Lin, H. C., Chien, C. W., & Ho, J. D. (2010). Herpes zoster ophthalmicus and the risk of stroke: a population-based follow-up study. *Neurology,* 74(10), 792–797. doi: 10.1212/WNL.0b013e3181d31e5c

Liu, J., Sui, X., Lavie, C. J., Hebert, J. R., Earnest, C. P., Zhang, J., & Blair, S. N. Association of Coffee Consumption With All-Cause and Cardiovascular Disease Mortality. *Mayo Clinic Proceedings(0).* doi: http://dx.doi.org/10.1016/j.mayocp.2013.06.020

Lopez-Garcia, E., Rodriguez-Artalejo, F., Rexrode, K. M., Logroscino, G., Hu, F. B., & van Dam, R. M. (2009). Coffee Consumption and Risk of Stroke in Women. *Circulation,* 119(8), 1116–1123. doi: 10.1161/circulationaha.108.826164

Mabuchi, H., Nohara, A., Kobayashi, J., Kawashiri, M. A., Katsuda, S., Inazu, A., . . . Hokuriku Lipid Research, G. (2007). Effects of CoQ10 supplementation on plasma lipoprotein lipid, CoQ10 and liver and muscle enzyme levels in hypercholesterolemic patients treated with atorvastatin: a randomized double-blind study. *Atherosclerosis,* 195(2), e182–189. doi: 10.1016/j.atherosclerosis.2007.06.010

Maki, K. C., Bays, H. E., Dicklin, M. R., Johnson, S. L., & Shabbout, M. (2011). Effects of prescription omega-3-acid ethyl esters, coadministered with atorvastatin, on circulating levels of lipoprotein particles, apolipoprotein CIII, and lipoprotein-associated phospholipase A2 mass in men and women with mixed dyslipidemia. *J Clin Lipidol,* 5(6), 483–492. doi: http://dx.doi.org/10.1016/j.jacl.2011.09.001

Marchioli, R., Barzi, F., Bomba, E., Chieffo, C., Di Gregorio, D., Di Mascio, R., . . . Investigators, o. b. o. t. G.-P. (2002). Early Protection Against Sudden Death by n-3 Polyunsaturated Fatty Acids After Myocardial Infarction: Time-Course Analysis of the Results of the Gruppo Italiano per lo Studio della Sopravvivenza nell'Infarto Miocardico (GISSI)-Prevenzione. *Circulation,* 105(16), 1897–1903. doi: 10.1161/01.cir.0000014682.14181.f2

Marik, P. E., & Varon, J. (2009). Omega-3 Dietary Supplements and the Risk of Cardiovascular Events: A Systematic Review. *Clinical Cardiology,* 32(7), 365–372. doi: 10.1002/clc.20604

Martínez-García, M.-A., Campos-Rodríguez, F., Catalán-Serra, P., Soler-Cataluña, J.-J., Almeida-Gonzalez, C., De la Cruz Morón, I., . . . Montserrat, J.-M. (2012). Cardiovascular Mortality in Obstructive Sleep Apnea in the Elderly: Role of Long-Term Continuous Positive Airway Pressure Treatment. *American Journal of Respiratory and Critical Care Medicine,* 186(9), 909–916. doi: 10.1164/rccm.201203-0448OC

Masaki, T. (2012). Sleep/wake cycle, circadian disruption and the development of obesity. *Nihon Rinsho,* 70(7), 1183–1187.

Mason, C. M., & Doneen, A. L. (2012). Niacin—a critical component to the management of atherosclerosis: contemporary management of dyslipidemia to prevent, reduce, or reverse atherosclerotic cardiovascular disease. *J Cardiovasc Nurs,* 27(4), 303–316. doi: 10.1097/JCN.0b013e31821bf93f

Matheson, E. M., Mainous, A. G., Everett, C. J., & King, D. E. (2011). Tea and Coffee Consumption and MRSA Nasal Carriage. *The Annals of Family Medicine,* 9(4), 299–304. doi: 10.1370/afm.1262

Max, W., Sung, H. Y., & Shi, Y. (2012). Deaths from secondhand smoke exposure in the United States: economic implications. *Am J Public Health,* 102(11), 2173–2180. doi: 10.2105/ajph.2012.300805

McKay, D. L., Chen, C.-Y. O., Saltzman, E., & Blumberg, J. B. (2010). Hibiscus Sabdariffa L. Tea (Tisane) Lowers Blood Pressure in Prehypertensive and Mildly Hypertensive Adults. *J Nutr,* 140(2), 298–303. doi: 10.3945/jn.109.115097

Mercer, J. R., Gray, K., Figg, N., Kumar, S., & Bennett, M. R. (2012). The Methyl Xanthine Caffeine Inhibits DNA Damage Signaling and Reactive Species and Reduces Atherosclerosis in ApoE$^{-/-}$ Mice. *Arterioscler Thromb Vasc Bio,* 32(10), 2461–2467. doi: 10.1161/atvbaha.112.251322

Michaelsson, K., Melhus, H., Warensjo Lemming, E., Wolk, A., & Byberg, L. (2013). Long term calcium intake and rates of all cause and cardiovascular mortality: community based prospective longitudinal cohort study. *Bmj,* 346(feb12 4), f228–f228. doi: 10.1136/bmj.f228

Miller, M., Beach, V., Mangano, C., Vogel, R. A. (2008, November 11). Positive Emotions and the Endothelium: Docs Joyful Music Improve Vascular Health?" Presented at the American Heart Association Scientific Sessions.

Mora-Ripoll, R. (2010). The therapeutic value of laughter in medicine. *Altern Ther Health Med,* 16(6), 56–64.

_____. (2011). Potential health benefits of simulated laughter: a narrative review of the literature and recommendations for future research. *Complement Ther Med,* 19(3), 170–177. doi: 10.1016/j.ctim.2011.05.003

Mora, S., Cook, N., Buring, J. E., Ridker, P. M., & Lee, I. M. (2007). Physical activity and reduced risk of cardiovascular events: potential mediating mechanisms. *Circulation,* 116(19), 2110–2118. doi: 10.1161/CIRCULATIONAHA.107.729939

Mozaffarian, D., Lemaitre, R. N., King, I. B., Song, X., Spiegelman, D., Sacks, F. M., . . . Siscovick, D. S. (2011). Circulating long-chain omega-3 fatty acids and incidence of congestive heart failure in older adults: the cardiovascular health study: a cohort study. *Ann Intern Med,* 155(3), 160–170. doi: 10.7326/0003-4819-155-3-201108020-00006

Musher, D. M., Rueda, A. M., Kaka, A. S., & Mapara, S. M. (2007). The Association between Pneumococcal Pneumonia and Acute Cardiac Events. *Clinical Infectious Diseases,* 45(2), 158–165. doi: 10.1086/518849

O'Keefe, J. H., Bhatti, S. K., Patil, H. R., Dinicolantonio, J. J., Lucan, S. C., & Lavie, C. J. (2013). Effects of Habitual Coffee Consumption on Cardiometabolic Disease, Cardiovascular Health, and All-cause Mortality. *J Am Coll Cardiol.* doi: 10.1016/j.jacc.2013.06.035

Oude Griep, L. M., Verschuren, W. M., Kromhout, D., Ocke, M. C., & Geleijnse, J. M. (2011). Colors of fruit and vegetables and 10-year incidence of stroke. *Stroke,* 42(11), 3190–3195. doi: 10.1161/STROKEAHA.110.611152

Park, Y., Subar, A. F., Hollenbeck, A., & Schatzkin, A. (2011). Dietary fiber intake and mortality in the nih-aarp diet and health study. *Arch Intern Med,* 171(12), 1061–1068. doi: 10.1001/archinternmed.2011.18

Planer, D., Lev, I., Elitzur, Y., Sharon, N., Ouzan, E., Pugatsch, T., . . . Lotan, C. (2011). Bupropion for smoking cessation in patients with acute coronary syndrome. *Arch Intern Med, 171*(12), 1055–1060. doi: 10.1001/archinternmed.2011.72

Rajpathak, S., Rimm, E. B., Li, T., Morris, J. S., Stampfer, M. J., Willett, W. C., & Hu, F. B. (2004). Lower toenail chromium in men with diabetes and cardiovascular disease compared with healthy men. *Diabetes Care, 27*(9), 2211–2216.

Rodondi, N., den Elzen, W. J., Bauer, D. C., et al. (2010). Subclinical hypothyroidism and the risk of coronary heart disease and mortality. *JAMA, 304*(12), 1365–1374. doi: 10.1001/jama.2010.1361

Rubinsztein, D. C., Marino, G., & Kroemer, G. (2011). Autophagy and aging. *Cell, 146*(5), 682–695. doi: 10.1016/j.cell.2011.07.030

Sawada, S. S., Lee, I.-M., Naito, H., Noguchi, J., Tsukamoto, K., Muto, T., . . . Blair, S. N. (2010). Long-Term Trends in Cardiorespiratory Fitness and the Incidence of Type 2 Diabetes. *Diabetes Care, 33*(6), 1353–1357. doi: 10.2337/dc09-1654

Sesso, H. D., Buring, J. E., Christen, W. G., et al. (2008). Vitamins e and c in the prevention of cardiovascular disease in men: The physicians' health study ii randomized controlled trial. *JAMA, 300*(18), 2123–2133. doi: 10.1001/jama.2008.600

Sesso, H. D., Christen, W. G., Bubes, V., et al. (2012). Multivitamins in the prevention of cardiovascular disease in men: The physicians' health study ii randomized controlled trial. *JAMA, 308*(17), 1751–1760. doi: 10.1001/jama.2012.14805

Smith, B., Wingard, D. L., Smith, T. C., Kritz-Silverstein, D., & Barrett-Connor, E. (2006). Does Coffee Consumption Reduce the Risk of Type 2 Diabetes in Individuals With Impaired Glucose? *Diabetes Care, 29*(11), 2385–2390. doi: 10.2337/dc06-1084

Stead, L. F., Perera, R., Bullen, C., Mant, D., Hartmann-Boyce, J., Cahill, K., & Lancaster, T. (2012). Nicotine replacement therapy for smoking cessation. *Cochrane Database Syst Rev, 11*, Cd000146. doi: 10.1002/14651858.CD000146.pub4

Sugawara, J., Tarumi, T., & Tanaka, H. (2010). Effect of mirthful laughter on vascular function. *Am J Cardiol, 106*(6), 856–859. doi: 10.1016/j.amjcard.2010.05.011

Suraj-Narayan, G., & Surajnarayan, S. (2011). Biopsychosocial impacts of laughter yoga and therapy on stroke survivors. *Journal of Critical Care, 26*(5), e37–e38.

Tahiri, M., Mottillo, S., Joseph, L., Pilote, L., & Eisenberg, M. J. (2012). Alternative smoking cessation aids: a meta-analysis of randomized controlled trials. *Am J Med, 125*(6), 576–584. doi: 10.1016/j.amjmed.2011.09.028

Tang, W. H., Wang, Z., Levison, B. S., Koeth, R. A., Britt, E. B., Fu, X., . . . Hazen, S. L. (2013). Intestinal microbial metabolism of phosphatidylcholine and cardiovascular risk. *N Engl J Med, 368*(17), 1575–1584. doi: 10.1056/NEJMoa1109400

Taubert, D., Roesen, R., Lehmann, C., Jung, N., & Schömig, E. (2007). Effects of low habitual cocoa intake on blood pressure and bioactive nitric oxide: A randomized controlled trial. *JAMA, 298*(1), 49–60. doi: 10.1001/jama.298.1.49

Teo, K. K., Ounpuu, S., Hawken, S., Pandey, M. R., Valentin, V., Hunt, D., . . . Yusuf, S. (2006). Tobacco use and risk of myocardial infarction in 52 countries in the INTER-HEART study: a case-control study. *The Lancet, 368*(9536), 647–658. doi: http://dx.doi.org/10.1016/S0140-6736(06)69249-0

Threapleton, D. E., Greenwood, D. C., Evans, C. E. L., Cleghorn, C. L., Nykjaer, C., Woodhead, C., . . . Burley, V. J. (2013). Dietary Fiber Intake and Risk of First Stroke: A Systematic Review and Meta-Analysis. *Stroke, 44*(5), 1360–1368. doi: 10.1161/strokeaha.111.000151

Thun, M. J., Carter, B. D., Feskanich, D., Freedman, N. D., Prentice, R., Lopez, A. D., . . . Gapstur, S. M. (2013). 50-year trends in smoking-related mortality in the United States. *N Engl J Med,* 368(4), 351–364. doi: 10.1056/NEJMsa1211127

Tjønna, A. E., Lee, S. J., Rognmo, Ø., Stølen, T. O., Bye, A., Haram, P. M., . . . Wisløff, U. (2008). Aerobic Interval Training Versus Continuous Moderate Exercise as a Treatment for the Metabolic Syndrome: A Pilot Study. *Circulation,* 118(4), 346–354. doi: 10.1161/circulationaha.108.772822

Trappe, H. J. (2010). The effects of music on the cardiovascular system and cardiovascular health. *Heart,* 96(23), 1868–1871. doi: 10.1136/hrt.2010.209858

The Tobacco, U., Dependence Clinical Practice Guideline, P., Staff, & Consortium, R. (2000). A clinical practice guideline for treating tobacco use and dependence: A us public health service report. *JAMA,* 283(24), 3244–3254. doi: 10.1001/jama.283.24.3244

Udell, J. A., Zawi, R., Bhatt, D. L., et al. (2013). Association between influenza vaccination and cardiovascular outcomes in high-risk patients: A meta-analysis. *JAMA,* 310(16), 1711–1720. doi: 10.1001/jama.2013.279206

Vaccari, C. S., Hammoud, R. A., Nagamia, S. H., Ramasamy, K., Dollar, A. L., & Khan, B. V. (2007). Revisiting niacin: reviewing the evidence. *J Clin Lipidol,* 1(4), 248–255. doi: 10.1016/j.jacl.2007.07.008

Vila-Corcoles, A., Ochoa-Gondar, O., Rodriguez-Blanco, T., Gutierrez-Perez, A., Vila-Rovira, A., Gomez, F., . . . Group, E. S. (2012). Clinical effectiveness of pneumococcal vaccination against acute myocardial infarction and stroke in people over 60 years: the CAPAMIS study, one-year follow-up. *BMC Public Health,* 12, 222. doi: 10.1186/1471-2458-12-222

Wang, J. C., & Bennett, M. (2012). Aging and atherosclerosis: mechanisms, functional consequences, and potential therapeutics for cellular senescence. *Circ Res,* 111(2), 245–259. doi: 10.1161/CIRCRESAHA.111.261388

Wang, L., Song, Y., Manson, J. E., Pilz, S., März, W., Michaëlsson, K., . . . Sesso, H. D. (2012). Circulating 25-Hydroxy-Vitamin D and Risk of Cardiovascular Disease: A Meta-Analysis of Prospective Studies. *Circ Cardiovasc Qual Outcomes,* 5(6), 819–829. doi: 10.1161/circoutcomes.112.967604

Wang, Z., Klipfell, E., Bennett, B. J., Koeth, R., Levison, B. S., Dugar, B., . . . Hazen, S. L. (2011). Gut flora metabolism of phosphatidylcholine promotes cardiovascular disease. *Nature,* 472(7341), 57–63. doi: 10.1038/nature09922

Willi, C., Bodenmann, P., Ghali, W. A., Faris, P. D., & Cornuz, J. (2007). Active smoking and the risk of type 2 diabetes: A systematic review and meta-analysis. *JAMA,* 298(22), 2654–2664. doi: 10.1001/jama.298.22.2654

Wolpowitz, D., & Gilchrest, B. A. (2006). The vitamin D questions: How much do you need and how should you get it? *Journal of the American Academy of Dermatology,* 54(2), 301–317. doi: http://dx.doi.org/10.1016/j.jaad.2005.11.1057

Wu, J. H., Lemaitre, R. N., King, I. B., Song, X., Sacks, F. M., Rimm, E. B., . . . Mozaffarian, D. (2012). Association of plasma phospholipid long-chain omega-3 fatty acids with incident atrial fibrillation in older adults: the cardiovascular health study. *Circulation,* 125(9), 1084–1093. doi: 10.1161/circulationaha.111.062653

Xia, S., Xu, S., Zhang, X., Zhong, F., & Wang, Z. (2009). Nanoliposomes Mediate Coenzyme Q10 Transport and Accumulation across Human Intestinal Caco-2 Cell Monolayer. *Journal of Agricultural and Food Chemistry,* 57(17), 7989–7996. doi: 10.1021/jf901068f

Yaemsiri, S., Sen, S., Tinker, L. F., Robinson, W. R., Evans, R. W., Rosamond, W., . . . He, K. (2013). Serum Fatty Acids and Incidence of Ischemic Stroke Among Postmenopausal Women. *Stroke.* doi: 10.1161/strokeaha.111.000834

Yokoyama, M., Origasa, H., Matsuzaki, M., Matsuzawa, Y., Saito, Y., Ishikawa, Y., . . . Shirato, K. (2007). Effects of eicosapentaenoic acid on major coronary events in hypercholesterol-aemic patients (JELIS): a randomised open-label, blinded endpoint analysis. *The Lancet,* 369(9567), 1090–1098. doi: http://dx.doi.org/10.1016/S0140-6736(07)60527-3

Zampelas, A., Panagiotakos, D. B., Pitsavos, C., Das, U. N., Chrysohoou, C., Skoumas, Y., & Stefanadis, C. (2005). Fish consumption among healthy adults is associated with decreased levels of inflammatory markers related to cardiovascular disease: the ATTICA study. *J Am Coll Cardiol,* 46(1), 120–124. doi: 10.1016/j.jacc.2005.03.048

Zomer, E., Owen, A., Magliano, D. J., Liew, D., & Reid, C. M. (2012). The effectiveness and cost effectiveness of dark chocolate consumption as prevention therapy in people at high risk of cardiovascular disease: best case scenario analysis using a Markov model. *Bmj,* 344, e3657. doi: 10.1136/bmj.e3657

Chapter Fourteen

The ACCORD Study Group. Effects of Combination Lipid Therapy in Type 2 Diabetes Mellitus. (2010). *N Engl J Med,* 362(17), 1563–1574.

Afilalo, J., Majdan, A. A., & Eisenberg, M. J. (2007). Intensive statin therapy in acute coronary syndromes and stable coronary heart disease: a comparative meta-analysis of randomised controlled trials. *Heart,* 93(8), 914–921. doi: 10.1136/hrt.2006.112508

Ahimastos, A. A., Walker, P. J., Askew, C., et al. (2013). Effect of ramipril on walking times and quality of life among patients with peripheral artery disease and intermittent claudication: A randomized controlled trial. *JAMA,* 309(5), 453–460. doi: 10.1001/jama.2012.216237

Antoniou, T., Gomes, T., Juurlink, D. N., Loutfy, M. R., Glazier, R. H., & Mamdani, M. M. (2010). Trimethoprim-sulfamethoxazole–induced hyperkalemia in patients receiving inhibitors of the renin-angiotensin system: A population-based study. *Arch Intern Med,* 170(12), 1045–1049. doi: 10.1001/archinternmed.2010.142

Baker, W. L., Coleman, C. I., Kluger, J., Reinhart, K. M., Talati, R., Quercia, R., . . . White, C. M. (2009). Systematic review: comparative effectiveness of angiotensin-converting enzyme inhibitors or angiotensin II-receptor blockers for ischemic heart disease. *Ann Intern Med,* 151(12), 861–871. doi: 10.7326/0003-4819-151-12-200912150-00162

Bangalore, S., Kumar, S., Wetterslev, J., & Messerli, F. H. (2011). Angiotensin receptor blockers and risk of myocardial infarction: meta-analyses and trial sequential analyses of 147,020 patients from randomised trials. *Bmj,* 342, d2234. doi: 10.1136/bmj.d2234

Barbalat, Y., Dombrovskiy, V. Y., & Weiss, R. E. (2012). Association between pioglitazone and urothelial bladder cancer. *Urology,* 80(1), 1–4. doi: 10.1016/j.urology.2012.03.032

Berger, J. S., Roncaglioni, M. C., Avanzini, F., Pangrazzi, I., Tognoni, G., & Brown, D. L. (2006). Aspirin for the primary prevention of cardiovascular events in women and men: A sex-specific meta-analysis of randomized controlled trials. *JAMA,* 295(3), 306–313. doi: 10.1001/jama.295.3.306

Bloch, M., Prock, A., Paonessa, F., Benz, V., Bahr, I. N., Herbst, L., . . . Kintscher, U. (2012). High-mobility group A1 protein: a new coregulator of peroxisome proliferator-activated receptor-gamma-mediated transrepression in the vasculature. *Circ Res,* 110(3), 394–405. doi: 10.1161/CIRCRESAHA.111.253658

Boden, W. E., O'Rourke, R. A., Teo, K. K., Hartigan, P. M., Maron, D. J., Kostuk, W. J., . . . Weintraub, W. S. (2007). Optimal Medical Therapy with or without PCI for Stable Coronary Disease. *N Engl J Med,* 356(15), 1503–1516. doi: 10.1056/NEJMoa070829

Borden, W. B., Redberg, R. F., Mushlin, A. I., Dai, D., Kaltenbach, L. A., & Spertus, J. A. (2011). Patterns and intensity of medical therapy in patients undergoing percutaneous coronary intervention. *JAMA,* 305(18), 1882–1889. doi: 10.1001/jama.2011.601

Brown, G., Albers, J. J., Fisher, L. D., Schaefer, S. M., Lin, J.-T., Kaplan, C., . . . Dodge, H. T. (1990). Regression of Coronary Artery Disease as a Result of Intensive Lipid-Lowering Therapy in Men with High Levels of Apolipoprotein B. *N Engl J Med,* 323(19), 1289–1298. doi: 10.1056/NEJM199011083231901

Campia, U., Matuskey, L. A., & Panza, J. A. (2006). Peroxisome Proliferator–Activated Receptor-γ Activation With Pioglitazone Improves Endothelium-Dependent Dilation in Nondiabetic Patients With Major Cardiovascular Risk Factors. *Circulation,* 113(6), 867–875. doi: 10.1161/circulationaha.105.549618

Cannon, C. P., Braunwald, E., McCabe, C. H., Rader, D. J., Rouleau, J. L., Belder, R., . . . Skene, A. M. (2004). Intensive versus Moderate Lipid Lowering with Statins after Acute Coronary Syndromes. *N Engl J Med,* 350(15), 1495–1504. doi: 10.1056/NEJMoa040583

Carroll, C. A., Coen, M. M., & Rymer, M. M. (2003). Assessment of the effect of ramipril therapy on direct health care costs for first and recurrent strokes in high-risk cardiovascular patients using data from the heart outcomes prevention evaluation (HOPE) study. *Clinical Therapeutics,* 25(4), 1248–1261. doi: http://dx.doi.org/10.1016/S0149-2918(03)80081-4

Cattaneo, M. (2007). Resistance to antiplatelet drugs: molecular mechanisms and laboratory detection. *J Thromb Haemost,* 5 Suppl 1, 230–237. doi: 10.1111/j.1538-7836.2007.02498.x

Chaitman, B. R., Hardison, R. M., Adler, D., Gebhart, S., Grogan, M., Ocampo, S., . . . Group, t. B. A. R. I. D. S. (2009). The Bypass Angioplasty Revascularization Investigation 2 Diabetes Randomized Trial of Different Treatment Strategies in Type 2 Diabetes Mellitus With Stable Ischemic Heart Disease: Impact of Treatment Strategy on Cardiac Mortality and Myocardial Infarction. *Circulation,* 120(25), 2529–2540. doi: 10.1161/circulationaha.109.913111

Collaborative meta-analysis of randomised trials of antiplatelet therapy for prevention of death, myocardial infarction, and stroke in high risk patients. (2002). *Bmj,* 324(7329), 71–86.

Collino, M., Aragno, M., Castiglia, S., Miglio, G., Tomasinelli, C., Boccuzzi, G., . . . Fantozzi, R. (2010). Pioglitazone improves lipid and insulin levels in overweight rats on a high cholesterol and fructose diet by decreasing hepatic inflammation. *British Journal of Pharmacology,* 160(8), 1892–1902. doi: 10.1111/j.1476-5381.2010.00671.x

Cooper, W. O., Hernandez-Diaz, S., Arbogast, P. G., Dudley, J. A., Dyer, S., Gideon, P. S., . . . Ray, W. A. (2006). Major Congenital Malformations after First-Trimester Exposure to ACE Inhibitors. *N Engl J Med,* 354(23), 2443–2451. doi: 10.1056/NEJMoa055202

Dagenais, G. R., Pogue, J., Fox, K., Simoons, M. L., & Yusuf, S. (2006). Angiotensin-converting-enzyme inhibitors in stable vascular disease without left ventricular systolic dysfunction or heart failure: a combined analysis of three trials. *The Lancet,* 368(9535), 581–588. doi: 10.1016/s0140-6736(06)69201-5

Daskalopoulou, S. S., Delaney, J. A. C., Filion, K. B., Brophy, J. M., Mayo, N. E., & Suissa, S. (2008). Discontinuation of statin therapy following an acute myocardial infarction: a population-based study. *Eur Heart J*. doi: 10.1093/eurheartj/ehn346

De Berardis, G., Lucisano, G., D'Ettorre, A., Pellegrini, F., Lepore, V., Tognoni, G., & Nicolucci, A. (2012). Association of aspirin use with major bleeding in patients with and without diabetes. *JAMA*, 307(21), 2286–2294. doi: 10.1001/jama.2012.5034

DeFronzo, R. A. (2009). From the Triumvirate to the Ominous Octet: A New Paradigm for the Treatment of Type 2 Diabetes Mellitus. *Diabetes*, 58(4), 773–795. doi: 10.2337/db09-9028

DeFronzo, R. A., Tripathy, D., Schwenke, D. C., Banerji, M., Bray, G. A., Buchanan, T. A., . . . Reaven, P. D. (2011). Pioglitazone for Diabetes Prevention in Impaired Glucose Tolerance. *N Engl J Med*, 364(12), 1104–1115. doi: 10.1056/NEJMoa1010949

Demmer, R. T., Desvarieux, M., Holtfreter, B., Jacobs, D. R., Jr., Wallaschofski, H., Nauck, M., . . . Kocher, T. (2010). Periodontal status and A1C change: longitudinal results from the study of health in Pomerania (SHIP). *Diabetes Care*, 33(5), 1037–1043. doi: 10.2337/dc09-1778

Dickstein, K., & Kjekshus, J. (2002). Effects of losartan and captopril on mortality and morbidity in high-risk patients after acute myocardial infarction: the OPTIMAAL randomised trial. *The Lancet*, 360(9335), 752–760. doi: 10.1016/s0140-6736(02)09895-1

Dietrich, T., Jimenez, M., Krall Kaye, E. A., Vokonas, P. S., & Garcia, R. I. (2008). Age-dependent associations between chronic periodontitis/edentulism and risk of coronary heart disease. *Circulation*, 117(13), 1668–1674. doi: 10.1161/CIRCULATIONAHA.107.711507

Dormandy, J. A., Charbonnel, B., Eckland, D. J. A., Erdmann, E., Massi-Benedetti, M., Moules, I. K., . . . Tato, J. (2005). Secondary prevention of macrovascular events in patients with type 2 diabetes in the PROactive Study (PROspective pioglitAzone Clinical Trial In macroVascular Events): a randomised controlled trial. *The Lancet*, 366(9493), 1279–1289. doi: http://dx.doi.org/10.1016/S0140-6736(05)67528-9

Dormuth, C. R., Hemmelgarn, B. R., Paterson, J. M., James, M. T., Teare, G. F., Raymond, C. B., . . . Ernst, P. (2013). Use of high potency statins and rates of admission for acute kidney injury: multicenter, retrospective observational analysis of administrative databases. *Bmj*, 346(mar18 3), f880–f880. doi: 10.1136/bmj.f880

Effect of Valsartan on the Incidence of Diabetes and Cardiovascular Events. (2010). *N Engl J Med*, 362(16), 1477–1490. doi: 10.1056/NEJMoa1001121

Effects of Combination Lipid Therapy in Type 2 Diabetes Mellitus. (2010). *N Engl J Med*, 362(17), 1563–1574. doi: 10.1056/NEJMoa1001282

Effects of Intensive Blood-Pressure Control in Type 2 Diabetes Mellitus. (2010). *N Engl J Med*, 362(17), 1575–1585. doi: 10.1056/NEJMoa1001286

Effects of Intensive Glucose Lowering in Type 2 Diabetes. (2008). *N Engl J Med*, 358(24), 2545–2559. doi: 10.1056/NEJMoa0802743

Effects of ramipril on cardiovascular and microvascular outcomes in people with diabetes mellitus: results of the HOPE study and MICRO-HOPE substudy. (2000). *The Lancet*, 355(9200), 253–259. doi: http://dx.doi.org/10.1016/S0140-6736(99)12323-7

Effects of the angiotensin-receptor blocker telmisartan on cardiovascular events in high-risk patients intolerant to angiotensin-converting enzyme inhibitors: a randomised controlled trial. (2008). *The Lancet*, 372(9644), 1174–1183. doi: 10.1016/s0140-6736(08)61242-8

Erdmann, E., Dormandy, J. A., Charbonnel, B., Massi-Benedetti, M., Moules, I. K., & Skene, A. M. (2007). The Effect of Pioglitazone on Recurrent Myocardial Infarction in 2,445

Patients With Type 2 Diabetes and Previous Myocardial Infarction: Results From the PROactive (PROactive 05) Study. *J Am Coll Cardiol,* 49(17), 1772–1780. doi: http://dx.doi.org/10.1016/j.jacc.2006.12.048

Escobar, C., Echarri, R., & Barrios, V. (2008). Relative safety profiles of high dose statin regimens. *Vasc Health Risk Manag,* 4(3), 525–533.

Feng, Q., Wilke, R. A., & Baye, T. M. (2012). Individualized risk for statin-induced myopathy: current knowledge, emerging challenges and potential solutions. *Pharmacogenomics,* 13(5), 579–594. doi: 10.2217/pgs.12.11

Forst, T., Karagiannis, E., Lubben, G., Hohberg, C., Schondorf, T., Dikta, G., . . . Pfutzner, A. (2008). Pleiotrophic and anti-inflammatory effects of pioglitazone precede the metabolic activity in type 2 diabetic patients with coronary artery disease. *Atherosclerosis,* 197(1), 311–317. doi: 10.1016/j.atherosclerosis.2007.05.006

Frye, R. L., August, P., Brooks, M. M., Hardison, R. M., Kelsey, S. F., MacGregor, J. M., . . . Sobel, B. E. (2009). A randomized trial of therapies for type 2 diabetes and coronary artery disease. *N Engl J Med,* 360(24), 2503–2515. doi: 10.1056/NEJMoa0805796

Fuster, V., & Sweeny, J. M. (2011). Aspirin: A Historical and Contemporary Therapeutic Overview. *Circulation,* 123(7), 768–778. doi: 10.1161/circulationaha.110.963843

Gasparyan, A. Y., Watson, T., & Lip, G. Y. (2008). The role of aspirin in cardiovascular prevention: implications of aspirin resistance. *J Am Coll Cardiol,* 51(19), 1829–1843. doi: 10.1016/j.jacc.2007.11.080

Geldmacher, D. S., Fritsch, T., McClendon, M. J., Lerner, A. J., Landreth, G. E. (2006, July 15–20). A double-blind, placebo-controlled, 18-month pilot study of the PPAR-gamma agonist pioglitazone in Alzheimer's disease. Program and abstracts of the 10th International Conference on Alzheimer's Disease and Related Disorders, Madrid, Spain. Abstract P2–408.

Goldstein, L. B., Bushnell, C. D., Adams, R. J., Appel, L. J., Braun, L. T., Chaturvedi, S., . . . Pearson, T. A. (2011). Guidelines for the Primary Prevention of Stroke: A Guideline for Healthcare Professionals From the American Heart Association/American Stroke Association. *Stroke,* 42(2), 517–584. doi: 10.1161/STR.0b013e3181fcb238

Golomb, B. A., Evans, M. A., Dimsdale, J. E., & White, H. L. (2012). Effects of statins on energy and fatigue with exertion: Results from a randomized controlled trial. *Arch Intern Med,* 172(15), 1180–1182. doi: 10.1001/archinternmed.2012.2171

Grau, A. J., Becher, H., Ziegler, C. M., Lichy, C., Buggle, F., Kaiser, C., . . . Dorfer, C. E. (2004). Periodontal disease as a risk factor for ischemic stroke. *Stroke,* 35(2), 496–501. doi: 10.1161/01.STR.0000110789.20526.9D

Green, L. A., & Seifert, C. M. (2005). Translation of Research Into Practice: Why We Can't "Just Do It". *The Journal of the American Board of Family Practice,* 18(6), 541–545. doi: 10.3122/jabfm.18.6.541

Grosser, T., Fries, S., Lawson, J. A., Kapoor, S. C., Grant, G. R., & FitzGerald, G. A. (2013). Drug resistance and pseudoresistance: an unintended consequence of enteric coating aspirin. *Circulation,* 127(3), 377–385. doi: 10.1161/CIRCULATIONAHA.112.117283

Gum, P. A., Kottke-Marchant, K., Welsh, P. A., White, J., & Topol, E. J. (2003). A prospective, blinded determination of the natural history of aspirin resistance among stable patients with cardiovascular disease. *J Am Coll Cardiol,* 41(6), 961–965. doi: http://dx.doi.org/10.1016/S0735-1097(02)03014-0

Hanefeld, M., Marx, N., Pfützner, A., Baurecht, W., Lübben, G., Karagiannis, E., . . . Forst, T. (2007). Anti-Inflammatory Effects of Pioglitazone and/or Simvastatin in High Cardiovascular Risk Patients With Elevated High Sensitivity C-Reactive Protein: The PIOSTAT

Study. *J Am Coll Cardiol,* 49(3), 290–297. doi: http://dx.doi.org/10.1016/j.jacc.2006.08.054

Hermida, R. C., Ayala, D. E., Mojon, A., & Fernandez, J. R. (2011). Bedtime dosing of anti-hypertensive medications reduces cardiovascular risk in CKD. *J Am Soc Nephrol,* 22(12), 2313–2321. doi: 10.1681/ASN.2011040361

Hlatky, M. A., Boothroyd, D. B., Melsop, K. A., Kennedy, L., Rihal, C., Rogers, W. J., . . . Group, f. t. B. A. R. I. D. S. (2009). Economic Outcomes of Treatment Strategies for Type 2 Diabetes Mellitus and Coronary Artery Disease in the Bypass Angioplasty Revascular-ization Investigation 2 Diabetes Trial. *Circulation,* 120(25), 2550–2558. doi: 10.1161/circulationaha.109.912709

Huck, O., Saadi-Thiers, K., Tenenbaum, H., Davideau, J. L., Romagna, C., Laurent, Y., . . . Roul, J. G. (2011). Evaluating periodontal risk for patients at risk of or suffering from atherosclerosis: recent biological hypotheses and therapeutic consequences. *Arch Cardiovasc Dis,* 104(5), 352–358. doi: 10.1016/j.acvd.2011.02.002

Investigators, H. H.-T. S. (2005). Long-Term Effects of Ramipril on Cardiovascular Events and on Diabetes: Results of the HOPE Study Extension. *Circulation,* 112(9), 1339–1346. doi: 10.1161/circulationaha.105.548461

Khera, A. V., & Rader, D. J. (2013). Cholesterol Efflux Capacity: Full Steam Ahead or a Bump in the Road? *Arterioscler Thromb Vasc Bio,* 33(7), 1449–1451. doi: 10.1161/atvbaha.113.301519

Koh, K. K., Quon, M. J., Han, S. H., Lee, Y., Kim, S. J., & Shin, E. K. (2010). Atorvastatin Causes Insulin Resistance and Increases Ambient Glycemia in Hypercholesterolemic Patients. *J Am Coll Cardiol,* 55(12), 1209–1216. doi: http://dx.doi.org/10.1016/j.jacc.2009.10.053

Kostis, W. J., Cheng, J. Q., Dobrzynski, J. M., Cabrera, J., & Kostis, J. B. (2012). Meta-analy-sis of statin effects in women versus men. *J Am Coll Cardiol,* 59(6), 572–582. doi: 10.1016/j.jacc.2011.09.067

Lalla, E., Kunzel, C., Burkett, S., Cheng, B., & Lamster, I. B. (2011). Identification of unrec-ognized diabetes and pre-diabetes in a dental setting. *J Dent Res,* 90(7), 855–860. doi: 10.1177/0022034511407069

Law, M. R., Morris, J. K., & Wald, N. J. (2009). Use of blood pressure lowering drugs in the prevention of cardiovascular disease: meta-analysis of 147 randomised trials in the context of expectations from prospective epidemiological studies. *Bmj,* 338, b1665. doi: 10.1136/bmj.b1665

Leeper, N. J., Ardehali, R., deGoma, E. M., & Heidenreich, P. A. (2007). Statin use in patients with extremely low low-density lipoprotein levels is associated with improved survival. *Circulation,* 116(6), 613–618. doi: 10.1161/CIRCULATIONAHA.107.694117

Lonn, E., Shaikholeslami, R., Yi, Q., Bosch, J., Sullivan, B., Tanser, P., . . . Yusuf, S. (2004). Effects of ramipril on left ventricular mass and function in cardiovascular patients with controlled blood pressure and with preserved left ventricular ejection fraction: A sub-study of the Heart Outcomes Prevention Evaluation (HOPE) trial. *J Am Coll Cardiol,* 43(12), 2200–2206. doi: http://dx.doi.org/10.1016/j.jacc.2003.10.073

Lonn, E. M., Yusuf, S., Dzavik, V., Doris, C. I., Yi, Q., Smith, S., . . . Teo, K. K. (2001). Effects of Ramipril and Vitamin E on Atherosclerosis: The Study to Evaluate Carotid Ultrasound Changes in Patients Treated With Ramipril and Vitamin E (SECURE). *Circulation,* 103(7), 919–925. doi: 10.1161/01.cir.103.7.919

Lonn, E. M., Yusuf, S., Jha, P., Montague, T. J., Teo, K. K., Benedict, C. R., & Pitt, B. (1994). Emerging role of angiotensin-converting enzyme inhibitors in cardiac and vascular protection. *Circulation,* 90(4), 2056–2069. doi: 10.1161/01.cir.90.4.2056

Mann, J. F. E., Schmieder, R. E., McQueen, M., Dyal, L., Schumacher, H., Pogue, J., . . . Yusuf, S. (2008). Renal outcomes with telmisartan, ramipril, or both, in people at high vascular risk (the ONTARGET study): a multicentre, randomised, double-blind, controlled trial. *The Lancet,* 372(9638), 547–553. doi: 10.1016/s0140-6736(08)61236-2

Mansi, I., F. C. R. P. M. M. U. M. E. M. (2013). Statins and musculoskeletal conditions, arthropathies, and injuries. *JAMA Intern Med,* 1–9. doi: 10.1001/jamainternmed.2013.6184

Massie, B. M., Carson, P. E., McMurray, J. J., Komajda, M., McKelvie, R., Zile, M. R., . . . Ptaszynska, A. (2008). Irbesartan in Patients with Heart Failure and Preserved Ejection Fraction. *N Engl J Med,* 359(23), 2456–2467. doi: 10.1056/NEJMoa0805450

Mazzone, T., Meyer, P. M., Feinstein, S. B., et al. (2006). Effect of pioglitazone compared with glimepiride on carotid intima-media thickness in type 2 diabetes: A randomized trial. *JAMA,* 296(21), 2572–2581. doi: 10.1001/jama.296.21.joc60158

Meier, C., Kraenzlin, M. E., Bodmer, M., Jick, S. S., Jick, H., & Meier, C. R. (2008). Use of thiazolidinediones and fracture risk. *Arch Intern Med,* 168(8), 820–825. doi: 10.1001/archinte.168.8.820

Mihaylova, B., Emberson, J., Blackwell, L., Keech, A., Simes, J., Barnes, E. H., . . . Baigent, C. (2012). The effects of lowering LDL cholesterol with statin therapy in people at low risk of vascular disease: meta-analysis of individual data from 27 randomised trials. *The Lancet,* 380(9841), 581–590. doi: 10.1016/s0140-6736(12)60367-5

Mohaupt, M. G., Karas, R. H., Babiychuk, E. B., Sanchez-Freire, V., Monastyrskaya, K., Iyer, L., . . . Draeger, A. (2009). Association between statin-associated myopathy and skeletal muscle damage. *Canadian Medical Association Journal,* 181(1–2), E11–E18. doi: 10.1503/cmaj.081785

Montecucco, F., & Mach, F. (2009). Update on statin-mediated anti-inflammatory activities in athcrosclerosis. *Semin Immunopathol,* 31(1), 127–142. doi: 10.1007/s00281-009-0150-y

Morikawa, A., Ishizeki, K., Iwashima, Y., Yokoyama, H., Muto, E., Oshima, E., . . . Haneda, M. (2011). Pioglitazone reduces urinary albumin excretion in renin-angiotensin system inhibitor-treated type 2 diabetic patients with hypertension and microalbuminuria: the APRIME study. *Clin Exp Nephrol,* 15(6), 848–853. doi: 10.1007/s10157-011-0512-3

Morris, Z. S., Wooding, S., & Grant, J. (2011). The answer is 17 years, what is the question: understanding time lags in translational research. *J R Soc Med,* 104(12), 510–520. doi: 10.1258/jrsm.2011.110180

MRC/BHF Heart Protection Study of cholesterol lowering with simvastatin in 20,536 high-risk individuals: a randomised placebocontrolled trial. (2002). *The Lancet,* 360(9326), 7–22. doi: 10.1016/s0140-6736(02)09327-3

Naci, H., Brugts, J., & Ades, T. (2013). Comparative Tolerability and Harms of Individual Statins: A Study-Level Network Meta-Analysis of 246,955 Participants From 135 Randomized Controlled Trials. *Circ Cardiovasc Qual Outcomes.* doi: 10.1161/circoutcomes.111.000071

Nakamura, T., Matsuda, T., Kawagoe, Y., Ogawa, H., Takahashi, Y., Sekizuka, K., & Koide, H. (2004). Effect of pioglitazone on carotid intima-media thickness and arterial stiffness in type 2 diabetic nephropathy patients. *Metabolism,* 53(10), 1382–1386. doi: http://dx.doi.org/10.1016/j.metabol.2004.05.013

Ni Chroinin, D., Asplund, K., Asberg, S., Callaly, E., Cuadrado-Godia, E., Diez-Tejedor, E., . . . Kelly, P. J. (2013). Statin therapy and outcome after ischemic stroke: systematic review and meta-analysis of observational studies and randomized trials. *Stroke,* 44(2), 448–456. doi: 10.1161/STROKEAHA.112.668277

Nicholls, S. J. (2013). Effect of Aliskiren on Progression of Coronary Disease in Patients With Prehypertension: The AQUARIUS Randomized Clinical Trial, Aliskiren and Coronary Disease in Prehypertension. *JAMA,* 310(11), 1135-1144. doi: 10.1001/jama.2013.277169

Nicholls, S. J., Tuzcu, E. M., Wolski, K., Bayturan, O., Lavoie, A., Uno, K., . . . Nissen, S. E. (2011). Lowering the Triglyceride/High-Density Lipoprotein Cholesterol Ratio Is Associated With the Beneficial Impact of Pioglitazone on Progression of Coronary Atherosclerosis in Diabetic Patients: Insights From the PERISCOPE (Pioglitazone Effect on Regression of Intravascular Sonographic Coronary Obstruction Prospective Evaluation) Study. *J Am Coll Cardiol,* 57(2), 153–159. doi: http://dx.doi.org/10.1016/j.jacc.2010.06.055

Nissen, S. E., Nicholls, S. J., Wolski, K., et al. (2008). Comparison of pioglitazone vs glimepiride on progression of coronary atherosclerosis in patients with type 2 diabetes: The periscope randomized controlled trial. *JAMA,* 299(13), 1561–1573. doi: 10.1001/jama.299.13.1561

O'Riordan, M. (2008, July 9). CASHMERE: No IMT Effect With Atorvastatin Over 12 Months. *Medscape.* http://www.medscape.com/viewarticle/577309

Paganini-Hill, A., White, S. C., & Atchison, K. A. (2011). Dental health behaviors, dentition, and mortality in the elderly: the leisure world cohort study. *J Aging Res,* 2011, 156061. doi: 10.4061/2011/156061

Parker, B. A., Capizzi, J. A., Grimaldi, A. S., Clarkson, P. M., Cole, S. M., Keadle, J., . . . Thompson, P. D. (2013). Effect of statins on skeletal muscle function. *Circulation,* 127(1), 96–103. doi: 10.1161/CIRCULATIONAHA.112.136101

Patrono, C., García Rodríguez, L. A., Landolfi, R., & Baigent, C. (2005). Low-Dose Aspirin for the Prevention of Atherothrombosis. *N Engl J Med,* 353(22), 2373–2383. doi: 10.1056/NEJMra052717

Pfützner, A., Marx, N., Lübben, G., Langenfeld, M., Walcher, D., Konrad, T., & Forst, T. (2005). Improvement of Cardiovascular Risk Markers by Pioglitazone Is Independent From Glycemic Control: Results From the Pioneer Study. *J Am Coll Cardiol,* 45(12), 1925–1931. doi: http://dx.doi.org/10.1016/j.jacc.2005.03.041

Phillips, P. S., Haas, R. H., Bannykh, S., Hathaway, S., Gray, N. L., Kimura, B. J., . . . England, J. D. (2002). Statin-associated myopathy with normal creatine kinase levels. *Ann Intern Med,* 137(7), 581–585.

Piccinni, C., Motola, D., Marchesini, G., & Poluzzi, E. (2011). Assessing the Association of Pioglitazone Use and Bladder Cancer Through Drug Adverse Event Reporting. *Diabetes Care,* 34(6), 1369–1371. doi: 10.2337/dc10-2412

Pignatelli, P., Carnevale, R., Pastori, D., Cangemi, R., Napoleone, L., Bartimoccia, S., . . . Violi, F. (2012). Immediate antioxidant and antiplatelet effect of atorvastatin via inhibition of Nox2. *Circulation,* 126(1), 92–103. doi: 10.1161/CIRCULATIONAHA.112.095554

Pignone, M., & Williams, C. D. (2010). Aspirin for primary prevention of cardiovascular disease in diabetes mellitus. *Nat Rev Endocrinol,* 6(11), 619–628. doi: 10.1038/nrendo.2010.169

Pilote, L., Abrahamowicz, M., Rodrigues, E., Eisenberg, M. J., & Rahme, E. (2004). Mortality rates in elderly patients who take different angiotensin-converting enzyme inhibitors after acute myocardial infarction: a class effect? *Ann Intern Med,* 141(2), 102–112.

Preiss, D., Seshasai, S., Welsh, P., et al. (2011). Risk of incident diabetes with intensive-dose compared with moderate-dose statin therapy: A meta-analysis. *JAMA,* 305(24), 2556–2564. doi: 10.1001/jama.2011.860

Reaven, P. D., Schwenke, D. C., Buchanan, T. Z., et al. (2009, June 7). Pioglitazone reduces long-term progression of carotid atherosclerosis in IGT. American Diabetes Association 2009 Scientific Sessions, New Orleans, LA. Abstract 15-LB.

Ridker, P. M. (2009). The JUPITER Trial: Results, Controversies, and Implications for Prevention. *Circ Cardiovasc Qual Outcomes,* 2(3), 279–285. doi: 10.1161/circoutcomes.109.868299

Rosenson, R. S., & Tangney, C. C. (1998). Antiatherothrombotic properties of statins: Implications for cardiovascular event reduction. *JAMA,* 279(20), 1643–1650. doi: 10.1001/jama.279.20.1643

Sacco, R. L., Diener, H.-C., Yusuf, S., Cotton, D., Ôunpuu, S., Lawton, W. A., . . . Yoon, B.-W. (2008). Aspirin and Extended-Release Dipyridamole versus Clopidogrel for Recurrent Stroke. *N Engl J Med,* 359(12), 1238–1251. doi: 10.1056/NEJMoa0805002

Sacks, F. M., Tonkin, A. M., Shepherd, J., Braunwald, E., Cobbe, S., Hawkins, C. M., . . . Group, f. t. P. P. P. P. I. (2000). Effect of Pravastatin on Coronary Disease Events in Subgroups Defined by Coronary Risk Factors: The Prospective Pravastatin Pooling Project. *Circulation,* 102(16), 1893–1900. doi: 10.1161/01.cir.102.16.1893

Saha, S. A., Molnar, J., & Arora, R. R. (2008). Tissue angiotensin-converting enzyme inhibitors for the prevention of cardiovascular disease in patients with diabetes mellitus without left ventricular systolic dysfunction or clinical evidence of heart failure: a pooled meta-analysis of randomized placebo-controlled clinical trials. *Diabetes, Obesity and Metabolism,* 10(1), 41–52. doi: 10.1111/j.1463-1326.2006.00688.x

Scannapieco, F. A., Papandonatos, G. D., & Dunford, R. G. (1998). Associations Between Oral Conditions and Respiratory Disease in a National Sample Survey Population. *Annals of Periodontology,* 3(1), 251–256. doi: 10.1902/annals.1998.3.1.251

Schneider, M. P., Hua, T. A., Bohm, M., Wachtell, K., Kjeldsen, S. E., & Schmieder, R. E. (2010). Prevention of atrial fibrillation by Renin-Angiotensin system inhibition: a meta-analysis. *J Am Coll Cardiol,* 55(21), 2299–2307. doi: 10.1016/j.jacc.2010.01.043

Sever, P. S., Dahlöf, B., Poulter, N. R., Wedel, H., Beevers, G., Caulfield, M., . . . Östergren, J. (2003). Prevention of coronary and stroke events with atorvastatin in hypertensive patients who have average or lower-than-average cholesterol concentrations, in the Anglo-Scandinavian Cardiac Outcomes Trial—Lipid Lowering Arm (ASCOT-LLA): a multicentre randomised controlled trial. *The Lancet,* 361(9364), 1149–1158. doi: http://dx.doi.org/10.1016/S0140-6736(03)12948-0

Siller-Matula, J. M. (2012). Hemorrhagic complications associated with aspirin: An under-estimated hazard in clinical practice? *JAMA,* 307(21), 2318–2320. doi: 10.1001/jama.2012.6152

Sipahi, I., Swaminathan, A., Natesan, V., Debanne, S. M., Simon, D. I., & Fang, J. C. (2012). Effect of Antihypertensive Therapy on Incident Stroke in Cohorts With Prehypertensive Blood Pressure Levels: A Meta-Analysis of Randomized Controlled Trials. *Stroke,* 43(2), 432–440. doi: 10.1161/strokeaha.111.636829

Snoep, J. D., Hovens, M. C., Eikenboom, J. J., van der Bom, J. G., & Huisman, M. V. (2007). Association of laboratory-defined aspirin resistance with a higher risk of recurrent cardiovascular events: A systematic review and meta-analysis. *Arch Intern Med,* 167(15), 1593–1599. doi: 10.1001/archinte.167.15.1593

Snow, V., Barry, P., Fihn, S. D., Gibbons, R. J., Owens, D. K., Williams, S. V., . . . Weiss, K. B. (2004). Primary care management of chronic stable angina and asymptomatic suspected or known coronary artery disease: a clinical practice guideline from the American College of Physicians. *Ann Intern Med,* 141(7), 562–567.

Spertus, J. A., Maron, D. J., Cohen, D. J., Kolm, P., Hartigan, P., Weintraub, W. S., . . . Mancini, G. B. J. (2013). Frequency, Predictors, and Consequences of Crossing Over to Revascularization Within 12 Months of Randomization to Optimal Medical Therapy in the Clinical Outcomes Utilizing Revascularization and Aggressive Drug Evaluation (COURAGE) Trial. *Circ Cardiovasc Qual Outcomes,* 6(4), 409–418. doi: 10.1161/circoutcomes.113.000139

Staniloae, C., Mandadi, V., Kurian, D., Coppola, J., Bernaski, E., El-Khally, Z., . . . Ambrose, J. (2007). Pioglitazone improves endothelial function in non-diabetic patients with coronary artery disease. *Cardiology,* 108(3), 164–169. doi: 10.1159/000096601

Sullivan, M. G. (2006, August 15). Diabetes drug class may lower risk of Alzheimer's. *The Free Library.* http://www.thefreelibrary.com/Diabetes drug class may lower risk of Alzheimer's.-a0171953302

Thomson Reuters ONE. Novartis announces termination of ALTITUDE study with Rasilez®/Tekturna® in high-risk patients with diabetes and renal impairment. (2011, December 20). www.reuters.com/article/2011/12/20/idUS48151 + 20-Dec-2011 + HUG20111220

Trelle, S., Reichenbach, S., Wandel, S., Hildebrand, P., Tschannen, B., Villiger, P. M., . . . Juni, P. (2011). Cardiovascular safety of non-steroidal anti-inflammatory drugs: network meta-analysis. *Bmj,* 342, c7086. doi: 10.1136/bmj.c7086

Tseng, C. H. (2012). Pioglitazone and bladder cancer in human studies: is it diabetes itself, diabetes drugs, flawed analyses or different ethnicities? *J Formos Med Assoc,* 111(3), 123–131. doi: 10.1016/j.jfma.2011.10.003

Ueno, M., Izumi, Y., Kawaguchi, Y., Ikeda, A., Iso, H., Inoue, M., & Tsugane, S. (2012). Prediagnostic plasma antibody levels to periodontopathic bacteria and risk of coronary heart disease. *Int Heart J,* 53(4), 209–214.

Wanner, C., Krane, V., März, W., Olschewski, M., Mann, J. F. E., Ruf, G., & Ritz, E. (2005). Atorvastatin in Patients with Type 2 Diabetes Mellitus Undergoing Hemodialysis. *N Engl J Med,* 353(3), 238–248. doi: 10.1056/NEJMoa043545

Watts, A., Crimmins, E. M., & Gatz, M. (2008). Inflammation as a potential mediator for the association between periodontal disease and Alzheimer's disease. *Neuropsychiatr Dis Treat,* 4(5), 865–876.

White, H. D., Simes, J., Stewart, R. A. H., Blankenberg, S., Barnes, E. H., Marschner, I. C., . . . Investigators, T. L. S. (2013). Changes in Lipoprotein-Associated Phospholipase A2 Activity Predict Coronary Events and Partly Account for the Treatment Effect of Pravastatin: Results From the Long-term Intervention with Pravastatin in Ischemic Disease Study. *J Am Heart Assoc,* 2(5). doi: 10.1161/jaha.113.000360

Wilcox, R., Kupfer, S., & Erdmann, E. (2008). Effects of pioglitazone on major adverse cardiovascular events in high-risk patients with type 2 diabetes: Results from PROspective pioglitAzone Clinical Trial In macro Vascular Events (PROactive 10). *Am Heart J,* 155(4), 712–717. doi: http://dx.doi.org/10.1016/j.ahj.2007.11.029

Wolff, T., Miller, T., & Ko, S. (2009). Aspirin for the primary prevention of cardiovascular events: an update of the evidence for the U.S. Preventive Services Task Force. *Ann Intern Med,* 150(6), 405–410.

Yamanouchi, T., Sakai, T., Igarashi, K., Ichiyanagi, K., Watanabe, H., & Kawasaki, T. (2005). Comparison of metabolic effects of pioglitazone, metformin, and glimepiride over 1 year in Japanese patients with newly diagnosed Type 2 diabetes. *Diabetic Medicine,* 22(8), 980–985. doi: 10.1111/j.1464-5491.2005.01656.x

Yang, H. B., Zhao, X. Y., Zhang, J. Y., Du, Y. Y., & Wang, X. F. (2012). Pioglitazone induces regression and stabilization of coronary atherosclerotic plaques in patients with impaired glucose tolerance. *Diabet Med,* 29(3), 359–365. doi: 10.1111/j.1464-5491.2011.03458.x

Yusuf, S., Gerstein, H., Hoogwerf, B., et al. (2001). Ramipril and the development of diabetes. *JAMA,* 286(15), 1882–1885. doi: 10.1001/jama.286.15.1882

Zhou, Z., Rahme, E., Abrahamowicz, M., Tu, J. V., Eisenberg, M. J., Humphries, K., . . . Pilote, L. (2005). Effectiveness of statins for secondary prevention in elderly patients after acute myocardial infarction: an evaluation of class effect. *CMAJ,* 172(9), 1187–1194. doi: 10.1503/cmaj.1041403

Zhou, Z., Rahme, E., & Pilote, L. (2006). Are statins created equal? Evidence from randomized trials of pravastatin, simvastatin, and atorvastatin for cardiovascular disease prevention. *Am Heart J,* 151(2), 273–281. doi: http://dx.doi.org/10.1016/j.ahj.2005.04.003

Zhu, Z., Shen, Z., Lu, Y., Zhong, S., & Xu, C. (2012). Increased risk of bladder cancer with pioglitazone therapy in patients with diabetes: a meta-analysis. *Diabetes Res Clin Pract,* 98(1), 159–163. doi: 10.1016/j.diabres.2012.05.006

Index

Bradley F. Bale, MD and Amy Doneen, MSN, ARNP are co-founders of the Bale/ Doneen Method, which they teach to healthcare providers in their American Academy of Family Medicine–accredited preceptorship program. They have given hundreds of lectures at leading medical conferences globally and have published their research in many peer-reviewed medical journals. They also co-founded the Heart Attack & Stroke Prevention Center in Spokane, Washington, of which Amy Doneen has been the Medical Director since 2003. She is also Adjunct Professor at Texas Tech Health Sciences School of Nursing and past Chair of the Pacific Northwest Preventative Cardiovascular Nurses Association. Dr. Bale serves as Medical Director of the Heart Health Program at Grace Clinic in Lubbock, Texas, and has a private practice in Nashville, Tennessee.

Bale and Doneen have also formed the Institute of Arteriology, a nonprofit organization aimed at promoting the study of arterial wall health with the mission to ensure all individuals have the opportunity to live their lives free of cardiovascular disease events.

Lisa Collier Cool is a bestselling author, blogger for Yahoo! Health, and winner of 19 medical journalism awards.